CURRENT MANAGEMENT OF MALIGNANT MELANOMA

Edited by **Ming Yu Cao**

INTECHOPEN.COM

Current Management of Malignant Melanoma

Edited by Ming Yu Cao

CBS, Edition **2016**

Published by InTech

Janeza Trdine 9, 51000 Rijeka, Croatia

Publishing Process Manager Davor Vidic

Technical Editor Teodora Smiljanic

Cover Designer InTech Design Team

Image Copyright SeDmi, 2011. Used under license from Shutterstock.com

Additional hard copies can be obtained from orders@intechopen.com

Current Management of Malignant Melanoma, Edited by Ming Yu Cao
p. cm.
ISBN 978-953-307-264-7

Contents

Preface

Melanoma is the deadliest form of skin cancer. The incidence of malignant melanoma has increased exponentially in recent decades. Although there are some available treatments for melanoma, the mortality rate is still high. The stage of melanoma at diagnosis is directly related to the treatment options and the survival rate. In the last decade, much more efforts have been made in the understanding and the management of the disease. This book has contributions from experts in the field, and provides the most recent perspectives of basic research and clinical development for the management of melanoma.

The purpose of this book is to provide a comprehensive source of information on melanoma, which includes the basic research, early diagnosis, prevention and treatment of melanoma, as well as development of new therapies or optimizing current treatments. The book should be especially useful for scientists and practicing physicians, to whom it offers an opportunity to keep abreast of recent advances in the field of melanoma.

The editor wishes to especially thank the contributing authors, whose efforts and expertise made this project a success. The editor would also like to acknowledge the contribution of Amy Cao for her assistance of the final editing of this book.

Dr. Ming Yu Cao, M.D., Ph.D.
CERB, BGTD, Health
Canada

Clinical Cytology in the Diagnosis and Management of Melanoma

Neelaiah Siddaraju
Jawaharlal Institute of Postgraduate Medical Education and Research (JIPMER)
India

1. Introduction

Melanoma, an aggressive tumor of the melanocytes is more prevalent among the white-skinned individuals with the highest incidence reported from Australia and New Zealand (Elwood M,2002). Primary melanomas usually involve the skin, mucosa, retina and leptomeninges. They are known to metastasize to lymph nodes, lung, liver and virtually any part of the body (Basler et al., 1997; Saqi et al., 2002; Ustün et al., 2002; De Las Casas et al., 2004; Parwani et al., 2004; Mohr et al., 2009). Surgical excision with adequate margins is the treatment of choice for cutaneous melanoma. The prognosis of melanoma varies with the site and stage of the disease (Damala et al., 2004; Mohr et al., 2009). Advanced disease with local recurrence, or distant metastasis carries a grave prognosis (Saqi et al., 2004). A variety of imaging techniques such as the chest and abdominal computed tomography (CT) scan, magnetic resonance imaging (MRI) of the brain and positron emission tomography (PET) are used in the staging work-up of patients with cutaneous melanoma, chiefly, for evaluating the potential metastatic sites such as the lungs, lymph nodes, liver and brain. An imaging work-up is generally not recommended in patients with a <1.0 mm thick lesion, as the cure rate in such cases is >90%. It is also not essential in patients with primary melanoma thicker than 1.0 mm, wherein a sentinel lymph node biopsy (SLNB) serves as a better staging tool (Mohr et al., 2009).

Justifiably, histologic examination of the surgical biopsies plays a major role in the diagnosis of primary and metastatic melanomas. Nonetheless, role of non-invasive/ minimally invasive cytologic techniques has also been adequately addressed (Rai, 2007). The cytologic techniques vary with the nature and location of the lesion and these include fine needle aspiration cytology (FNAC), imprint cytology (IC), scrape cytology, as well as, the examination of exfoliative samples such as the serous body fluids, sputum, cerebrospinal fluid (CSF) and synovial fluid (Paridaens et al., 1992; Deshpande et al., 2001; Saqi et al., 2002; Ali et al., 2005). Of these, FNAC is widely employed and its primary role is to confirm the metastatic or recurrent melanoma lesions (Saqi et al., 2002; Mágori, 2003; Siddaraju et al., 2007). By cytologic means, various authors have been able to detect metastatic melanoma deposits in a wide variety of sites inclusive of adrenal, kidney, omentum, pancreas, parotid, soft tissue, spine, breast, thyroid and brain (Saqi et al., 2002; Artal et al., 2004; Hernandez et al., 2004; Gombos et al., 2004; Bozbora et al., 2005; Kung et al., 2009; Kaneko et al., 2009). Not infrequently, cytology is used for diagnosing primary melanoma as well (Layfield et al., 1993; Dey et al., 1996; Gupta et al., 2003; Mágori, 2003; Kotoulas et al., 2007). A significant literature is also available with regard to the cytologic diagnosis of ocular melanomas (Paridaens et al., 1992; Kashyap et al., 2002; Augsburger et al., 2002; Char et al., 2006; Young et al., 2007, 2008; Solo et al., 2009). Ultrasound (US) or computed tomography (CT) guided FNAC is particularly valuable for visceral metastases. More recently, lymph node ultrasound (US) with fine needle aspiration cytology (FNAC) is considered a potential cost effective alternative for an SLNB (Voit et al., 2006; van Akkooi et al., 2010). Although, rare studies have reported very low sensitivity which is attributed to tiny and necrotic lesions (Voit et al., 1999; van Rijk et al., 2006); most authors have emphasized the importance of US-guided FNAC in the detection of sentinel lymph node metastasis (Voit et al., 1999, 2002, 2006 & 2010). With a positive cytology of the sentinel node, surgeons can proceed with the direct radical lymph node dissection in patients with melanoma. Significantly, attempts have also been made to apply molecular- based techniques on the material obtained by FNA, as well as on exfoliative samples (Angeletti et al., 2004; Kalogeraki 2006; Maat et al., 2007; Savoia et al., 2008; McCannel et al., 2010).

The present chapter deals chiefly with the role of cytology in the clinical management of melanoma patients. A careful evaluation of cytologic samples is of critical importance for a variety of reasons, going to be addressed subsequently in this chapter. Despite the considerable, current knowledge about the cytomorphology of melanoma, owing to its inherent histomorphologic variation; a cytologic diagnosis is often difficult, especially, when the lesions are encountered in unusual locations, or with amelanotic presentation. Apparently, such situations necessitate the need for ancillary tests like immunocytochemistry (ICC) and ultrastructural examination (Mágori, 2003; Rosai, 2005). The importance of clinical history need not be overemphasized when interpreting cytologic specimens; for example, a known history of melanoma can significantly contribute to a cytodiagnosis of recurrent and metastatic melanoma (Mágori, 2003).

2. Histopathology of melanoma

Melanoma is well-known for its widely varied histomorphologic pattern. The major histologic forms include superficial spreading melanoma, nodular melanoma, acral lentigenous melanoma and desmoplastic melanoma (Piris et al., 2010). The histologic patterns include pseudo-glandular, pseudo-papillary, peritheliomatous, hemangiopericytoma-like, trabecular and alveolar. The tumor may be associated with fibroblastic response, formation of metaplastic or neoplastic cartilage, osteoclast-like giant cells and pseudo-epitheliomatous hyperplasia of the overlying dermis (Rosai, 2005). Also described are the cases of psammomatous, myxoid, balloon cell and signet ring cell melanomas (Eckert et al., 1992; Mowat et al., 1994; Hitchcock et al., 1999; Monteagudo et al., 2001). Individual melanoma cells can be epithelioid, spindle shaped or extremely bizarre with their size ranging from that of a small lymphocyte to giant multinucleate forms. The cytoplasm may be eosinophilic, basophilic, foamy, rhabdoid, oncocytic, or completely clear. Melanin can be abundant or absent (amelanotic). Malignant melanoma is readily diagnosed by the presence of melanin granules. Although amelanotic melanoma can also contain a few melanin granules, it is often difficult to differentiate it from non-melanotic tumors (Rosai, 2005). Currently, the criteria considered for the histologic diagnosis of cutaneous melanoma include the asymmetry and poor circumscription of the lesion; predominance of single melanocytes; irregular confluent nests; suprabasal melanocytes; hair follicle involvement and absence of maturation; cytologic atypia; dermal lymphocytic infiltrate and necrosis.

However, the diagnostic process should not just involve the mechanical use of these histologic parameters; as a study by Urso et al. has clearly established that, one or more of these histologic features are often present in benign melanocytic nevi as well. Of these, absence of maturation, mitoses and necrosis are never encountered in benign nevi (Urso et al., 2005). The versatile histologic patterns and responses of melanoma are apparently reflected on the cytologic materials as well.

3. Cytologic evaluation of melanoma

3.1 Technical aspects

The most commonly used cytologic technique is the fine needle aspiration (FNA); however, exfoliative and imprint cytology are also used depending on the clinical situation (Paridaens et al., 1992; Deshpande et al., 2001; Saqi et al., 2002). The technique of FNAC is as per that described in any of the standard text books (Orell & Vielh, 1999). Orbital FNA is performed via transcleral, transcorneal or transvitreal approach using 25-30guage needle (Augsburger et al., 2002; Char et al., 2006; Young et al., 2007, 2008). For tiny and vascular lesions, non-aspiration technique is preferable (Solo et al., 2009). In case of suspected conjunctival melanoma, imprint cytology using cellulose acetate strips has been found to be very useful (Paridaens et al., 1992). Imprint cytology of sentinel node can give a quicker and reliable result (Badgwell et al., 2011). Touch imprints taken from the edge of the primary cutaneous/ mucosal ulcerative lesion can often assist in distinguishing a carcinoma from melanoma. Figure 1 is that of a touch imprint taken from the ulcer edge in one of our cases of melanoma.

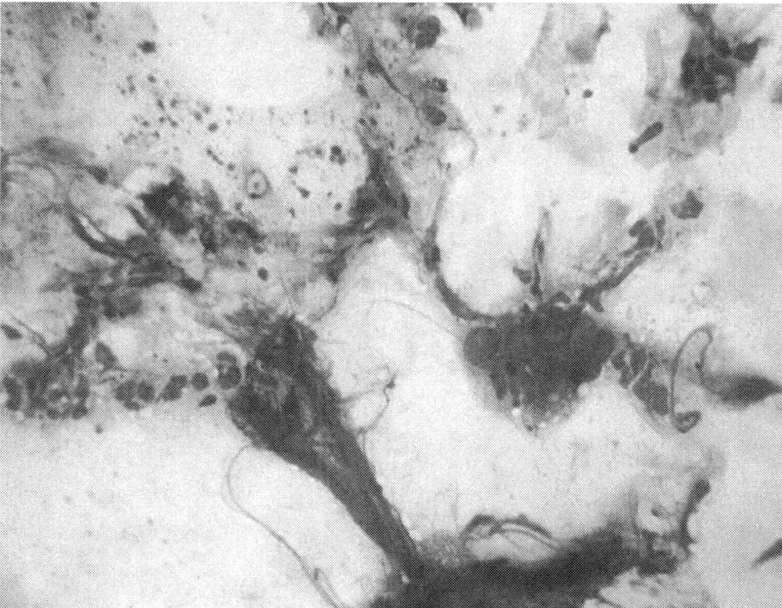

Fig. 1. An imprint taken from the ulcer edge showing pigmented cells; a few characteristic extracellular melanin granules are also appreciated (MGG stain, X400)

3.2 Naked eye examination of cytologic samples

Gross nature of the cytologic material in cases of pigmented melanoma is usually blackish and often fluid-like (Artal et al., 2004). With respect to melanotic melanomas, this is our experience as well. Rare cases of metastatic melanoma manifesting with blackish pleural effusion have been documented. Naked eye examination of such fluid material should serve as a 'clue' to the metastatic involvement of the thorax by melanoma. However, clinicians, as well as, the pathologists should be aware of the fact that a blackish effusion is often related to bacterial and fungal infections, or to hemorrhage (Liao et al., 2010).

3.3 Microscopic examination of cytologic samples

As for the microscopic picture, irrespective of primary, recurrent, metastatic, melanotic or amelanotic melanomas; a striking cytomorphologic feature documented by most authors is its high cell-yield with a predominant population of dissociated cells (Woyke et al., 1980; Perry et al., 1986; Nasiell et al., 1991 Deshpande et al., 2001; Saqi et al., 2002; De Las Casas et al., 2004; Parwani et al., 2004; Damala et al., 2004; Siddaraju et al., 2007). Marked cellularity and nuclear pleomorphism; with plasmacytoid (cells with eccentrically placed nuclei), polygonal or spindle cells; inclusion-like prominent nucleoli; intra-nuclear cytoplasmic inclusions; increased mitotic activity; and variable number of bi- and multinucleated cells are the other features frequently observed in melanoma (Woyke et al., 1980; Perry et al., 1986; Kapila et al., 1991; Layfield et al., 1993; Dey et al., 1996; Deshpande et al., 2001; Saqi et al., 2002; Kashyap et al., 2002; Gupta et al., 2003; Artal et al., 2004; Gombos et al., 2004; Siddaraju et al., 2007). Melanotic melanomas show a variable amount of pigment. Even the cases of amelanotic melanomas often exhibit coarse or fine pigment granules in rare or, a few cells which can be picked up on careful cytologic examination (Perry et al., 1986; Kapila et al., 1991; Deshpande et al., 2001). The cytologic diagnosis of amelanotic melanoma is challenging; because, in the absence of pigment, the tumor cells may mimic those of carcinoma or sarcoma in cytologic samples, particularly those obtained by fine needle aspiration. Irregular nuclear outline and coarse chromatin are the features common to any of the malignant lesions, which is also applicable for melanoma cells (Woyke et al., 1980; Layfileld et al., 1993; Deshpande et al., 2001).

Of the general cytomorphologic features elaborated above, intranuclear cytoplasmic inclusions (INCIs) are of diagnostic importance, only in conjunction with other cytomorphologic and clinical features. Their occurrence in papillary (PTC), medullary (MTC) and anaplastic thyroid carcinomas (ATC); bronchioloalveolar carcinoma (BAC), hepatocellular carcinoma (HCC) and renal cell carcinoma (RCC) is well known (Orell, Silverman, Leiman, 1999). Interestingly, we have also documented a rare case of embryonal rhabdomyosarcoma manifesting with frequent INCIs on FNAC (Kumar et al., 2009). Often, we have observed them as artifactual change in the cervicovaginal smears (perhaps due to air drying artefact) and in degenerated cells on FNAC. Uncommonly, they have also been noticed in certain benign lesions such as pigmented villonodular synovitis and inflammatory psedotumors (Gangane et al., 2003; Hosler et al., 2004). The table1 highlights some of the common, as well as, rare conditions that manifest with INCIs along with the clinical and cytologic features that assist in their distinction from each other. This aspect is of importance, particularly, while dealing with the metastatic lesions.

Serial no.	Condition	Incidence	Major cytologic / clinical features assisting in accurate diagnosis
1	Melanoma	Frequent	High cell-yield, dissociated pleomorphic cells, melanin pigment, inclusion-like nucleoli, intranuclear cytoplasmic inclusions (INCIs), expression of melanoma markers
2	Papillary thyroid carcinoma (PTC)	Frequent	Papillary pattern, metaplastic epithelial cells, nuclear grooves and other associated features
3	Medullary thyroid carcinoma (MTC)	Less frequent than PTC	Amyloid, cytoplasmic red granules
4	Anaplastic thyroid carcinoma (ATC)	Less frequent than PTC	Rapid clinical course, absent expression of melanoma markers
5	Bronchioloalveolar carcinoma (BAC)	Common	Prominent clustering, papillary and adeno pattern
6	Hepatocellular carcinoma (HCC)	Common	Sinusoidal pattern, cords of cells, naked nuclei, intracellular bile pigment (well differentiated), Elevated serum alpha-feto protein (AFP)
7	Renal cell carcinoma (RCC)	Common	Single cells, cohesive fragments, sheet-like pattern, finely vacuolated/granular cytoplasm, bland nuclei in low grade RCC
8	Embryonal rhabdomyosarcoma (ERMS)	Extremely unusual	Small round cell tumor, strap cells, expression of muscle markers
9	Artifactual (our unpublished observation)	Due to processing defect or degenerative change	Poor quality smears
Benign lesions			
1	Inflammatory pseudotumor (Hosler et al., 2004)	Uncommon	Prominent inflammatory component, features identifiable as reactive changes
2	Pigmented villonodular synovitis (Gangane et al., 2003)	Uncommon	Joint involvement, demonstration of hemosiderin pigment by Perl's stain
3	Epithelioid angiomyolipoma (orell, 1999)	Well known	Associated adipocyte component

Table 1. Showing differential diagnosis of intranuclear cytoplasmic inclusions (INCIs)

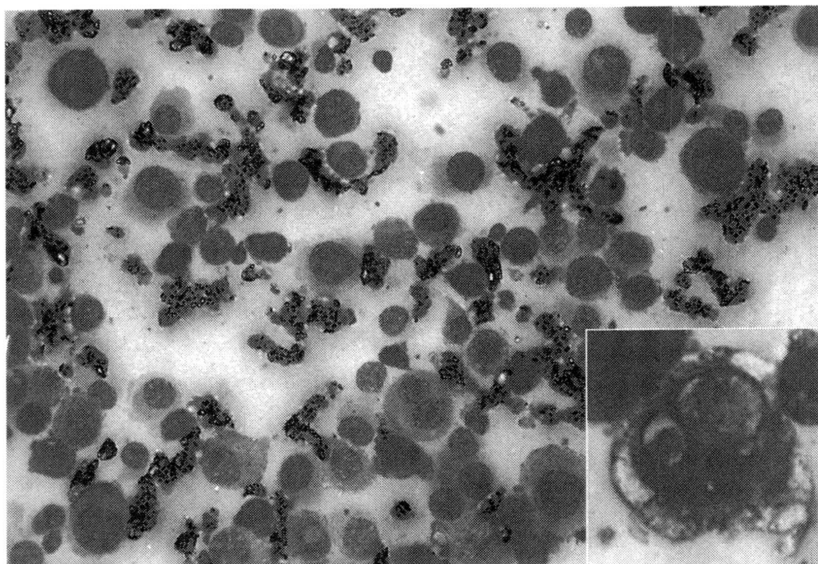

Fig. 2. Our case of recurrent amelanotic melanoma showing plasmacytoid cells; inset highlights distinct INCIs (MGG stain, X400)

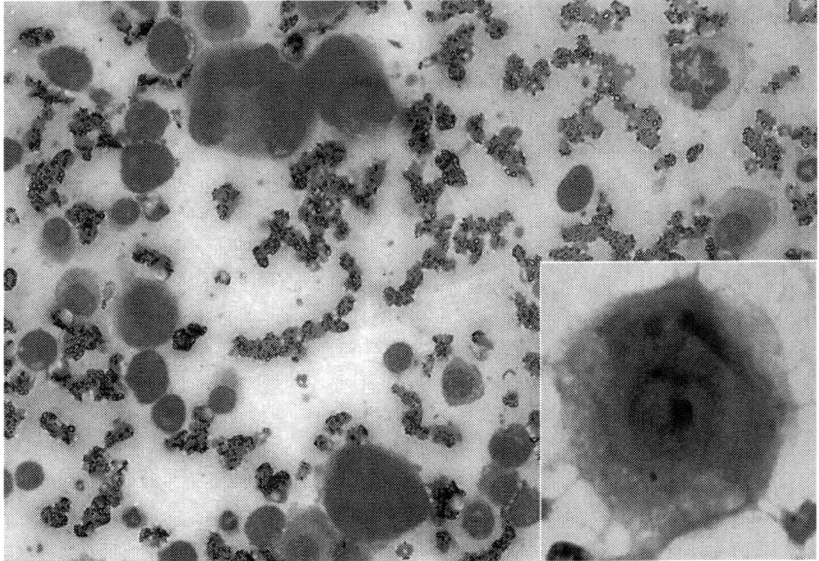

Fig. 3. Another microscopic field from the same case showing multinucleated giant cells with a mitosis (MGG stain, X400); inset shows a digitally magnified cell with an ecto-endocytoplasmic differentiation and prominent inclusion-like nucleoli (PAP stain, x400)

Reviewing further literature on cytology of melanoma is perhaps; of immense help to the clinicians in understanding the diagnostic difficulties encountered, especially by the cytopathologists. In fact, there is a genuine need for the close interaction between the clinicians and pathologists for the proper management of patients with melanoma. Naseill et al. (1991) categorized 81 metastatic melanomas on cytology into classic, carcinoma-like, spindle cell, lymphoma-like, myxoid, clear cell and undifferentiated melanomas. This clearly explains why melanoma has a varied differential diagnosis consisting of a variety of carcinomas, sarcomas and hematolymphoid malignancies that often comprise also of non-Hodgkin's lymphoma (NHL) (Naseill et al., 1991) and plasmacytoma/ myeloma (Siddaraju et al., 2007). In this context, we like to share one of our interesting cases of a recurrent melanoma that manifested with 3 different swellings (axilla, chest wall and back) exhibiting features of a pleomorphic malignant tumor on FNAC. At presentation, the patient's requisition carried a diagnosis of recurrent soft tissue sarcoma, with which the cytologic findings did not match. Cytomorphology varied so widely, with most of the cells displaying plasmacytoid appearance (figure 2). At one stage, owing to the elderly age of the patient, we had a suspicion of plasmacytoma/ myeloma, although, cytologic and clinical features were not very typical. Numerous bizarre bi-nucleate and multi-nucleate giant cells (figure 3); variable chromatin pattern; prominent inclusion-like nucleoli; frequent intra-nuclear cytoplasmic inclusions (figure 2: inset); varied cytoplasmic features (figure 4) such as intensely eosinophilic, as well as, basophilic cytoplasm; cytoplasmic vacuolations; rare signet ring cells and cells with ecto-endoplasmic differentiation (figure 3: inset) were noted. There were also a few strands of fibrocollagenous tissue, to which the tumor cells were adherent (figure 4: inset); this corresponded with the distinct alveolar pattern observed on the later review of the histologic sections. Some of the cytologic features suggested an

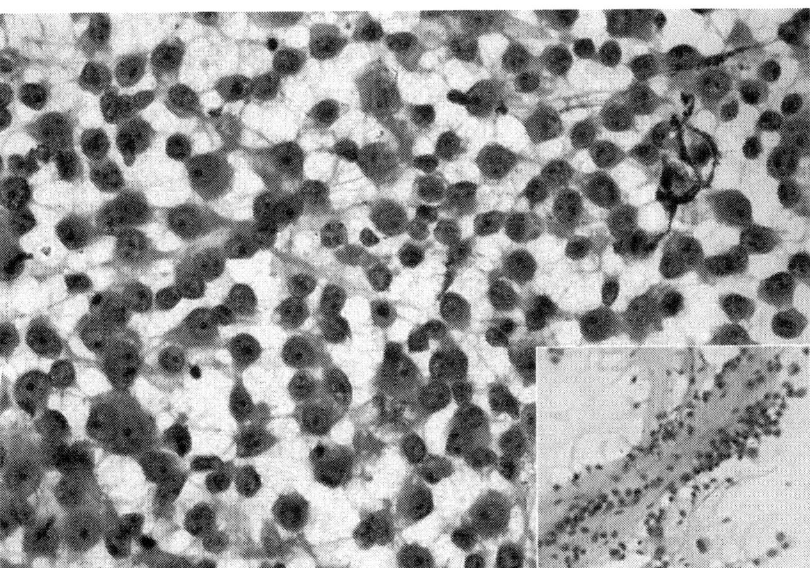

Fig. 4. A smear showing cells with varied cytoplasmic features; inset shows a fibrocollagenous strand with adherent neoplastic cells (PAP stain, x400)

amelanotic melanoma; however, in view of the clinical diagnosis of recurrent soft tissue sarcoma, we offered a diagnosis of an undifferentiated malignant tumor with a possibility of amelanotic melanoma. Subsequently, we learnt that it was diagnosed elsewhere, as a malignant peripheral nerve sheath tumor (MPNST), based on its immunoexpression of S-100. Histologically, the sections revealed a prominent alveolar pattern, vaguely simulating an alveolar rhabdomyosarcoma with a tiny focus displaying junctional activity. We procured the paraffin tissue blocks of this case and performed IHC with desmin, S100, and Melan-A, of which the latter two markers were strongly positive (figures 5&6), confirming our cytologic suspicion of melanoma (Siddaraju et al., 2007).

Other unusual cytologic features described by the various authors are the papillary fragments with fibrovascular cores (Baloch et al., 1999), myxoid stroma (Elliot et al., 2001) ballon cells (Friedman et al., 1982), signet ring cells (Siddaraju et al., 2007) with pseudolipoblastic appearance (Holck et al., 2002), cells with rhabdoid features (Slagel et al., 1997) and cells arranged in alveolar pattern (Gupta et al., 2003). Although rare, a divergent differentiation such as chondroid, neural, myofibroblastic, and osteocartilagenous differentiation is well known in melanomas; and the lack of awareness of this fact can create serious diagnostic problems to the evaluator. Such an instance is well exemplified by a rare case of anal melanoma that also manifested with a mass in the groin. The FNA of the groin mass in that particular case revealed a neoplasm rich in chondroid matrix, raising the possibility of a second primary mesenchymal tumor. However, a review of the histologic slides from the primary growth showed divergent chondroid differentiation in the anal melanoma, establishing the metastatic nature of the groin mass (Hanley et al., 2009). Some of the variants of melanoma are discussed separately.

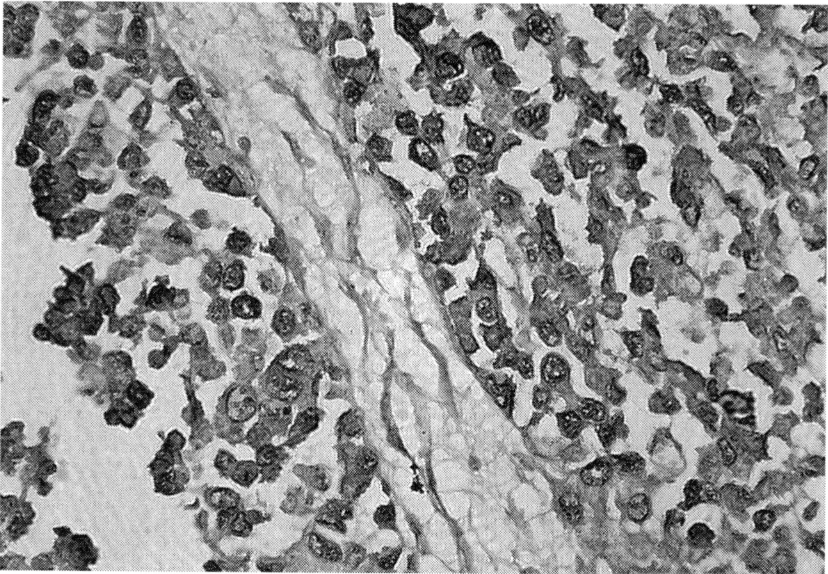

Fig. 5. Melanoma cells exhibiting cytoplasmic and nuclear expression of S-100 on histologic section (IHC stain, X400)

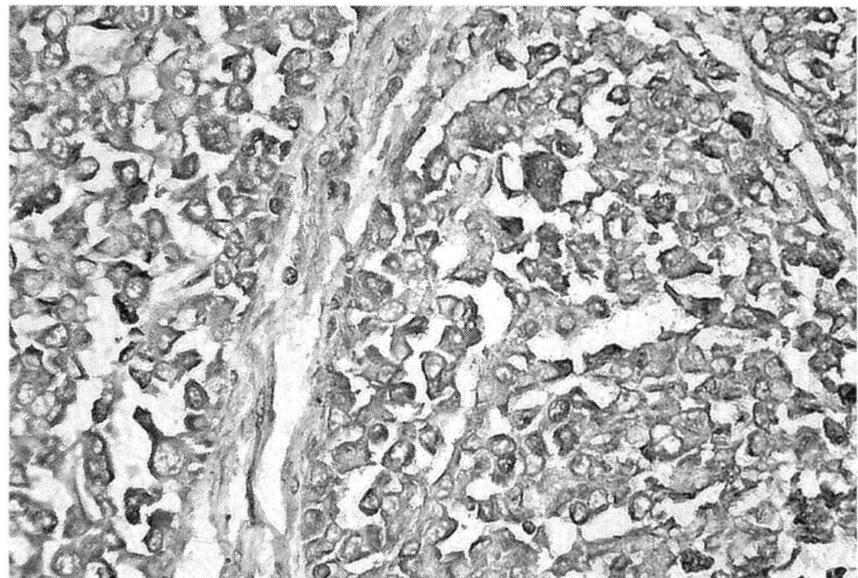

Fig. 6. Neoplastic cells with cytoplasmic Melan-A expression on histologic section (IHC stain, X400)

3.3.1 Spindle cell melanoma

Spindle cell melanoma is a morphologic variant of melanoma which is difficult to diagnose on specimens obtained by fine-needle aspiration (FNA). Piao et al. (2008) studied a large series (67 patients) of metastatic spindle cell melanomas on FNAC (all primaries were histologically proven). The smears were cellular and comprised predominantly of spindle cells that frequently formed cohesive fascicles, or whorls intermingled with scattered epithelioid tumor cells. Significantly, the common features of melanoma such as dishesive cellular distribution, cytoplasmic melanin pigment, intranuclear cytoplasmic inclusions, macronucleoli, and binucleation or multinucleation were infrequent in these cases. When present, they were found in cells with epithelioid morphology. Remarkably, 9% of the cases totally lacked the classic characteristics of melanoma. Spindle cells displayed variable cytologic atypia that ranged from deceptively bland cells resembling the reactive fibroblasts to those indistinguishable from pleomorphic high-grade sarcomas. When the morphologic features were compared with those of the primary tumor, the discrepant cell type was observed in 20% of the cases with the previous primary lesions displaying the epithelioid morphology. Interestingly, the spindle cells also tended to lose immunoexpression of melanoma markers. In such cases, familiarity with cytologic features combined with clinical and immunoperoxidase findings are required to avoid misinterpretation (Piao et al., 2008). Prominent inclusion-like nucleoli are highly characteristic of melanomas; however, we have seen rare cases of pure spindle cell melanoma metastasizing to inguinal nodes that almost completely lacked nucleoli. The classic clinical history of pigmented lesion in the sole of foot, with cells exhibiting melanin pigment facilitated an easy diagnosis in such instances.

On FNAC, in the absence of a reliable clinical history, an amelanotic spindle cell melanoma is likely to be mistaken for spindle cell sarcomas, or, in a location like inguinal region, for a metastatic squamous cell carcinoma with spindle cell morphology.

3.3.2 Desmoplastic melanoma

Desmoplastic melanoma (DM) is an unusual, non-pigmented, sclerosing variant of spindle cell malignant melanoma that can range in appearance from sarcomatoid to scar-like lesion. Cytomorphologic features described on FNA include a moderate cellularity with pleomorphic spindle cells occurring singly and in small aggregates. The spindle cells exhibit plump nuclei with deep grooves and folds, coarse and clumped chromatin, and inconspicuous to multiple, prominent nucleoli, along with naked spindly nuclei. Intranuclear cytoplasmic inclusions are rare. Generally, cytoplasm is scanty to moderate in amount with a fine wispy character, clinging to the nuclear poles. Often, a variable amount of dense stromal material associated with a few spindle cells is seen. Point to be remembered is that immunohistochemically, most desmoplastic melanomas are positive for S-100 and negative for specific melanoma markers (van Ells et al., 2007).

3.3.3 Balloon cell melanoma

Balloon cell melanoma is a histologic variant composed predominantly, or entirely of large cells with abundant, vacuolated cytoplasm. It shares the common cytologic features of melanoma, such as discohesion, nuclear pleomorphism and intranuclear cytoplasmic pseudoinclusions, but generally lacks melanin pigment; however, it is positive for S-100, HMB-45 and Melan-A (Baehner et al., 2005). The entity needs to be distinguished from metastatic adenocarcinoma, liposarcoma and other clear cell tumors.

3.3.4 Signet ring cell melanoma

Although rare, cytology of signet ring cell melanoma has been on record. Tsang et al. (1993) documented a case that manifested as a groin mass in a patient who had undergone below knee amputation for superficial spreading melanoma of the right foot. FNA smears in this case showed poorly cohesive, large cells with eccentric nuclei, most of which exhibited signet ring morphology. Only a small proportion of cells displayed melanin pigment clinching the right diagnosis. In the absence of melanin pigment and the clinical history, such cases are likely to be misdiagnosed as metastatic signet ring cell adenocarcinoma. Appropriate history and application of ICC can avoid misinterpretation of such cases. The case reported by Tsang et al was histologically proven to be a 'metastatic signet ring cell melanoma' with positive expression of HMB-45 and S-100, and negativity for cytokeratin.

3.3.5 Myxoid melanoma

Myxoid melanoma is an extremely rare variant with only a limited number of cases documented. Initial FNA cytologic description of this distinct variant of melanoma was given by Rocomora et al. in 1988. The lesion needs to be distinguished from other myxoid tumors such as myxoid liposarcoma (myxoid LPS), extraskeletal myxoid chondrosarcoma (extraskeletal MCS), myxoid malignant fibrous histiocytoma (myxoid MFH), chordoma and malignant peripheral nerve sheath tumor (MPNST). Although certain cytomorphologic features assist distinguishing these lesions from each other, a cytopathologist may have to depend on ICC in difficult situations. The table 2 shows the salient clinical, cytologic and immunocytochemical features that help distinguishing these lesions. It's worth noting that myxoid melanoma is usually HMB-45 negative, but strongly positive for S-100, along with a positive melanoma marker like NK1/C3 (Elliot et al., 2001).

Tumor	Average age (yrs)	Commonest site	Salient cytology	ICC
Myxoid LPS	46	Deep seated tissues- thigh, buttock, extremities	Round to spindle cells with lipoblasts and chicken-wire capillary network; lacy myxoid background	S-100 + Vimentin + Keratin – HMB45 –
Extra skeletal MCS	65	Deep seated soft tissue of extremities	Small, round to oval cells, pleomorphic mesenchymal cells in an abundant loose myxoid stroma	S-100 + Vimentin + Keratin + HMB45 –
Myxoid MFH	65	Thigh, trunk, head and neck	Large, pleomorphic, bizarre cells in a myxoid background	S-100 + Vimentin + Keratin + HMB45 –
Chordoma	Any age for spheno-palatine site	Sacrococcygeal, spheno-palatine	Small round to oval cells and and physaliphorous cells in a loose myxoid stroma	S-100 + Vimentin + Keratin + EMA + HMB45 –
MPNST	3-35		Epithelioid variant: large pleomorphic cells, INCI +/-, melanin +/-	S-100+ (focal) Vimentin + Keratin – Desmin – HMB45 +/–

Table 2. Cytologic differential diagnosis of myxoid melanoma

3.4 Location-based cytologic interpretation of melanoma

Differential diagnosis of melanoma depends not only on the overlapping cytomorphologic features or patterns, but also on the site of primary or metastatic involvement. For example, an amelanotic melanoma of the cervix may have a differential diagnosis of rhabdomyosarcoma, mixed malignant mullerian tumor (MMMT), adenocarcinoma and poorly differentiated squamous cell carcinoma (Deshpande et al., 2001). An amelanotic melanoma (epithelioid type) involving the glandular organs like salivary gland and breast is likely to be misinterpreted as an adenocarcinoma (Cangiarella et al., 1998; Bangerter, 2009). Similarly, a primary or metastatic spindle cell (amelanotic) melanoma of the breast may have a differential diagnosis of a variety of sarcomas such as leiomyosarcoma, malignant fibrous histiocytoma (MFH), neurogenic sarcoma, or dermatofibrosarcoma protuberans (DFSP) (Artal et al., 2004) and also a malignant phylloides, when epithelial component is absent. There also has been a rare case report of mediastinal spindle cell melanoma which was misinterpreted as 'spindle cell thymoma' owing to its location in the anterior mediastinum. Cytologic smears of this case were hemorrhaghic with a loosely dispersed population of spindle cells having prominent nucleoli. A rare situation as this, stresses the need for cytopathologists to be cautious when interpreting mediastinal spindle cell lesions. Melanoma in the mediastinum is extremely rare and both physicians and pathologists should be aware of this remote possibility (Bavi et al. 2005).

With the fact that melanoma can mimic a wide variety of neoplasms, one also needs to be careful while dealing with the aspirates from multiple sites; particularly, in the absence of a reliable history, as it is not infrequent to find a coexisting second lesion with melanoma. In this context, we share the experience of one of our recent cases with a previous history of melanoma of foot. This patient presented with inguinal lymphadenopathy, as well as, an intra-abdominal mass. FNA from the inguinal node yielded blackish material, which on microscopic examination showed abundant melanin pigment that obscured the morphology of neoplastic cells (figure 7); while, the aspirate from the abdominal mass showed well preserved cellular elements, with loosely clustered and dissociated population of pleomorphic malignant cells (figure 8). Although, variation in cytomorphology of the two different aspirates raised suspicion of a dual malignancy, considering the clinical history, a thorough search for melanin pigment was made; and rare pigmented malignant cells, as well as, a few melanophages were detected, confirming the diagnosis of metastatic melanoma in both the sites.

3.5 Interpretation of melanotic melanoma and its differentiation from other pigmented lesions

Often a cytopathologist needs to be cautious, when interpreting melanotic melanoma as well. Appearance of melanin pigment in cytologic smears varies according the stain used. Most cytology laboratories use one of the Romanowsky stains (in our laboratory it is May-Grünwald- Giemsa) along with the Papanicolou (PAP) and haematoxylin-eosin (H-E) stains. Various authors describe melanin pigment to be yellow to brown-black, and bluish-black in the Papanicolaou/ H-E stained, and dark-brown to black on the May-Grünwald-Giemsa (MGG) stained smears (Saqi et al., 2002; Kashyap et al., 2002). In our experience, melanin pigment takes up shades of brown colour with the Papanicolaou (figure 10), and bottle-green hue with MGG stain (figure 7). The intensity of color varies with the amount of intra or extracellular melanin pigment. An abundant pigment obscures the cytomorphologic details, necessitating the need for a careful search for cells with preserved morphology (figure 7). Owing to the overlapping shades of color, the melanin pigment needs to be differentiated from other endogenous pigments such as lipofuscin, hemosiderin and bile; special stains such as Perl's, periodic-acid-Schiff (PAS), Fontana-Masson and Ziehl-Neelsen (Z-N) stains are useful in this regard (Perry et al., 1986). Melanin is positive with Fontana-Masson; lipofuscin with PAS and Z-N stains; and hemosiderin with Perl's stain. Bile pigment is generally identified by its greenish-black and yellowish-green appearance in MGG and Papanicolaou stains respectively (Orell, 1999). Gathering appropriate history is also of relevance in differentiating melanin pigment from that of tattooing. Tattooing (intradermal injection of an exogenous pigment) is known to cause discoloration of the draining lymph nodes resulting in so called 'tattoo lymphadenitis' (Bordea et al., 2009). Anthracotic pigment, the other exogenous pigment, generally does not cause diagnostic difficulty, as it is confined to the alveolar macrophages of the respiratory cytologic samples;

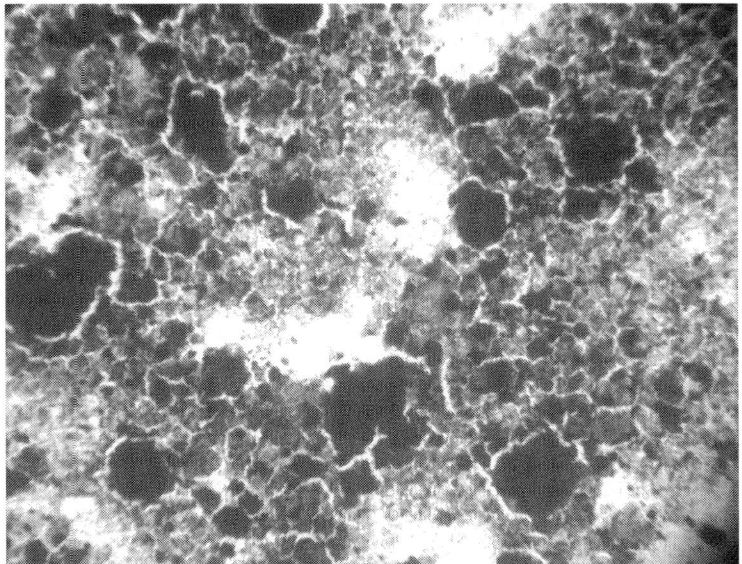

Fig. 7. FNA smear from inguinal node showing an abundant bottle-greenish pigment obscuring the cell morphology (MGG stain, x400)

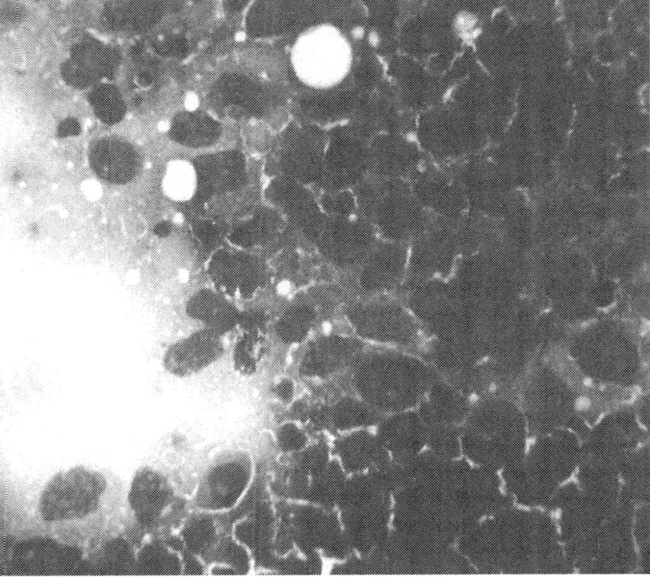

Fig. 8. Aspirate from the intra-abdominal mass of the same case showing pleomorphic melanoma cells with a rare cell displaying melanin pigment (MGG stain, x400)

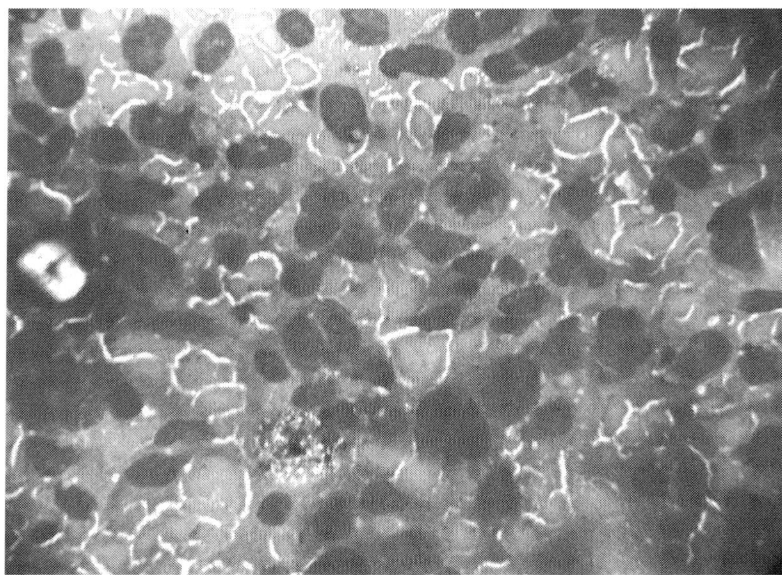

Fig. 9. Another microscopic field from the abdominal aspirate showing dissociated, pleomorphic, non-pigmented melanoma cells

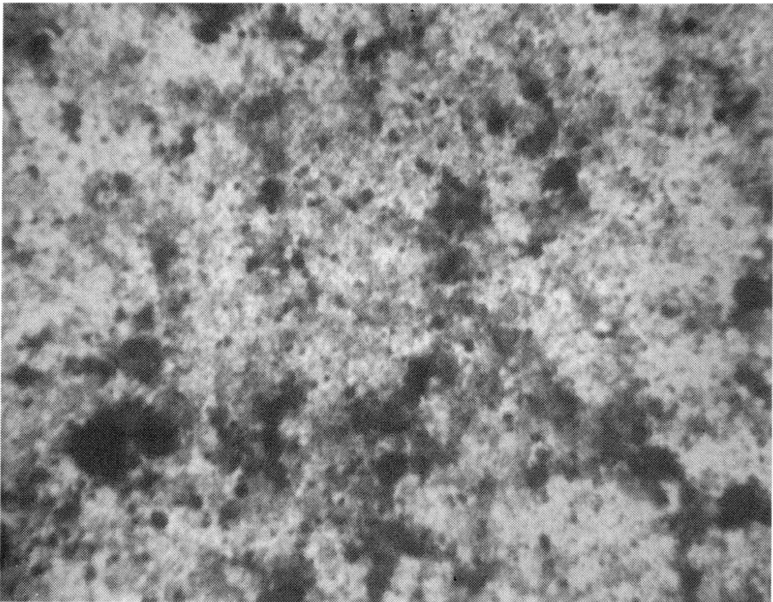

Fig. 10. Abundant melanin pigment with shades of browinish color (PAP stain, X400)

their absence in epithelial/ epithelial-like cells is of help in excluding a melanoma, or, other pigmented neoplasms. Although, the pigment can also be seen in an anthracotic node, it is rarely sampled for cytologic examination. There has been a case report of exaggerated pigmented granulomatous reaction to the artificial joint implant in a 72-year-old man who had undergone bilateral total hip arthroplasty, in whom, aspirate from the inguinal region was misinterpreted as metastatic melanoma from an unknown primary. Microscopically, the smears of this patient showed both intracellular and extracellular black pigment with obscured cytomorphology; although, appreciable cells were reported to be pleomorphic with prominent nucleoli. The patient had no evidence of primary cutaneous melanoma. On surgical exploration and histologic examination, what was presumed to be the bulky enlarged lymph nodes was found to be the soft tissue with pigment-laden macrophages and granulomatous reaction that occurred as a response to metallic prosthetic material. This rare case further emphasizes the need for critical attention to the clinical details and also a careful cytologic evaluation in the presence of pigmented debris obscuring the cytomorphology (Xin et al., 2004). Table 3 shows various types of pigments and their distinguishing features.

Pigment	History, location and microscopic appearance	Fontana-Masson	Perl's stain	PAS stain	Z-N stain
Melanin	Shades of brown on Papanicolau & bottle greenish-blackish on MGG stains	Positive	Negative	Negative	Negative
Hemosiderin	Golden-brown on Papanicolaou & greenish-brown/blackish on MGG	Negative	Positive	Negative	Negative
Lipofuscin	Golden-yellow to brown, autofluorescence	Negative	Negative	Positive	Positive
Blie	Cytologic samples from liver, greenish black with MGG and yellowish green with PAP stain	Negative	Negative	Negative	Negative
Carbon (anthracotic)	Alveolar macrophages in the respiratory samples	Negative	Negative	Negative	Negative
Tattoo	History of tattooing	Negative	Negative	Negative	Negative

Table 3. Showing features distinguishing various pigments

In the context of the pigmented lesions, we would like to share our experience of a pigmented pulmonary neoplasm in which we suggested the possibility of pulmonary melanoma. Unfortunately, due to the patient's refusal to undergo further FNAC / biopsy, work-up of this case was incomplete; however, based on the available clinical data and a careful cytomorphologic evaluation of the intra-thoracic FNA material from the lung, we could suggest a diagnosis of 'primary pulmonary melanoma'. A solitary lung lesion in the absence of swelling or lesion elsewhere (skin, GIT and eye); and a predominant population of dissociated or loosely clustered cells (figs 11 & 12), made us consider the possibility of a primary pulmonary melanoma, rather than the metastatic deposit. Here, the point noteworthy is that a pigmented neoplasm in the intra-thoracic location need not necessarily be a melanoma and should be differentiated from other rare pigmented tumors like melanocytic carcinoid, melanotic paraganglioma and melanotic schwannoma (Dountsis et al., 2003). Morphologically our case did not fit into any of these lesions. To our knowledge, melanocytic carcinoid and melanotic paraganglioma have not been documented on cytology, but there have been rare case reports of melanotic schwannoma diagnosed on FNAC, as well as on exfoliative cytology. In all these cases the authors found it highly difficult to distinguish melanoma vs. schwannoma, not only due to the morphologic overlap, but also due to its immunophenotypic and ultrastructural resemblance (Jaffer et al., 2000; Schmitz et al., 2005). Melanotic schwannoma most frequently occurs in the paraspinal region and less commonly at locations such as the intestines, heart, bronchus, liver, skin, soft tissue and bone (Jaffer et al., 2000). The table 4 shows the differential diagnosis of an intra-thoracic melanotic lesion.

Pigmented lesion	Number/location	Evidence of extra-primary site	Cytology
Primary melanoma	Usually solitary/lung	Nil	High cell yield; dispersed/ loosely clustered, pleomorphic malignant cells; inclusion-like nucleoli; intra-nuclear cytoplasmic inclusions
Metstatic melanoma	Usually multiple/ lung	Detectable on further work-up: eg. Skin, GIT or eye	Same as that of primary melanoma
Melanocytic carcinoid	Usually solitary/ lung	Nil	Depends on the type of carcinoid (classic, atypical, spindle cell or, adenocarcinoid)
Melanotic schwannoma	Usually solitary/ mediastinal		Usually, a spindle cell population with other features such as Verocay bodies
Melanotic paraganglioma	Usually solitary/ mediastinal		Evidence of cells with red cytoplasmic granularity

Table 4. Differential diagnosis of an intra-thoracic melanotic lesion on FNAC

Melanoma of lung is extremely rare accounting for 0.01% of all lung tumors. Clinically, it is confused with other conventional types of lung cancer (Wilson et al., 1997). The tumor is frequently endobronchial in origin and 30% of the cases are diagnosed incidentally on chest radiography (Ost et al., 1999). A preoperative computed tomography guided FNAC is of great help in its detection; this was how it was detected in our patient as well. The proposed criteria for diagnosing the primary pulmonary melanoma comprise clinical detection of a solitary lung tumor; absence of melanoma of the skin, mucous membrane and eye or, any other detectable tumor at the time of diagnosis; histologically demonstrable junctional changes like "dropping off" or "nesting" of melanoma cells just beneath the bronchial

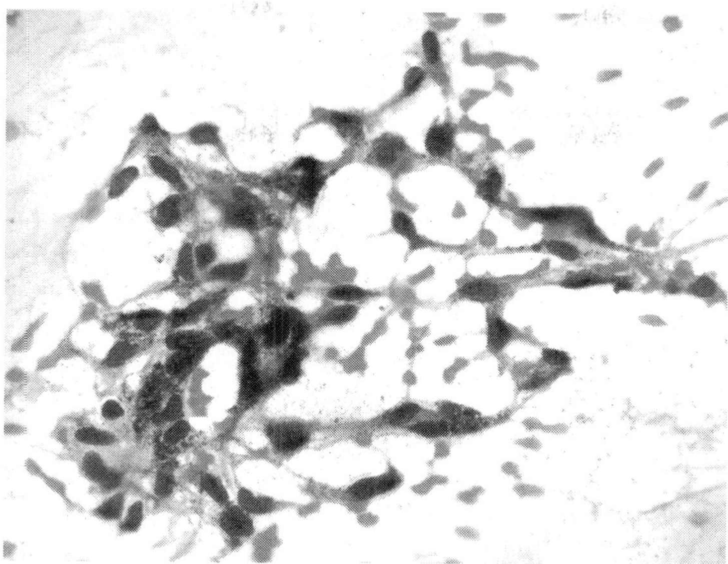

Fig. 11. The aspirate smear from primary pulmonary melanoma showing a microscopic field with a predominant spindle cell population (PAP stain, X400)

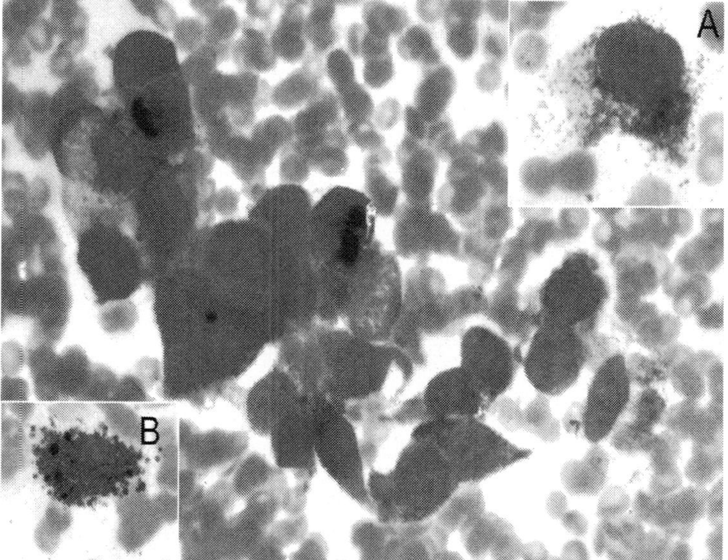

Fig. 12. Another microscopic field from the same case showing loosely cohesive pigmented melanoma cells with epithelioid morphology; Inset A- a pigmented neoplastic cell (MGG stain, X400); Inset B- a melanophage (MGG stain, X400)

epithelium; and invasion of the bronchial epithelium by melanoma cells. Although, more than 30 cases of the primary pulmonary melanomas are documented, not all of them have met the required criteria. Due to the small number of cases reported, experience with respect to the management and the prognosis of the disease is also limited (Dountsis et al., 2003). However, the surgical treatment includes resection of the tumor with an oncologically adequate margin; lobectomy, or pneumonectomy (Rosai, 2001). As for the occurrence of pulmonary melanoma, one of the hypotheses says that melanocytes exist throughout the body as cells of a dispersed neuroendocrine system. Normally, these melanocytes migrate to the epidermis and the dermoepidermal junction of the skin, but they may also migrate to the viscera during embryogenesis. This hypothesis suggested for locations like esophagus and larynx may also be applicable for lung (Pomeranz et al., 1995).

The other melanotic lesions to be considered by the cytopathologists are dermatopathic lymphadenopathy, pigmented basal cell carcinoma (BCC) and Bednar tumor. Dermatopathic lymphadenopathy is easily differentiated from metastatic melanoma not only by the clinical history, but also by the distinct cytomorphologic features. Smears from a case of dermatopathic lymphadenitis show a spectrum of reactive lymphoid cells along with cohesive (usually) clusters of melanin-laden histiocytes, in contrast to characteristically discohesive melanoma cells. We have documented a case of pigmented BCC which displayed basaloid, as well as, spindle cell population seen as cohesive fragments, and clusters on cytologic smears. Cytologically, the absence of cell-dissociation easily excluded a melanoma, while a combination of basaloid and spindle cells excluded a Bednar tumor. Cohesive clusters of basaloid cells at places exhibiting peripheral palisading favored a definitive diagnosis of pigmented BCC. (Siddaraju et al., 2008)

The incidence of melanoma in India is low as compared to that of the western population (Nair et al., 1998). Most cases of melanoma we encounter in our institute (JIPMER, which is a referral center) are those involving the soles of the feet. Many of these patents are males who present with inguinal lymphadenopathy. In the last two years, we encountered 27 metastatic melanomas, most of them with primaries in the soles of the feet. The morphologic aspects we recorded were similar to those already described in the indexed literature. Personally, I have not come across the variants such as pure balloon cell, myxoid and signet ring cell melanomas. In our experience, diagnosing pigmented melanoma is not much of a problem (although, care needs to be taken with the pigmented lesions as well); but diagnostic difficulties are common with amelanotic melanomas and the problem should be resolved with an extreme attention to the clinical details, as well as, by the application of ancillary tests. In my personal experience, the cytomorphologic features of great assistance in the accurate cytodiagnosis of amelanotic melanoma are a high cell-yield; dispersed, pleomorphic cell population; inclusion-like prominent nucleoli and the presence of intranuclear cytoplasmic inclusions.

3.6 Ancillary tests for melanoma

Immunocytochemistry is the most useful ancillary test in difficult situations. Specific immunomarkers for melanoma include HMB-45, Melan-A, tyrosinase and microphthalmia transcription factor. S-100, although least specific, is of great practical importance, as it is more consistently positive in melanoma than any other specific markers. Also, the entities that enter the differential diagnosis of melanoma are generally negative for S-100. Melanoma antigen recognized by T cells (MART-1) is another sensitive as well as specific marker for melanoma. Between melan A and MART-1, Melan A has a tendency to stain more cells (Fetsch et al., 2001). Not just the melanoma markers, but also a panel of markers need to be used depending on the differential diagnosis. Thus, one may have to use various epithelial (such as cytokeratin), mesenchymal (such as vimentin) and hematolymphoid (B and T, as well as CD68) markers depending on the clinical and cytomorphologic manifestations (Pelayes et al., 2010). Some authors have shown liquid-based cytology (LBC) preparations to be superior to conventional smears for ICC (Pelayes et al., 2010). Very rarely ultrastructural features need to be evaluated for diagnosing melanomas and the features include the presence of premelanosomes and melanosomes. Melanoma of soft parts or Clear cell sarcoma of soft parts (CCSSP) is phenotypically and immunohistochemically indistinguishable from cutaneous melanoma. Although, clinical features and certain cytomorphologic findings are of some value in distinguishing between the two, a definitive diagnosis may require the cytogenetic evaluation. This may be of particular importance with metastatic/ recurrent lesions with inadequate history (Tong et al., 2002; Kumar et al., 2003; Salem Shabb et al., 2003).

3.7 Role of cytology in ocular melanomas

Clinical diagnosis of ocular melanoma is difficult, especially, when the lesion is amelanotic. Ocular cytology, in particular FNAC can assist in its accurate diagnosis, especially with the ancillary aids (Kashyap et al., 2002; Augsburger et al., 2002; Char et al., 2006; Young et al., 2007 & 2008; Solo et al., 2009). FNAC, when done with essential precaution under the supervision of an ophthalmologist and under CT/ US guidance, provides highly accurate results (Solo et al., 2009). Studies have found no evidence of local tumor dissemination or recurrence following FNA (Faulkner-Jones et al., 2005; Pelayes et al., 2010). Young et al. in their study of 25 patients with macular choroidal melanoma, could obtain diagnostic material in 74% of the cases. Although, complications such as retinal perforation, submacular/ vitreous hemorrhage occurred in some cases, none of them required treatment. Submacular and vitreous hemorrhages cleared spontaneously within a month's period (Young et al., 2008). Augsburger et al. (2002) reported their experience of transvitreal FNAC of 34 small, non-invasive, melanocytic choroidal tumors. The cell-yield was diagnostic in 64.7% the cases. Of these, 47.1% were diagnosed as melanoma and the rest were interpreted as intermediate lesions (11.8%) and benign nevi (5.9%) respectively. The cases with insufficient FNA material (12 lesions) were designated as "nevus versus melanoma" for facilitating a further FNA follow-up. Four of these "nevus versus melanoma" cases were eventually reclassified as small choroidal melanomas and treated; while the others turned out to be benign nevi. Thus, considerable numbers of small melanocytic choroidal tumors that were likely to be categorized as 'choroidal melanoma' were shown to be benign nevi or intermediate lesions on FNA follow-up (Augsburger et al., 2002).

Iris ring melanomas are rare. In the initial stage, either they are not diagnosed or misdiagnosed as 'pigmentary glaucoma'. The patients with iris ring melanomas may not have an obvious mass lesion and, present usually with a subtle heterochromia or marked pigmentation, visible only in the trabecular meshwork. Most series have described an iris ring melanoma as a tumor involving the 360 degrees of the anterior chamber angle, although it can sometimes present as an apparently focal iris mass. Char et al. (2006) could accurately diagnose 11 of 16 cases (69%) on FNAC, performed using a 25 gauge needle going through a transcorneal route into the iris - corneal angle 180 degrees away from the main tumour mass. In cases of heterochromia without a distinct mass, an area of angle pigmentation was aspirated in the same manner. Morphologically, most cases were either of spindle cell, or, mixed spindle/ epithelioid morphology. The limitation of FNAB in diagnosing iris ring melanomas is that, even in an optimal setting, the specimens are paucicellular, often leaving the cytopathologists in a diagnostic dilemma (Char et al., 2006).

Cytology has a significant role in distinguishing pigmented lesions of the conjunctiva which can be benign, pre-malignant, or frankly malignant (melanoma). Conjunctival melanomas are potentially lethal and they arise in association with pre-existing primary acquired melanosis (PAM). It is important to recognise and monitor this precursor lesion owing to its malignant potential. Follow-up of suspicious conjunctival lesions by repeated biopsies may cause symblepharon, lid deformities, and discomfort to the patient. Conjunctival impression cytology using cellulose acetate paper has been in use for diagnosing various ocular surface disorders. Being less distressing to the patients, this quick, simple, non-invasive and inexpensive technique has proven useful for neoplastic lesions as well. The technique involves pressing a 2 x 6 mm cellulose acetate filter paper (millipore) held by forceps onto the conjunctival surface with the aid of a small solid rod for 3 to 5 seconds. The cellulose acetate imprint strip (obtained without using topical anaesthesia) is placed in a fixative containing glacial acetic acid, 37% formaldehyde, absolute ethyl alcohol and distilled water. Subsequently, the specimen is stained with PAS/ Papanicolaou stains and mounted on glass slides.

The topographic distribution and relative proportion of atypical melanocytes are better appreciated on impression cytology. Benign conditions such as conjunctival nevus and primary acquired melanosis (PAM) without atypia are not associated with the ascent of atypical melanocytes through the conjunctival epithelium; while the late stages of PAM and obvious melanomas are associated with the ascent. This is the basis for the interpretation of conjunctival impression cytology (Paridaens., 1992). Paridaens et al. (1992) evaluated conjunctival imprint cytology in differentiating melanocytic tumours of the bulbar conjunctiva in 24 patients. Impression cytology predicted the histologic diagnosis by detection of superficial atypical melanocytes and their proportion relative to benign epithelial cells in 73% of the cases (Paridaens et al., 1992). One should remember that the benign nevi, PAM without atypia, and early stages of PAM with atypia can only be diagnosed by histology, with cytology being 'negative' in such instances. Repeated examinations may increase the sensitivity of impression cytology. A disadvantage of touch imprint cytology, in comparison to exfoliative cytology, is the difficulty in focusing due to the thickness of the filter paper, which affects the cytologic assessment. Another limitation is its inability to sample the lesions located in the fornix and tarsal conjunctiva; in these cases, one can opt for exfoliative cytology with the use of cotton wool swab after topical anaesthesia. In general, although a diagnostic biopsy remains necessary for determination of the origin and extent of the lesions; the use of imprint cytology can minimise the frequency of biopsy in recurrent tumors and suspicious areas (Paridaens et al., 1992).

Our experience with ocular melanomas is limited. In one of our studies that evaluated the use of fine needle cytology in orbital and eyelid lesions, we had a single case of recurrent choroidal melanoma, which was diagnosed with the non-aspiration needling technique. Although grossly, material obtained appeared scanty, presence of obvious malignant cells with melanin pigment facilitated an easy diagnosis (Solo et al., 2009).

3.8 Melanoma of soft parts

"Melanoma of the soft parts (MSP)" or "clear cell sarcoma of the soft parts (CCSSP)" is a distinct entity with unique genetic rearrangement (t12;22) (q13;q12). Its morphologic, immunohistochemical and ultrastructural resemblance to cutaneous melanoma is well established. This phenotypic resemblance between the two necessitates the need for distinguishing CCSSP from the metastatic deposits of cutaneous melanoma (Kumar et al., 2003). Morphologhic features shared by these tumors on FNA smears include high cell yield; a predominant population of dissociated cells with plasmacytoid, polygonal and rarely spindle shapes; hyperchromasia (in some cases); prominent, round nucleoli and intranuclear cytoplasmic inclusions (INCIs). Mitoses are rare or variable and intracellular melanin is extremely rare (Tong et al., 2002; Kumar et al., 2003; Salem Shabb et al., 2003). Features such as 3-D clusters with microacinar pattern (Tong et al., 2002; Kumar et al., 2003); pale, blue, fragile or vacuolated and clear cytoplasm; a few bi- and multinucleated cells, vesicular nuclei (Tong et al., 2002; Kumar et al., 2003); extreme pleomorphism with bizarre giant cells and frequent mitoses have also been described in CCSSP (Tong et al., 2002; Kumar et al., 2003; Salem Shabb et al., 2003). As in melanoma, tumor cells exhibit positivity with histochemIcal stains such as Fontana-Masson and Schmorl's stains (Tong et al., 2002; Kumar et al., 2003) and immunohistochemically express melanoma markers such as S-100, HMB-45 and melan-A (Tong et al., 2002; Kumar et al., 2003). Ultrastructurally, often they show melanocytic differentiation with melanosomes (Tong et al., 2002; Kumar et al., 2003). However, clinically, the tumor differs from cutaneous melanoma by its younger age group (median age 30), female predilection and a general tendency to involve the tendons and fascia of the upper and lower extremities. Prognostically, in comparison to cutaneous melanoma, it runs an indolent course, although bigger tumors are likely to show a rapid deterioration (Tong et al., 2002) with multiple local recurrences, distant metastasis and poorer prognosis (Kumar et al.2003). Owing to the considerable morphologic overlap, a variety of cytologic differential diagnoses are considered, of which the important ones comprise alveolar soft part sarcoma, carcinomas, synovial sarcoma and epithelioid sarcoma (Kumar et al., 2003). Chong et al. (1997) documented a case of CCSSP of the gluteal region in a 12-year-old child, manifesting as a small round cell sarcoma on FNAC. The case exhibited cohesive cell balls, rossettes and dissociated cells in a clean background. Many cells had eccentric nuclei with irregularly dispersed chromatin, occasional intranuclear vacuoles and eosinophilic nucleoli; the later features in an aspirate from the deep seated mass, in a child should suggest the possibility of CCSSP and prompt an ICC demonstration of melanoma markers (Chong et al., 1997).

3.9 Further advances in cytology of melanoma

In situations where routine cytomorphology and immunomarkers fail to contribute to the diagnosis of melanoma, certain other ancillary studies on cytologic samples (some of which are molecular-based) have shown to provide useful diagnostic and prognostic information. Angeletti et al (2004) performed a novel tyramide-based tyrosinase assay (a simple in-situ biochemical test) on FNA material obtained from a small series of melanoma patients. For standardization, the authors used YUGEN8 melanoma cell lines and the HeLa cells as positive and negative controls respectively. They showed this simple, quick and inexpensive assay to be a sensitive and specific method for diagnosing melanoma on cytologic samples. At molecular level, HSP-70 protein, C-myc oncogene, and HLA-DR antigen are said to play a significant role in the metastasis and prognosis of cutaneous melanomas. Kalogeraki et al. (2006) studied immunoexpression of these proteins on cytologic material by ICC, and found it to be significantly associated with 'Clark levels'. In particular, HSP-70 expression is believed to be of value in the identification of melanoma patients with poor prognosis

(Kalogeraki et al., 2006). Studies also have shown tyrosinase reverse transcription polymerase chain reaction (RT-PCR) on fine-needle aspirates (FNA-PCR) to increase the diagnostic sensitivity of cytology, when US/ FNAC fails to detect the sentinel node metastasis in melanoma (Voit et al., 1999). Such studies have been performed on exfoliative samples as well. In a study involving 79 urine samples from patients with metastatic melanoma, Savoia et al. (2008) demonstrated that RT-PCR studies on exfoliative samples increased the sensitivity of cytology. The authors emphasized its utility as an additional tool in cases of negative or suspicious conventional urinary cytology.

Also being performed is the cytogenetic analysis on FNA material for detection of monosomy 3, an abnormality, associated with the adverse outcome in patients with uveal melanomas. Young et al. (2008) successfully carried out fluorescent-in-situ-hybridization (FISH) and/ or GeneChip 500k NspI Mapping array analysis on cytologic samples from 24 patients with macular choroidal melanoma and based on their results, emphasized its importance in the detection of chromosomal aberrations on cytologic material. However, Maat et al. (2007) demonstrated the heterogeneity for copy of chromosome 3 on FISH analysis performed on paraffin sections and felt that assigning patients to risk categories based on FNA samples for cytogenetic studies (for monosomy3) may be subject to error. Another significant study on FNA material by McCannel et al. (2010) demonstrated 2 cytogenetically distinct groups of choroidal melanomas characterized by chromosome 3 loss, or chromosome 6p gain. These findings may provide new insight into the biologic nature of choroidal melanoma and are likely to contribute to the development of targeted therapies (McCannel et al., 2010).

4. Conclusion

A variety of cytologic techniques are available to aid clinical evaluation of patients with melanoma, of which fine needle aspiration cytology (FNAC) is the frontrunner. The techniques have a significant role, particularly in the detection of potential metastatic sites and the recurrent lesions. They have a major role in the pre-therapeutic diagnosis of primary ocular melanomas and their recurrence. Though, specifically not indicated, it is often useful for incidental detection of primary cutaneous melanomas and also, the primary melanomas occurring elsewhere. With adequate and appropriate clinical details, an experienced cytopathologist, acquainted with the varied cytomorphologic spectrum, in particular of amelanotic melanomas can provide a reasonable diagnosis in most cases. The use of ancillary aids such as immunocytochemistry (ICC) and electron microscopy (EM) are of critical value in the diagnostically challenging cases. The care also needs to be taken when interpreting the pigmented lesions, to exclude the rare lesions simulating melanotic melanomas. Currently, the ultrasound (US) examination of sentinel node with fine needle aspiration cytology (FNAC) is under consideration as a potential, cost-effective alternative to sentinel lymph node biopsy (SLNB). Also, being attempted is the use of cytologic material for the molecular and cytogenetic evaluation to provide useful prognostic information with the possible therapeutic implication. Clinicians should make judicious use of the simple, non-invasive/ minimally invasive cytologic techniques in the management of melanoma patients.

5. Acknowledgements

I express my sincere thanks to Dr. Sara Grace Priyadarshini, the first year Junior Resident in Pathology, JIPMER, Pondicherry, for her timely help in gathering our recent cytologic data on cases of melanoma. I also thank Dr. Shramana Mandal, Assistant Professor of Pathology, JIPMER, Pondicherry, for providing one of her interesting cases of melanoma, which has been included in the present chapter. I am also thankful to Dr. Bhawana A. Badhe and Dr. Debdatta Basu, Professors of Pathology, JIPMER, Pondicherry, for their assistance in the final editing of the chapter.

6. References

Ali TZ, Zakowski MF, Yung RC, Burroughs FH, Ali SZ. Exfoliative sputum cytology of cancers metastatic to the lung. *Diagn Cytopathol*. 2005;33:147-51.

Angeletti C, Khomitch V, Halaban R, Rimm DL. Novel tyramide-based tyrosinase assay for the detection of melanoma cells in cytological preparations. *Diagn Cytopathol*. 2004;31:33-7.

Artal AE, Gómez-Aracil V, Alvira RM, Azua-Romeo J, Arraiza A. Spindle cell malignant melanoma metastatic to the breast from a pigmented lesion on the back. A case report. *Acta Cytol*. 2004;48:387-90.

Augsburger JJ, Corrêa ZM, Schneider S, Yassin RS, Robinson-Smith T, Ehya H, Trichopoulos N. Diagnostic transvitreal fine-needle aspiration biopsy of small melanocytic choroidal tumors in nevus versus melanoma category. *Trans Am Ophthalmol Soc*. 2002;100:225-32; discussion 232-4.

Badgwell BD, Pierce C, Broadwater JR, Westbrook K, Korourian S, Davis D, Hiatt K, Lee J, Cheung WL, Klimberg VS. Intraoperative sentinel lymph node analysis in melanoma. *J Surg Oncol*. 2011;103:1-5.

Baehner FL, Ng B, Sudilovsky D. Metastatic balloon cell melanoma: a case report. *Acta Cytol*. 2005;49:543-8.

Baloch ZW, Sack MJ, Yu GH, Gupta PK. Papillary formations in metastatic melanoma. *Diagn Cytopathol* 1999;20:148-51

Bargenter M. Cytomorphologic pitfall of primary malignant melanoma of the parotid gland. *Acta Cytol* 2009;53:435-6

Basler GC, Fader DJ,Yahanda A, Sondak VK, Johnson TM. The utility of fine needle aspiration in the diagnosis of melanoma metastasis to lymph nodes. *J Am Acad Dermatol* 1997;36:403-8

Bavi P, Shet T, Gujral S. Malignant melanoma of mediastinum misdiagnosed as a spindle cell thymoma in a fine needle aspirate: a case report. *Acta Cytol*. 2005;49:424-6.

Bordea C, Latifaj B, Jaffe W. Delayed presentation of tattoo lymphadenopathy mimicking malignant melanoma lymphadenopathy. *J Plast Reconstr Aesthet Surg*. 2009; 62(8):e283-5.

Bozbora A, Barbaros U, Kaya H, Erbil Y, Kapran Y, Ozbey N, Ozarmagan S. Thyroid metastasis of malignant melanoma. *Am J Clin Oncol*. 2005;28:642-3.

Cangiarella J, Symmans F, Cohen JM, Goldenberg A, Shapiro RL, Waisman J. Malignant melanoma metastatic to breast. Cancer Cytopathology 1998;84:160-2

Chong SM, Nilsson BS, Quah TC, Wee A. Malignant melanoma: an uncommon cause of small round cell malignancy in childhood. Acta Cytol 1997;41:609-10

Char DH, Kemlitz AE, Miller T, Crawford JB. Iris ring melanoma: fine needle biopsy. *Br J Ophthalmol* 2006;90:420-2

Damala K, Tsanou E, Pappa L, Sintou-Mantela E, Peschos D, Agnantis NJ, Malamou-Mitsi V. A rare case of primary malignant melanoma of the scrotum diagnosed by fine-needle aspiration. *Diagn Cytopathol*. 2004;31:413-6.

De Las Casas LE, Gokden M, Baker SJ, Korourian S, Hermonat PL, You H, Miranda RN, Shalkham JE, O'Brien LA, Mukunyadzi P. Malignant melanoma metastatic to the liver. A cytomorphologic comparative study to identify reproducible diagnostic criteria. *Acta Cytol.* 2004;48:32-8

Deshpande AH, Munshi MM. Primary malignant melanoma of the uterine cervix: report of a case diagnosed by cervical scrape cytology and review of the literature. *Diagn Cytopathol* 2001;25:108-11

Dey P, Das A, Radhika S, Nijhawan R. Cytology of primary skin tumors. *Acta cytol* 1996;40:708-13

Dountsis A, Zisis C, Karagianni E, Dahabreh J. Primary malignant melanoma of the lung: a case report. *World J Surg Oncol.* 2003:1:26

Eckert F, Baricevic B, Landthaler M, Schmidt U. Metastatic signet ring cell melanoma in a patient with an unknown primary tumor. Histologic, immunohistochemical, and ultrastructural findings. *J Am Acad Dermatol* 1992;26:870-5

Elliot D, Pittman MB. Malignant melanoma with a myxoid stroma: a diagnostic pitfall on fine needle aspiration cytology. *Diagn Cytopathol* 2001;25:185-90

Elwood M. What are the prospects for population screening for melanoma? In: Eds.Bishop Jn, GoreM. Melanoma: Critical debates, First edition. Blackwell science. Great Britain. 2002;pp107-20

Faulkner-Jones BE, Foster WJ, Harboue JW, Smith ME, Davila RM. Fine needle aspiration biopsy with adjunct Immunohistochemistry in intraocular tumor management. *Acta Cytol* 2005;49:297-308

Fetsch PA, Filie AC, Steinberg SM, Abati A. Comparison of antibodies to MART-1 and Melan A in fine needle aspiration samples of metastatic malignant melanoma. *Diagn Cytopathol* 2001;25:78-9

Friedman M, Rao U, Fox S. Cytology of metastatic balloon cell melanoma. *Acta Cytol* 1982;26:39-43

Gangane N, Anshu, Shivkumar VB, Sharma SM. Intranuclear inclusions in a case of pigmented villonodular synovitis of the ankle. *Diagn Cytopathol.* 2003;29:349-51.

Gombos EC, Esserman LE, Dacosta D, Odzer-Umlas SL, Weisberg S, Poppiti RJ Jr. "Cystic" metastatic melanoma of the breast diagnosed by fine-needle aspiration: imaging and pathologic findings. *Breast J.* 2004;10:449-51.

Gupta S, Sodhani P, Jain S. Primary malignant melanoma of uterine cervix: a rare entity diagnosed on fine needle aspiration cytology--report of a case. *Cytopathology.* 2003;14:153-6.

Hanley KZ, Weiss SW, Logani S. Melanoma with cartilaginous differentiation: Diagnostic challenge on fine-needle aspiration with emphasis on differential diagnosis. *Diagn Cytopathol.* 2009;37:51-5.

Hernandez O, Zagzag D, Kelly P, Golfinos J, Levine PH. Cytological diagnosis of cystic brain tumors: a retrospective study of 88 cases. Diagn Cytopathol. 2004 ;31:221-8.

Hitchcock MG, McCalmont TH, White WL. Cutaneous melanoma with myxoid features: twelve cases with differential diagnosis. *Am J Surg Pathol* 1999;23:1506-13

Holck S, Siemsen M, Jensen DB, Mogensen AM. Endoscopic ultrasonography-guided fine needle aspiration biopsy for staging malignant melanoma of the esophagus. A case report. *Acta Cytol.* 2002;46:744-8.

Hosler GA, Steinberg DM, Sheth S, Hamper UM, Erozan YS, Ali SZ. Inflammatory pseudotumor: a diagnostic dilemma in cytopathology. *Dian Cytopathol* 2004; 31:267-70

Jaffer S, Woodruff JM. Cytology of melanotic scwannoma in a fine needle aspirate and pleural effusion. *Acta Cytol* 2000;44:1095-1100

Kalogeraki A, Garbagnati F, Darivianaki K, Delides GS, Santinami M, Stathopoulos EN, Zoras O. HSP-70, C-myc and HLA-DR expression in patients with cutaneous malignant melanoma metastatic in lymph nodes. *Anticancer Res.* 2006;26:3551-4.

Kaneko C, Kosuge Y. Cytodiagnosis of metastatic amelanotic melanomas to lymph node by fine needle aspiration cytology: adjunctival value of immunohistochemical staining and electron microscopy. *Journal of Analytical Bioscience* 2009;32:340-4

Kapila K, Kharbnda K, Verma K. Cytomorphology of metastatic melanoma-use of S-100 protein in the diagnosis of amelanotic melanoma. *Cytopathology* 1991;2:229-37

Kashyap S, Sen S, Sharma MC, Sethi A. Diagnostic intraocular aspiration cytology of choroidal melanoma. *Diagn Cytopathol.* 2002;26:389-91.

Kotoulas C, Skagias L, Konstantinou G, Tsilalis T, Tsintiris K, Laoutidis G, Sambaziotis D. Primary pulmonary melanoma diagnosis: the role of immunohistochemistry and immunocytochemistry. *J BUON.* 2007;12:543-5.

Kumar N, Das PM, Jain S, Sodhani P, Gupta S. Melanoma of the soft parts: diagnosis of metastatic and recurrent tumors by aspiration cytology. *Diagn Cytopathol.* 2003;28:295-300.

Kumar S, Siddaraju N, Singh N, Basu D, Srinivasan R: "Intrnuclear Cytoplasmic inclusions"- an extremely unusual finding in embryonal rhabdomyosarcoma: a report of a rare case in a young female child presenting with an orbital mass. *Diagn Cytopathol.*2009; 37:740-3

Kung B, Aftab S, Wood M, Rosen D. Malignant melanoma metastatic to the thyroid gland: a case report and review of the literature. *Ear Nose Throat J.* 2009;88(1):E7.

Layfield LJ, Glasgow BJ. Aspiration biopsy cytology of primary cutaneous tumors. *Acta Cytol* 1993;37:679-88

Liao W-H, Chen C-H, Chih-Yen Tu C-Y. Black pleural effusion in melanoma. CMAJ 2010; 182(8)

Maat W, Jordanova ES, van Zelderen-Bhola SL, Barthen ER, Wessels HW, Schalij-Delfos NE, Jager MJ. The heterogeneous distribution of monosomy 3 in uveal melanomas: implications for prognostication based on fine-needle aspiration biopsies. *Arch Pathol Lab Med.* 2007;131:91-6.

Mágori A. The role of fine needle aspiration biopsy in the diagnosis of melanoma. *Magy Onkol.* 2003;47:41-3.

McCannel TA, Burgess BL, Rao NP, Nelson SF, Straatsma BR. Identification of candidate tumor oncogenes by integrative molecular analysis of choroidal melanoma fine-needle aspiration biopsy specimens. *Arch Ophthalmol.* 2010;128:1170-7.

Mohr P, Eggemont AMM, Hauschild A, Buzaid A. Staging of cutaneous melanoma. *Annals of Oncology* 2009;20(supple 6):vi14-vi21

Monteagudo C, Ferrandez A, Gondalez-Davesa M, Lombart Bosch A. Psammomatous malignant melanoma arising in an intradermal naevus. *Histopathology* 2001;39:493-7

Mowat A, Reid R, Mackie R. Balloon cell metastatic melanoma: an important differential in the diagnosis of clear cell tumors. *Histopathology* 1994;24:469-72

Nair MK, Varghese C, Mahadevan S, Cherian T, Joseph F. Cutaneous malignant melanoma-clinical epidemiology and survival. *J Indian Med Assoc* 1998;96:19-20, 28

Nasiell K, Tani E, Skoog L. Fine needle aspiration cytology and immunocytochemistry of metastatic melanoma. *Cytopathology* 1991;2:137-47

Orell SR, Vielh P. The techniques of cytology. In Eds.Orell SR, Sterrett GF, Walters MN-I, Whitaker D. Manual and atlas of fine needle aspiration cytology. Third edition. Churchil Livingstone. London. 1999; Pp10-27

Orell SR. The thyroid gland. In Eds. Orell SR, Sterrett GF, Walters MN-I, Whitaker D. Manual and atlas of fine needle aspiration cytology. Third edition. Churchil Livingstone. London. 1999; Pp110-44

Orell SR, Silverman JF. Lung, chest wall and pleura. In Eds. Orell SR, Sterrett GF, Walters MN-I, Whitaker D. Manual and atlas of fine needle aspiration cytology. Third edition. Churchil Livingstone. London. 1999; Pp202-50

Orell SR, Leiman G. Liver and spleen. In Eds.Orell SR, Sterrett GF, Walters MN-I, Whitaker D. Manual and atlas of fine needle aspiration cytology. Third edition. Churchil Livingstone. London. 1999; Pp268-90

Orell SR. Kidney, adrenal and retroperitoneum proper. In Eds. Orell SR, Sterrett GF, Walters MN-I, Whitaker D. Manual and atlas of fine needle aspiration cytology. Third edition. Churchil Livingstone. London. 1999; Pp310-36

Ost D, Joseph C, Sogoloff H, Melezes G. Primary pulmonary melanoma: case report and literature review. *Mayo Clin Proc.* 1999;74:62-6

Paridaens AD, McCartney AC, Curling OM, Lyons CJ, Hungerford JL. Impression cytology of conjunctival melanosis and Melanoma. *Brit J of Ophthalmol*, 1992;76: 198-201.

Parwani AV, Chan TY, Mathew S, Ali SZ. Metastatic malignant melanoma in liver aspirate: cytomorphologic distinction from hepatocellular carcinoma. *Diagn Cytopathol.* 2004;30:247-50.

Pelayes DE, Zárate JO. Fine needle aspiration biopsy with liquid-based cytology and adjunct immunohistochemistry in intraocular melanocytic tumors. *Eur J Ophthalmol.* 2010;20:1059-65.

Perry MD, Gore M, Seigler HF, Johnston WW. Fine needle aspration biopsy of metastatic melanoma. A morphologic analysis of 174 cases. *Acta Cytol* 1986;30:385-96

Piao Y, Guo M, Gong Y. Diagnostic challenges of metastatic spindle cell melanoma on fine-needle aspiration specimens. *Cancer.* 2008;114:94-101

Piris A, Prieto-Granada N, Imber MJ, Mihm Jr MC. Melanocytic lesions. In: Eds. Mills SE. Carter D, Greenson JK, Reuter VE, Stoler MH. Sternberg's diagnostic surgical pathology. 5th edition. Vol 1. Lippincott Williams & Wilkins. Philadelphia. 2010;30:77-98

Pomeranz AA, Garlook JH. Primary melanocarcinoma of the esophagus. *Ann Surg.*1955;142:297-301

Rai NN. Symposium on ophthalmic cytology: held during the 36th Annual Conference of Indian Academy of cytologists at Ranchi on 5th November 2006. Introduction to ophthalmic cytology- modalities and classification of neoplasms. JOC 2007;24:11-15

Rocomora A, Carrillo R, Vives R, Solera JC. Fine needle aspiration biopsy of myxoid metastasis of malignant melanoma. *Acta Cytol* 1988;32:94-100

Rosai J. Malignant melanoma. In: Eds. Rosai J, Rosai and Ackerman's Surgical Pathology. Vol 1. Ninth Edition. Mosby. St. Louis. 2005:pp164-76

Rosai J. The continuing role of morphology in the molecular age. *Mod pathol*. 2001;14:258-60

Salem Shabb SN, Boulos F, Tawil A, Hussein M, Hourani M. Clear cell sarcoma (malignant melanoma of soft parts): fine-needle aspiration cytology of a highly pigmented tumor. *Diagn Cytopathol*. 2003;28:313-5.

Saqi A, McGrath CM, Skovronsky D, Yu GH. Cytomorphologic features of fine-needle aspiration of metastatic and recurrent melanoma. *Diagn Cytopathol*. 2002;27:286-90.

Savoia P, Osella-Abate S, Comessatti A, Nardò T, Marchiò C, PacchioniD , Quaglino P, Bernengo MG. Traditional urinary cytology and tyrosinase RT-PCR in metastatic melanoma patients: correlation with clinical status. *J Clin Pathol* 2008;61:179-83

Schmitz KJ, Unkel C, Grabellus F, Baba HA, Dirsch O, Neumann A. Melanotic schwannoma of the neck mimicking a malignant melanoma. *Eur Arch Otorhinolaryngol*. 2005;262:182-5.

Siddaraju N, Solo S, Soundararaghavan J, Srinivasan R. Fine needle aspiration biopsy in pigmented basal cell carcinoma. Acta cytol 2008;52:509-11

Siddaraju N, Yaranal PJ, Mishra MM, Soundararaghavan J. Fine needle aspiration cytology in recurrent amelanotic melanoma. *Acta Cytol* 2007;51:829-32

Slagel DD, Rabb SS, silverman JF. Fine needle aspiration biopsy of metastatic malignant melanoma with rhabdoid features,. Pitfalls,and ancillary studies. *Acta Cytol* 1997;4:1426-1430

Solo S, Siddaraju N, Srinivasan R. Use of fine needle cytology in the diagnosis of orbital and eyelid lesions. *Acta Cytol* 2009;53:41-52

Tong TR, Chow TC, Chan OW, Lee KC, Yeung SH, Lam A, Yu CK. Clear-cell sarcoma diagnosis by fine-needle aspiration: cytologic, histologic, and ultrastructural features; potential pitfalls; and literature review. *Diagn Cytopathol*. 2002;26:174-80.

Tsang WY, Chan JK, Chow LT. Signet ring cell melanoma mimicking adenocarcinoma. A case report. *Acta Cytol* 1993;37:559-62

Urso C, Rongioletti F, Innocenzi D, Batolo D, Chimenti S, Fanti PL, Filotico R, Gianotti R, Lentini M, Tomasini C, Pippione M. Histological features used in the diagnosis of melanoma are frequently found in benign melanocytic naevi. *J Clin Pathol* 2005;58:409-12

Ustün M, Risberg B, Davidson B, Berner A. Cystic change in metastatic lymph nodes: a common diagnostic pitfall in fine-needle aspiration cytology. *Diagn Cytopathol*. 2002;27:387-92.

van Akkooi AC, Voit CA, Verhoef C, Eggermont AM. New developments in sentinel node staging in melanoma: controversies and alternatives. *Curr Opin Oncol*. 2010;22:169-77.

van Ells BL, Madory JE, Hoda RS. Desmoplastic melanoma morphology on Thinprep: A report of two cases. *CytoJournal* 2007, 4:18

van Rijk MC, Teertstra HJ, Peterse JL, Nieweg OE, Olmos RA, Hoefnagel CA, Kroon BB. Ultrasonography and fine-needle aspiration cytology in the preoperative evaluation of melanoma patients eligible for sentinel node biopsy. *Ann Surg Oncol*. 2006;13:1511-6.

Voit C, Kron M, Schäfer G, Schoengen A, Audring H, Lukowsky A, Schwürzer-Voit M, Sterry W, Winter H, Rademaker J. Ultrasound-guided fine needle aspiration cytology prior to sentinel lymph node biopsy in melanoma patients. *Ann Surg Oncol*. 2006;13:1682-9.

Voit C, Schoengen A, Schwürzer M, Weber L, Meyer T, Proebstle TM. Detection of regional melanoma metastases by ultrasound B-scan, cytology or tyrosinase RT-PCR of fine needle aspirates. *Brit J Cancer* 1999;80:1672-7

Voit C, Schoengen A, Schwürzer-Voit M, Weber L, Ulrich J, Sterry W, Proebstle TM. The role of ultrasound in detection and management of regional disease in melanoma patients. *Semin Oncol.* 2002;29:353-60.

Voit C, van Akkooi AC, Schäfer-Hesterberg G, Schoengen A, Kowalczyk K, Roewert JC, Sterry W, Eggermont AM. Ultrasound morphology criteria predict metastatic disease of the sentinel nodes in patients with melanoma. *Clin Oncol.* 2010;28:847-52.

Wilson RW, Joseph C, Moran CA. Primary melanoma of the lung: a Clinicopathologic and immunohistochemical study of eight cases. *Am J Surg Pathol.* 1997;21:1196-1202

Woyke S, Domagala W, Czerniak B, Strokowska M. Fine needle cytology of malignant melanoma of the skin. *Acta Cytol* 1980;24:529-38

Xin W, Davenport RD, Chang AE, Michael CW. Exaggerated pigminted granulomatous reaction to the artificial joint implant mimics metastatic melanoma. *Diagn Cytopathol* 2004;30:198-200

Young TA, Rao NP, Glasgow BJ, Moral JN, Straatsma BR. Fluorescent in situ hybridization for monosomy 3 via 30-gauge fine-needle aspiration biopsy of choroidal melanoma in vivo. *Ophthalmology.* 2007;114:142-6.

Young TA, Burgess BL, Rao NP, Glasgow BJ, Straatsma BR. Transscleral fine-needle aspiration biopsy of macular choroidal melanoma. *Am J Ophthalmol.* 2008;145:297-302.

Non-Invasive Determination of Breslow Index

Amouroux Marine and Blondel Walter
Centre de Recherche en Automatique de Nancy (CRAN)
UMR 7039 CNRS – Nancy University,
2 avenue de la Forêt de Haye, 54516 Vandoeuvre-lès-Nancy cedex
France

1. Introduction

1.1 Current melanoma diagnosis

1.1.1 Histopathology is the current gold standard technique of melanoma diagnosis

Although histopathologic examination remains the gold standard for cancer diagnosis, melanoma has the potential to be diagnosed through noninvasive approaches because of its cutaneous location (Rigel, Russak et al. 2010). Whenever a suspicious skin lesion is removed a histological examination is warranted (Garbe, Peris et al. 2009). The histopathologic report should include the following information (Ruiter, Spatz et al. 2002):
- Diagnosis and clinicopathologic type; when there is uncertainty about malignancy it should be clearly stated in the report conclusion,
- Tumour thickness in mm (Breslow depth),
- Presence or absence of ulceration,
- Level of invasion (Clark level), especially for thin melanomas <1mm in thickness,
- Microsatellites (if present), and
- Lateral and deep excision margins.

Besides these absolutely necessary histologic features, additional informations can be provided, including:
- Number of mitoses per mm^2 (in hot spots). The mitotic activity can inform about the risk of relapse and, in some series, the probability of sentinel node positivity,
- Growth phase (horizontal or vertical),
- Presence or absence of established regression,
- Presence or absence of a dense tumour infiltrating lymphocytes (TIL) infiltrate,
- Lymphatic emboli, and
- Vascular or perineural involvement.

In some instances, when the histologic diagnosis is unclear, immunohistochemical stains may be helpful (i.e. S-100 protein, HMB45 and Melan-A for the confirmation of the melanocytic nature of the tumour, HMB45 as an additional feature of malignancy when there is an inverted positive gradient, MIB-1 as a proliferation marker). It is advised to use standardised pathology worksheets. An example of such a standardised pathology worksheet can be downloaded at www.melanomagroup.eu.

1.1.2 American Joint Committee on Cancer (AJCC) Tumor-Node-Metastasis (TNM) classification of melanomas

Tables 1 and 2 display most recent (2009) classification as well as clinical and pathological staging recommended by the American Joint Committee on Cancer (AJCC) (Balch, Gershenwald et al. 2009).

Classification	Thickness (mm)	Ulceration Status/Mitoses
Tis	NA	NA
T1	≤ 1.00	a: without ulceration and mitoses < 1/mm² b: with ulceration or mitoses > 1/mm²
T2	1.01-2.00	a: without ulceration b: with ulceration
T3	2.01-4.00	a: without ulceration b: with ulceration
T4	> 4.00	a: without ulceration b: with ulceration
	Number of metastatic nodes	Nodal metastatic burden
N0	0	NA
N1	1	a: micrometastasis b: macrometastasis
N2	2-3	a: micrometastasis b: macrometastasis c: In transit metastases/staellites without metastatic nodes
N3	4 + metastatic nodes, or matted nodes, or in transit metastases/satellites with metastatic nodes	
	Site	Serum LDH
M0	No distant metastases	NA
M1a	Distant skin, subcutaneous, or nodal metastases	Normal
M1b	Lung metastases	Normal
M1c	All other visceral metastases	Normal
	Any distant metastases	Elevated
Abbreviations: T, tumor; N, node; M, metastasis; is, in situ; NA, not applicable; LDH, lactate deshydrogenase. Micrometastases are diagnosed after sentinle lymph node biopsy Macrometastases are defined as clinically detectable nodal metastases confirmed patholoically		

Table 1. TNM staging categories of cutaneous melanoma

	Clinical staging				Pathologic staging		
	T	N	M		T	N	M
0	Tis	N0	M0	0	Tis	N0	M0
IA	T1a	N0	M0	IA	T1a	N0	M0
IB	T1b	N0	M0	IB	T1b	N0	M0
	T2a	N0	M0		T2a	N0	M0
IIA	T2b	N0	M0	IIA	T2b	N0	M0
	T3a	N0	M0		T3a	N0	M0
IIB	T3b	N0	M0	IIB	T3b	N0	M0
	T4a	N0	M0		T4a	N0	M0
IIC	T4b	N0	M0	IIC	T4b	N0	M0
III	Any T	N > N0	M0	IIIA	T1-4a	N1a	M0
					T1-4a	N2a	M0
				IIIB	T1-4b	N1a	M0
					T1-4b	N2a	M0
					T1-4a	N1b	M0
					T1-4a	N2b	M0
					T1-4a	N2c	M0
				IIIC	T1-4b	N1b	M0
					T1-4b	N2b	M0
					T1-4b	N2c	M0
					Any T	N3	M0
IV	Any T	Any N	M1	IV	Any T	Any N	M1

Clinical staging includes microstaging of the primary melanoma and clinical/radiologic evaluation for metastases. By convention, it should be used after complete excision of the primary melanoma with clinical assessment for regional and distant metastases.
Pathologic staging includes microstaging of the primary melanoma and pathologic information about the regional lymph nodes after partial (IE, sentinel node biopsy) or complete lymphadnectomy. Pathologic stage 0 or stage IA patients are the exception; they do not require pathologic evaluation of their lymph nodes.

Table 2. Anatomic stage groupings for cutaneous melanoma

1.2 Breslow index

Among the aforementioned pathologic features to be determined in a histopathologic report of a melanoma diagnosis, tumour thickness also mentioned as Breslow index, is the basic criterion for staging a melanoma, once malignancy is confirmed.

1.2.1 Definition of Breslow index

By means of an ocular micrometer, the maximal thickness of the lesion is measured in several slides from the top of the granular cell layer to the deepest point of invasion. If the lesion is ulcerated, the ulcer base over the deepest point of invasion is used rather than the top of the granular cell layer (Breslow 1975). Such maximal thickness is called "Breslow index".

1.2.2 Breslow index plays several roles in melanoma management

As soon as in 1970, Alexander Breslow proposed tumour thickness as a valuable tool in prognosing patients' survival as well as in selecting patients for prophylactic lymph node dissection (Breslow 1970). Breslow index is also used for recommendations of melanoma excision margins (Lens, Nathan et al. 2007).

1.2.2.1 Breslow index as a prognostic factor

Melanoma prognosis is based on several clinical and histopathological criteria (Tichy, Ditrichova et al. 2007). As seen in Table 2, the most significant and independant one is Breslow index. In 1975, Breslow explains that a serious problem in using Clark's levels of invasion as a prognostic factor is the difficulty in differentiating between an advanced level II and a level III lesion as the difference is somewhat subjective unless instruction was given by Dr. Clark himself. By contrast, measurement of tumor thickness is objective, and good agreement among pathologists is to be expected (Breslow 1975). Last recommendations by the AJCC mention that for thinnest melanomas (i.e. Breslow index < 1 mm), the mitotic rate histologically defined as mitoses per mm² replaces Clark level for defining T1b stage melanomas compared to the 2002 edition of the AJCC melanoma staging system.

1.2.2.2 Breslow index as the determination factor of excision margins

The primary treatment of melanoma is surgical excision. An excisional biopsy is preferred, both to give the dermatopathologist/pathologist an optimal specimen and to allow evaluation of the excision margins for residual tumour. Incisional biopsies should not be performed when an excisional biopsy is technically possible. The definitive surgical excision should be performed with safety margins preferentially within 4–6 weeks after initial diagnosis. The recommendations mentioned in table 3 are consistent with the evidence that smaller excision margins are appropriate; the values given in table 3 are in concordance with the American and Australian recommendations. The current recommendations are based on both prospective, randomised studies and international consensus conferences. There are limited data to suggest that margin has an effect on loco-regional recurrence, but there are no data to support an impact of margin on survival (Garbe, Peris et al. 2009).

Tumour thickness (Breslow index)	Excision margin (cm)
In situ	0.5
≤ 2 mm	1
> 2 cm	2

Table 3. Recommended excision margins of melanomas

1.2.2.3 Breslow index as the primary predictive factor of sentinel lymph node status

Sentinel Lymph Node Biopsy (SLNB) is a minimally invasive technique developed to identify patients with nodal metastases and who could be candidates for complete lymph node dissection (Johnson, Sondak et al. 2006). A positive SLNB has been shown to be the best predictor of recurrence and survival in patients with clinically node-negative cutaneous melanoma (Wagner, Ranieri et al. 2003). Patient mean charges for SLNB and wide excision alone respectively are $12,193 and $1,466 (Agnese, Abdessalam et al. 2003). In the Multicenter Selective Lymphadenectomy Trial, an overall complication rate of 10% after lymphatic mapping and sentinel lymph node biopsy was reported (46% wound infection) (Cascinelli, Bombardieri et al. 2006). Allergic reactions to the blue dye have also been rarely reported

(Daley, Norman et al. 2004). Thus selection of patients for SLNB is an area of debate. Breslow index is a validated, reproducible factor that is predictive of SLN status, and it currently is the primary criterion used to determine whether or not SLN biopsy is considered (Paek, Griffith et al. 2007). National Comprehensive Cancer Network recommendations are to perform SLNB on appropriate patients defined as patients with stage IA thin melanomas (1.0 mm or less) with adverse prognostic factors such as thickness over 0.75 mm, positive deep margins, lymphovascular invasion, or young patient age. Ranieri et al (Ranieri, Wagner et al. 2006) mention Breslow thickness, Clark level of invasion and mitotic index as statistically significant criterions in disease subset <1 mm in predicting the SLNB result. In the disease subset .75 to 1.0 mm thick, only mitotic index was predictive of the SLNB result.

2. Interest of non-invasive determination of Breslow index

The objective of this current chapter is to review the techniques whose potential to non-invasively determine Breslow index has been studied. Basic and technical principles of each technique will be mentioned as well as their accuracy in the determination of a factor whose importance in the clinical management of melanoma is so important as previously demonstrated. Currently Breslow index is measured by the anatomo-pathologist after incisional or excisional biopsy of the suspected lesion. So why non invasive determination of Breslow index would be of utmost clinical value?

The accuracy of a biopsy depends on the expertise of the clinician. If a decision not to do a complete excision is made, partial biopsy specimens are usually taken from the most deeply pigmented, elevated, nodular, or other clinically suspect area. However, as a result of sampling error or a lack of correlation between the clinical and histological features, the portion biopsied may not be the most histologically representative portion of the lesion (Ng, Barzilai et al. 2003). Ng et al (Ng, Barzilai et al. 2003) found that in 95 of 108 initial shave or punch biopsies (88%), the physicians' clinical assessment of the melanoma for biopsy was accurate. A majority (84.8%) of the latter physicians were dermatologists with a median time of 11 years of post residency clinical experience. Khorshid et al found that general practitioners made a confident clinical diagnosis of melanoma 17% of the time and that the rate of incomplete excisions was significantly higher among general practioners (Khorshid, Pinney et al. 1998).

Moreover SLNB can be affected by the surgical resection of the primary lesion. When the primary lesion is intact or excised with a narrow margin, the lymphatic vessels draining the lesion remain intact, making SLNB a highly accurate method of identifying the lymph node basins at risk and the lymph nodes most likely to harbor metastatic disease. Although SLNB and wide local excision (WLE) are usually performed during a single operation, some patients are referred for SLN identification after a WLE has been performed. There is concern that the patterns of afferent lymphatic flow from a primary tumour site in this setting may be altered as a result of a WLE's disruption of the lymphatic vessels. This disruption may negatively impact the ability to identify SLNs and/or render SLNB less accurate in reflecting the pathologic status of the draining lymph node basins in these patients, since the remaining drainage pathways identified may no longer represent the primary tumour's actual drainage. Theoretically, SLNB could misidentify the true SLNs, leaving patients at greater risk for lymph node basin failure and denying some patients the potential benefit of early therapeutic lymph node dissection and early adjuvant therapy (Gannon, Rousseau et al. 2006). Studies are controversial on whether or not prior WLE impairs SLN status. Lesion location bias and rotational flap closure have been proposed as explanations to such controversies (McCready, Ghazarian et al. 2001; Gannon, Rousseau et al. 2006).

In conclusion to such clinical problems associated with invasive determination of Breslow index, we think that non-invasive determination of Breslow index would be a great advance in every day clinical management of melanoma. What techniques have been proposed to do so?

3. Non-invasive determination of Breslow index

Techniques for non-invasive Breslow determination use either mechanical or electromagnetic waves. A wave is the propagation of a perturbation inducing reversible variations of local physical properties. It transports energy but no matter. Ultrasounds and optical waves are used mainly because of their innocuousness.

In the next paragraphs, ultrasonography then several optical techniques will be developed. Basic physical principles of each type of wave interaction with skin will be described then accuracy of Breslow index determination by such techniques will be given. One paragraph will talk about techniques that have already given promising results in a clinical environment *in vivo*, namely ultrasonography and dermoscopy. A second paragraph will address Diffuse Reflectance Spectroscopy (DRS) that has been tested on phantoms mimicking melanoma. A third paragraph will talk about two techniques that have given preliminary results on potential Breslow index determination: the first one, infrared microimaging, performed on fixed and paraffin-embedded tissues (i.e. after excision of the tumour) and the second one, photoacoustic microscopy, performed *in vivo* on mice on which melanoma human cells were xenografted. Finally a fourth paragraph will address the topic of two techniques that have already shown excellent results in the area of skin thickness determination but for which no studied has yet been carried out to determine Breslow thickness although they do have the potential of doing so at least for thin melanoma (<1 mm): Optical Coherent Tomography (OCT) and Confocal Microscopy (CM).

3.1 In vivo techniques already available in clinics
3.1.1 Ultrasonography

3.1.1.1 Technical basis

Ultrasound is a longitudinal mechanical pressure wave. It is characterized by its velocity which has been reported for human skin, ranging from 1498 up to 1710 m/s (Agache and Humbert 2004). According to the information reported by Weichenthal (Weichenthal, Mohr et al. 2001), in the tissue of human skin affected by melanoma the ultrasound velocity deviates only by 1% from the value obtained in the case of healthy skin. If the ultrasound velocity is known, it is possible to calculate skin and/or tumour thickness *in vivo*, from the expression $l = v \cdot t/2$, where t is the time separating echoes generated by the external medium-epidermis interface and the dermis-subcutis interface, and v is ultrasonic velocity (Jasaitiene, Valiukeviciene et al. 2011).

3.1.1.2 Ultrasounds and skin interactions

Ultrasounds are characterized by frequencies between 20 kHz and 20 MHz. The choice of frequency impacts maximum penetration depth as well as axial resolution. Indeed ultrasound attenuation A is proportional to frequency f: $A = A_0 \cdot f^\beta$ ($\beta \sim 1$ for soft tissues). Maximum thickness of human skin is 300 μm for epidermis and 2.5 mm for dermis (Moore, Lunt et al. 2003). Axial resolution λ is calculated as follows: $\lambda = v / f$. In the next paragraph several studies use different ultrasound frequencies that therefore influence measurements accuracy of Breslow index. To give the reader a rough idea of such possible axial resolutions: 79 μm and 21 μm using 20 MHz and 75 MHz ultrasounds respectively.

3.1.1.3 Non-invasive determination of Breslow index using ultrasonography (Guitera, Li et al. 2008; Machet, Belot et al. 2009; Vilana, Puig et al. 2009; Kaikaris, Samsanavicius et al. 2010)

In most studies evaluating sonography for measuring cutaneous lesions in the published literature, investigators used frequencies of 20 MHz or higher. However 20-MHz scanners are not available in many clinics or dermatology practices. But such studies using 10 MHz are as important as studies using 75 MHz ultrasounds even though they do not have the same goal. On the one hand, 10-MHz ultrasonography aims at distinguishing between thick (> 1 mm) and thin (< 1 mm) melanomas. Such a boundary is important in every day clinical practice for determining safety margins and for indication for SLNB in a potential one-time procedure; on the other hand, by increasing transducer frequency and as it increases axial resolution, technological advances can be expected to improve the accuracy of sonometric measurements of melanoma thinner than 1 mm. Another piece of information to keep in mind is that maximum penetration depth of 20- and 100-MHz ultrasounds is 7.6 mm and 1.5 mm respectively. Therefore, highest ultrasound frequencies may not be used to estimate melanomas thicker than 1.5 mm.

In order to evaluate the ability of ultrasonography to determine Breslow index, sonometric measurements are compared to the current gold-standard type of measurement: histometry, following a methodology described in previous paragraphs.

Correlation between sonometric and histometric results shows the relationship between investigation methods but not the sameness of separate examination results. Thus Bland and Altman (Bland and Altman 1986) created the Band and Altman graph that includes the numerical identity between the test results of two different methods. It uses the differences between the paired measurements and is suggested to be a more useful indication as to whether one method can be a valid substitution for another.

Melanomas generally appear as solid homogeneous hypoechoic lesions and naevi have a more irregular distributed internal echo. Dermis appears hyperechoic. When the tumours extend beyond the dermis-subcutis border, the demarcation may become difficult because apart from connective tissue septae, the subcutaneous fatty tissue is also hypoechoic. Also when lesions are that thin that they do not infiltrate the dermis, they can be invisible to ultrasonography. Other causes of discrepancies between sonometry and histometry are:
- Nevus cell collection beneath the melanoma,
- Hyperkeratosis that may cause overestimation,
- Anatomical location: strongest correlation for head and neck regions and overestimation for ear, genitalia or nail,
- Histological type: strongest correlation for nodular and superficial melanomas,
- Peritumoral reaction such as inflammatory infiltrate, fibrosis, neovascularisation and elastosis in the surrounding dermis are believed to overestimate thickness when measured with ultrasound since all these dermal modifications appear as hypoechoic, and

- Actinic damage (such as on face) resulting in subepidermal hypoechoic band result in overestimation.

General overestimation of sonometric results compared to histometric results may also be due to excision processing:

- Natural shrinkage of the skin occurring after excision, particularly evident for the dermis, and
- Routine histology using conventional formalin-paraffin processing frequently distorts the anatomy of the horny layer and may result in artefacts including shrinkage of the tissue.

Table 4 gives three examples of published results of comparison between histometry and sonometry in evaluating Breslow index.

Reference	Ultrasound frequency	Mean difference between histometry and sonometry
(Pellacani and Seidenari 2003)	20 MHz	6 µm
(Gambichler, Moussa et al. 2007)	20 MHz *vs.* 100 MHz	71 µm *vs.* 16.9 µm
(Vilana, Puig et al. 2009)	14 MHz < 1 mm *vs.* < 2 mm > 2 mm	60 µm 30 µm

Table 4. Mean difference between histometric and sonometric measurements of melanoma thickness

3.1.1.4 Conclusion

The use of higher transducer frequencies (75-100 MHz) may further improve not only thickness measurements (particularly for melanomas < 1 mm) but also differentiate between malignant and benign melanocytic lesions. However limited availability of the high frequency ultrasound devices still precludes their widespread use. Rallan (Rallan, Dickson et al. 2006; Rallan, Bush et al. 2007) report that ultrasound imaging may help to differentiate benign pigmented lesions such as seborrheic keratosis, pigmented basal cell carcinoma or dermal nevus from melanoma but not atypical nevi from thin melanoma which is the main problem. Since accurate diagnosis of melanoma is mandatory before clinical management according to Breslow index determination, Doppler tool may be used to detect abnormal vascularisation which may help for differential diagnosis. Contrast agents may be used as well as other types of techniques based on light and that will be described in the next paragraphs: dermoscopy or confocal microscopy.

3.1.2 Dermoscopy

3.1.2.1 Light-skin interactions

Light is defined as electromagnetic waves that can be detected by human eye. Therefore light commonly includes electromagnetic waves whose wavelengths are between 380 and 760 nm long. Oftentimes ultraviolet (UV) as well as infrared (IR) radiation are included into so-called "light". Although such radiations are not visible they behave the same way as light from a geometrical optics point of view. As seen in Table 5, the International Commission on

Illumination (*Commission Internationale de l'Eclairage*, CIE) defines colours as spectral ranges within the light bandwidth.

Colours	Spectral ranges (nm)
UVC	250 – 280
UVB	280 – 315
UVA	315 – 380
Violet	380 – 439
Blue	439 – 498
Green	498 – 568
Yellow	568 – 592
Orange	592 – 631
Red	631 – 760
Infrared	760 – 25,000

Table 5. Spectral ranges defined by the International Commission on Illumination within the optical bandwidth

Skin is an optically inhomogeneous and absorbing media whose average refractive index is higher than that of air. This is responsible for partial reflection of the radiation at the tissue / air interface. Reflection from the surface of any flat material, where the angle of reflection is equal to the angle of incidence, is known as "specular reflection". When the reflective surface is a bulk material, the reflection spectrum is governed by the Fresnel equations: as a result this type of reflection has been called Fresnel reflection (Griffiths and Haseth 2007). Bulk scattering is a major cause of dispersion of approximately 5 - 7% of the incident radiation (over the entire spectrum) in the backward direction.

The remaining part of the radiation penetrates the tissue. Multiple scattering and absorption are responsible for radiation broadening and decay as it travels through the tissue.

Two types of subsurface scattering occur within skin layers: Mie and Rayleigh scattering (Jacques 1996).

The first and outermost section of human skin is the stratum corneum, which is a stratified structure approximately 10 – 20 μm thick mainly composed of dead cells, called corneocytes, embedded in a particular lipid matrix. Light absorption is low in this tissue, with the amount of transmitted light being relatively uniform in the visible region of the light spectrum.

The epidermis is a 30 – 300 μm thick structure in which four layers can be distinguished from a cellular point of view. From bottom to top, keratinocytes start from undifferenciated cells (unipotent stem cells) to become specialized cells (corneocytes). The four layers each correspond to a different maturation step of keratinocytes along their ascension to the top:

- stratum basale includes unipotent stem cells that are each responsible for the renewal of a portion of the epidermis; they undergo asymmetric division: each stem cell gives rise to one daughter stem cell and another daughter cell that undergoes differentiation in starting its way towards the skin surface; besides keratinocytes stratum basale includes melanocytes but such cells' main role in light – skin interaction will be in explaining light absorption;
- stratum spinosum are given this name because keratinocytes look like spines,
- stratum granulosum; this name was given because of the keratin dots within the keratinocytes cytoplasm, and

- stratum lucidum that can be distinguished in thick skin (e.g. palm) composed of transparent epidermal cells with traces of nuclei.

The epidermis propagates and absorbs light. The absorption properties come from a natural chromophore: melanin produced by melanocytes then transmitted to melanosomes that lie within the stratum spinosum. Typically the volume fraction of the epidermis occupied by melanosomes varies from 1.3% (Fitzpatrick skin type I) to 43% (Fitzpatrick skin type VI).

The dermis is a 600 – 2,500 μm thick structure which also propagates and absorbs light. It can be divided into two layers based on histological appearance:

- papillary dermis, and
- reticular dermis.

These layers are composed of connective tissue made of type I and III collagen and elastin, with nerves and blood vessels. Haemoglobin is a natural chromophore found in blood cells. In the arteries and in veins, 90-95% and 47% respectively of haemoglobin is oxygenated. These two types of haemoglobin, namely oxygenated and deoxygenated haemoglobin, have slightly different absorption spectra. Two other blood-derived pigments are found in the dermis: bilirubine and β–carotene (that may be found in the epidermis as well).

The hypodermis is a subcutaneous adipose tissue characterized by a negligible absorption of light (Technical report of A. Krishnaswamy and G.V.G. Baranowski, A study on skin optics, CS-2004-01).

3.1.2.2 Dermoscopy

Dermoscopy, also called dermatoscopy, epiluminescence microscopy or skin surface microscopy, was developed in the 1990s in order to augment the early diagnosis of melanoma. First technologies allowed the observer to examine pigmented skin lesions covered by a drop of oil and a glass slide through a stereo microscope. Then dermoscopy developed into a hand-held lighted magnifier to analyze skin lesions by observing newly defined and descriptively named subsurface structures: eg, dots, streaks, veils, and networks. The initial instruments used an oil or alcohol interface to decrease light reflection, refraction, and diffraction. This made the epidermis essentially translucent and allowed *in vivo* visualization of subsurface anatomic structures of the epidermis and papillary dermis that are otherwise not discernable to the unaided eye. Dermoscopes usually facilitate a 10-fold magnification of the skin. Newer instruments make the process easier to use by using cross-polarizing light filters which eliminate the need for oil or alcohol. Computer-based polarized light dermoscopes were lately commercialized (Rigel, Russak et al. 2010).

3.1.2.3. Breslow index determination based on dermoscopy

As described on the dermoscopy.org web site (Dermoscopy), dermoscopic criteria for the *in vivo* detection of melanoma depth are:

- pigment network: its occurrence inversely correlates with melanoma thickness,
- blue-whitish veil corresponds to an acanthotic epidermis with focal hypergranulosis above sheets of heavily pigmented melanocytes in the dermis. A blue-whitish veil is observed in 78% of melanomas > 0.75 mm thick and only in 21% of melanomas < 0.76 mm thick.
- Atypical vascular patterns are defined as vascular structures irregularly distributed throughout a given melanoma. Under this definition, atypical vascular patterns are seen in 66% of melanomas > 0.75 mm thick and only in 14% of melanomas < 0.76 mm thick.

Combinations of dermoscopic criteria along with clinical criteria such as clinical elevation, assessed as flat, palpable, or nodular and largest diameter have subsequently been proven to increase accuracy in the preoperative evaluation of melanoma thickness. By subdividing all melanomas into two groups of less than, or greater than, 0.75 mm thickness, these combinations allow correct thickness predictions in 93% of thin non-metastazing (TnM) melanomas and 82% of melanomas > 0.75 mm for a total of 89% of cases (Argenziano, Fabbrocini et al. 1999). Carli et al showed that a 6.8 dermatoscopic score allowed a 79%-positive predictive value for classification of melanomas into two groups of Breslow index less than or greater than 0.55 mm (Carli, de Giorgi et al. 2000). However Haenssle (Haenssle, Korpas et al. 2009) chose to use the 7-point checklist as this algorithm can be learned and applied more easily by nonexperts (e.g., residents in dermatology) while still allowing a high sensitivity. They carried out a 10 year–prospective clinical study on 688 patients at increased melanoma risk detecting a total of 127 melanomas. This study showed no statistical significance in lower 7-point checklist score in melanoma *in situ* compared to invasive melanoma.

3.2 Diffuse Reflectance Spectroscopy (DRS)

Optical spectroscopy methods are based on interactions of light with biological tissues. During the past twenty years, Diffuse Reflectance (DR) and AutoFluorescence (AF) spectroscopies have been the most investigated spectroscopy modalities. DR spectroscopy is based on elastic scattering of photons within biological tissues. Elastic scattering is caused by variations in the refractive index of small particles in the medium, resulting in dispersion of light in all directions, without loss of energy, i.e. no wavelength shift between incident and reflected light. Different types and sizes of scattering centres can be found within the

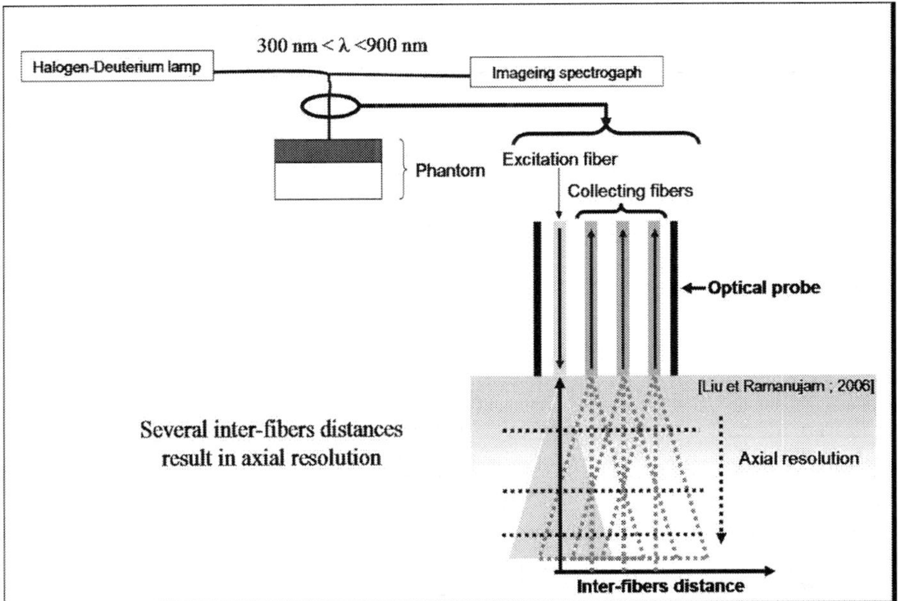

Fig. 1. Principle of axial resolution obtained thanks to several collecting optical fibres at several distances from the excitation optical fibre in Diffuse Reflectance Spectroscopy

tissue: collagen fibres, cellular membranes and subcellular structures (nuclei, mitochondria). As seen in figure 1, in order to use DR spectroscopy for Breslow index determination, Amouroux (Amouroux, Blondel et al. 2008) used several collecting optical fibres at different distances from the excitation optical fibre. Because of numerical aperture of optical fibres, the probing depth (different from the penetration depth) increases with inter-fibre distance. Of course this has limitation due to decreasing intensity with inter-fibre increase. It has been reported that excitations in the wavelength range 337 – 400 nm allow for probing depth of 225 – 250 μm in skin tissues with inter-fibres distance of 250 μm (Katika and Pilon 2006).

To our knowledge, the only study on Breslow index determination using DRS was carried out on phantoms as a preliminary study prior to a clinical trial. Two-layer phantoms mimicking dermis (6.3 mm thick) for the bottom layer and melanoma (2, 3, 4, 5 and 6 mm) for the upper layer were made of gelatine as a solid 3D-matrix, intralipids for the scattering properties and coffee for the absorbing properties of melanoma. Based on the slopes of decreasing intensities recorded at the 5 different inter-fibre distances (271, 536, 834, 1076 and 1341 μm), the five different top layers' thicknesses could be discriminated. Further works need to discriminate thicknesses less than 1 mm which is at stake in clinical practice: 0.5, 1 and 1.5 mm for instance.

3.3 Techniques that have shown preliminary results

3.3.1 Infrared-microimaging

Absorption and scattering (Raman) infrared vibrational spectroscopies consist in determining vibrational frequencies of atoms within molecules giving access to information on that molecule's state and further on its environment for instance. Fourier Transform Infrared (FTI) spectroscopy can be performed directly on fixed and paraffin-embedded tissues without staining. Reports have shown the possibility to discriminate between melanoma and normal epidermis or between melanoma and benign nevi. In 2010, Ly (Ly, Cardot-Leccia et al. 2010), carried out the first study on the possibility by FTI spectroscopy to distinguish between the different types of melanoma and to identify IR specific signatures of dermatopathological parameters: ulceration, Breslow index, Clark level and number of mitoses per mm^2. In each colour-coded image, pixels assigned to the same cluster represent an area of similar biochemical composition, producing an automated and objective digital staining of the sample. Ly et al found out that only one tumour cluster was observed for good prognosis melanomas whereas two or three clusters were simultaneously present for bad prognosis melanoma. However they still could not correlate such findings to Breslow index, even though Breslow index can be related to prognosis. Further studies will probably have to be carried out in order to determine whether or not it is possible to have an automated Breslow index determination through FIT extracted features. Such determination would spare a lot of time and would avoid Breslow index misdetermination if the section of the excised tumour is not made along the thickest part of the tumour.

3.3.2 Photoacoustic microscopy

Photoacoustic is a non-invasive imaging modality for imaging biological tissue structures by means of laser-induced ultrasound. Structures with optical absorption, such as blood vessels for instance, can be imaged with the spatial resolution of ultrasound. Lateral and axial resolutions as well as penetration depth were reported to be 45 μm, 15 μm and 3 mm respectively. Oh et al report good agreement with histometric measurements of melanomas obtained on mice after human melanoma cells xenografted subcutaneously (Oh, Li et al. 2006).

3.4 Techniques that may have the potential to be used for Breslow index determination

Optical Coherence Tomography (OCT) as well as Confocal Microscopy (CM) are widely used techniques used for skin thicknesses (epidermis, dermis, etc.) measurements. However, probably because of their low penetration depth (1 mm and 0.3 mm respectively), they have not been studied in the context of Breslow index determination yet. But as we will see in the next paragraph, they could potentially address determination of thin melanomas especially since they provide good accuracy in differential diagnosis of pigmented skin lesions.

3.4.1 Optical Coherence Tomography (OCT)

Different terms are employed in the literature to specify this method on investigations: dual-beam coherent interferometry or laser Doppler interferometry, optical coherence tomography (OCT) or optical coherence reflectometry. OCT is analogous to ultrasonic imaging, which measures the intensity of reflected infrared light rather than reflected sound waves from the sample. Time gating is employed so that the time for the light to be reflected back (or echo delay time) is used to assess the intensity of back-reflection as a function of depth. Unlike ultrasound, the echo time delay on the order of femtoseconds cannot be measured electronically due to the high speed associated with the propagation of light. Therefore, a time-of-flight technique has to be engaged to measure such an ultrashort time delay of light back-reflected from the different depth of a sample. OCT uses an optical interferometer illuminated by a low-coherent-light source so solve this problem (Tuchin 2007).

To our knowledge, no study has yet addressed the issue of Breslow index determination using OCT. Only one study tried to determine OCT specific features of benign and malignant melanocytic skin lesions. OCT of benign nevi demonstrated correlates of typical histological features including the finger-shaped elongation of rete ridges and dense cell clusters in the dermoepidermal junction zone and/or dermis. OCT features of malignant melanoma were large vertically arranged icicle-shaped structures, which mainly corresponded to dense dermal infiltrates of melanocytes as confirmed by histology. However Gambichler (Gambichler, Regeniter et al. 2007) were not able to detect any definitive features in OCT images enabling to differentiate tumour subtypes and tumour stages, e.g. thin *vs.* thick melanomas. The latter observation is, however, not surprising because the penetration depth of current OCT techniques is limited to about 1 mm in highly turbid media such as human skin. However, the greatest challenge in the diagnosis of malignant melanoma represents the discrimination of early melanomas (<1 mm) from benign nevi, for example. OCT techniques that provide a depth of penetration of approximately 1 mm potentially address the aforementioned diagnostic issue.

3.4.2 Confocal microscopy (CM)

Confocal Scanning Laser Microscopy (CLSM) is a non-invasive technique that provides real-time *in vivo* imaging of skin lesions at variable depths in horizontal planes equivalent to the resolution of conventional microscopes. With this technique, a beam splitter separates the light mixture from the laser by allowing only laser light to pass through while reflecting fluorescence light onto a detection apparatus with a pinhole-sized spatial filter. Scattered photons can be selected from a given volume. The great advantage of a confocal microscope is that axial resolution is enhanced, which results in the "optical sectioning" capability. Reflectance Confocal Microscopy (RCM) allows a higher resolution analysis of dermoscopic features than does CLSM but is more technically sensitive and expensive to use and is not as effective in analyzing deeper structures. RCM can assess microanatomical structures to a depth of only 300 μm (Tuchin 2007; Rigel, Russak et al. 2010).

In a study aiming at evaluating RCM as a secondary source of information for pigmented skin lesions after clinical (naked eye) and dermoscopic evaluations, Guitera (Guitera, Pellacani et al. 2009) found out RCM examination was particularly accurate for light-colored lesions. This is of utmost medical value since such lesions are well-known clinical and dermoscopy challenges. RCM helps improve specificity thus dramatically reducing the rate of benign lesions excisions by 23% for the current study. A 98%-sensitivity is reached when clinically suspicious lesions were assessed for diagnosis by combining dermoscopy and RCM.

4. Conclusion

Non-invasive Breslow index determination would allow one-time procedure for melanoma clinical management which would be of utmost medical interest for several reasons: unimpaired sentinel lymph node status, low morbidity, pain and stress associated to surgical excision margins. However, as explained throughout the current chapter, such a determination requires melanoma diagnosis prior to Breslow determination. As a result, all techniques reported in this chapter (based on ultrasounds, optical waves or both), not only demonstrate their ability to determine Breslow thickness but also how they increase diagnosis accuracy. Therefore, as previously mentioned (studies combining confocal microscopy and dermoscopy or ultrasounds and optical microscopy), the key for an optimal melanoma management in a clinical environment might be to combine different of the aforementioned techniques and see which combination would allow not only an accurate melanoma diagnosis but also a precise Breslow index determination. Studies should now be carried out in this philosophy.

5. References

Agache, P. and P. Humbert (2004). Measuring the skin. Berlin, Spring-Verlag.

Agnese, D. M., S. F. Abdessalam, et al. (2003). "Cost-effectiveness of sentinel lymph node biopsy in thin melanomas." Surgery 134(4): 542-7; discussion 547-8.

Amouroux, M., W. C. Blondel, et al. (2008). "A preliminary study on skin phantoms to test spatially resolved-Diffuse Reflectance Spectroscopy as a tool to help diagnose cutaneous melanoma: A non-invasive measurement of Breslow index." Biomed Mater Eng 18(4-5): 339-43.

Argenziano, G., G. Fabbrocini, et al. (1999). "Clinical and dermatoscopic criteria for the preoperative evaluation of cutaneous melanoma thickness." J Am Acad Dermatol 40(1): 61-8.

Balch, C. M., J. E. Gershenwald, et al. (2009). "Final version of 2009 AJCC melanoma staging and classification." J Clin Oncol 27(36): 6199-206.

Bland, J. M. and D. G. Altman (1986). "Statistical methods for assessing agreement between two methods of clinical measurement." Lancet 1(8476): 307-10.

Breslow, A. (1970). "Thickness, cross-sectional areas and depth of invasion in the prognosis of cutaneous melanoma." Ann Surg 172(5): 902-8.

Breslow, A. (1975). "Tumor thickness, level of invasion and node dissection in stage I cutaneous melanoma." Ann Surg 182(5): 572-5.

Carli, P., V. de Giorgi, et al. (2000). "Preoperative assessment of melanoma thickness by ABCD score of dermatoscopy." J Am Acad Dermatol 43(3): 459-66.

Cascinelli, N., E. Bombardieri, et al. (2006). "Sentinel and nonsentinel node status in stage IB and II melanoma patients: two-step prognostic indicators of survival." J Clin Oncol 24(27): 4464-71.

Daley, M. D., P. H. Norman, et al. (2004). "Adverse events associated with the intraoperative injection of isosulfan blue." J Clin Anesth 16(5): 332-41.

Dermoscopy, I. S. o. "Dermoscopy tutorial: measurement of melanoma thickness, http://www.dermoscopy.org/atlas/5step/description_d.htm." Retrieved March, 29, 2011.

Gambichler, T., G. Moussa, et al. (2007). "Preoperative ultrasonic assessment of thin melanocytic skin lesions using a 100-MHz ultrasound transducer: a comparative study." Dermatol Surg 33(7): 818-24.

Gambichler, T., P. Regeniter, et al. (2007). "Characterization of benign and malignant melanocytic skin lesions using optical coherence tomography in vivo." J Am Acad Dermatol 57(4): 629-37.

Gannon, C. J., D. L. Rousseau, Jr., et al. (2006). "Accuracy of lymphatic mapping and sentinel lymph node biopsy after previous wide local excision in patients with primary melanoma." Cancer 107(11): 2647-52.

Garbe, C., K. Peris, et al. (2009). "Diagnosis and treatment of melanoma: European consensus-based interdisciplinary guideline." Eur J Cancer 46(2): 270-83.

Griffiths, P. R. and J. A. D. Haseth (2007). Fourier Transform infrared spectrometry. Canada, John Wiley and Sons.

Guitera, P., L. X. Li, et al. (2008). "Melanoma histological Breslow thickness predicted by 75-MHz ultrasonography." Br J Dermatol 159(2): 364-9.

Guitera, P., G. Pellacani, et al. (2009). "In vivo reflectance confocal microscopy enhances secondary evaluation of melanocytic lesions." J Invest Dermatol 129(1): 131-8.

Haenssle, H. A., B. Korpas, et al. (2009). "Seven-point checklist for dermatoscopy: performance during 10 years of prospective surveillance of patients at increased melanoma risk." J Am Acad Dermatol 62(5): 785-93.

Jacques, S. (1996). "Origins of tissue optical properties in the uva visible and nir regions." OSA TOPS on Advances in Optical imaging and Photon Migration 2: 364-369.

Jasaitiene, D., S. Valiukeviciene, et al. (2011). "Principles of high-frequency ultrasonography for investigation of skin pathology." J Eur Acad Dermatol Venereol 25(4): 375-82.

Johnson, T. M., V. K. Sondak, et al. (2006). "The role of sentinel lymph node biopsy for melanoma: evidence assessment." J Am Acad Dermatol 54(1): 19-27.

Kaikaris, V., D. Samsanavicius, et al. (2010). "Measurement of melanoma thickness - comparison of two methods: ultrasound versus morphology." J Plast Reconstr Aesthet Surg.

Katika, K. M. and L. Pilon (2006). "Steady-state directional diffuse reflectance and fluorescence of human skin." Appl Opt 45(17): 4174-83.

Khorshid, S. M., E. Pinney, et al. (1998). "Melanoma excision by general practitioners in north-east Thames region, England." Br J Dermatol 138(3): 412-7.

Lens, M. B., P. Nathan, et al. (2007). "Excision margins for primary cutaneous melanoma: updated pooled analysis of randomized controlled trials." Arch Surg 142(9): 885-91; discussion 891-3.

Ly, E., N. Cardot-Leccia, et al. (2010). "Histopathological characterization of primary cutaneous melanoma using infrared microimaging: a proof-of-concept study." Br J Dermatol 162(6): 1316-23.

Machet, L., V. Belot, et al. (2009). "Preoperative measurement of thickness of cutaneous melanoma using high-resolution 20 MHz ultrasound imaging: A monocenter prospective study and systematic review of the literature." Ultrasound Med Biol 35(9): 1411-20.

McCready, D. R., D. M. Ghazarian, et al. (2001). "Sentinel lymph-node biopsy after previous wide local excision for melanoma." Can J Surg 44(6): 432-4.

Moore, T. L., M. Lunt, et al. (2003). "Seventeen-point dermal ultrasound scoring system--a reliable measure of skin thickness in patients with systemic sclerosis." Rheumatology (Oxford) 42(12): 1559-63.

Ng, P. C., D. A. Barzilai, et al. (2003). "Evaluating invasive cutaneous melanoma: is the initial biopsy representative of the final depth?" J Am Acad Dermatol 48(3): 420-4.

Oh, J. T., M. L. Li, et al. (2006). "Three-dimensional imaging of skin melanoma in vivo by dual-wavelength photoacoustic microscopy." J Biomed Opt 11(3): 34032.

Paek, S. C., K. A. Griffith, et al. (2007). "The impact of factors beyond Breslow depth on predicting sentinel lymph node positivity in melanoma." Cancer 109(1): 100-8.

Pellacani, G. and S. Seidenari (2003). "Preoperative melanoma thickness determination by 20-MHz sonography and digital videomicroscopy in combination." Arch Dermatol 139(3): 293-8.

Rallan, D., N. L. Bush, et al. (2007). "Quantitative discrimination of pigmented lesions using three-dimensional high-resolution ultrasound reflex transmission imaging." J Invest Dermatol 127(1): 189-95.

Rallan, D., M. Dickson, et al. (2006). "High-resolution ultrasound reflex transmission imaging and digital photography: potential tools for the quantitative assessment of pigmented lesions." Skin Res Technol 12(1): 50-9.

Ranieri, J. M., J. D. Wagner, et al. (2006). "The prognostic importance of sentinel lymph node biopsy in thin melanoma." Ann Surg Oncol 13(7): 927-32.

Rigel, D. S., J. Russak, et al. (2010). "The evolution of melanoma diagnosis: 25 years beyond the ABCDs." CA Cancer J Clin 60(5): 301-16.

Ruiter, D. J., A. Spatz, et al. (2002). "Pathologic staging of melanoma." Semin Oncol 29(4): 370-81.

Tichy, M., D. Ditrichova, et al. (2007). "Double skin tumors with an atypical clinical picture." Acta Dermatovenerol Alp Panonica Adriat 16(2): 63-6.

Tuchin, V. V. (2007). Tissue optics: light scatterig methods and instruments for medical diagnosis. Bellingham (WA), SPIE.

Vilana, R., S. Puig, et al. (2009). "Preoperative assessment of cutaneous melanoma thickness using 10-MHz sonography." AJR Am J Roentgenol 193(3): 639-43.

Wagner, J. D., J. Ranieri, et al. (2003). "Patterns of initial recurrence and prognosis after sentinel lymph node biopsy and selective lymphadenectomy for melanoma." Plast Reconstr Surg 112(2): 486-97.

Weichenthal, M., P. Mohr, et al. (2001). "The velocity of ultrasound in human primary melanoma tissue - implications for the clinical use of high resolution sonography." BMC Dermatol 1: 1.

3

Current Controversies in the Surgical Management of Melanoma

Joyce DP, Prichard RS and Hill ADK
Beaumont Hospital, Dublin
Ireland

1. Introduction

The incidence of malignant melanoma has increased exponentially in recent decades (Jemal et al., 2001). Indeed it has been estimated that the incidence worldwide doubles every 10 to 15 years (Cascinelli & Marchesini, 1989). The American Cancer Society projected over 38,000 new cases of melanoma in males and 29,000 in females in 2009 (American Cancer Society, 2009). Currently, melanoma accounts for 3% of cancer diagnoses annually and although this is fewer than the reported incidence of other skin cancers the prognosis is unfortunately significantly worse. Melanoma accounts for 2% of cancer deaths in men and 1% in women (Boring et al., 1994). Survival is directly related to stage at diagnosis. Recent years have seen improvements in overall survival with 87% survival at five years for all patients, and 94% in patients with localized disease (Parker et al., 1996; Kopf, 1988). However, survival for patients with stage IV disease remains low at 25% at 2 years (Balch et al., 2001).

Public awareness of melanoma has increased in parallel with this increasing incidence. The most important risk factor is intermittent high exposure to ultraviolet radiation. However, despite this increasing awareness, the practice of ultraviolet radiation protection behaviour is low. Worryingly, in a 2005 survey in the US up to 14% of adults, primarily women and young adults, reported the use of indoor tanning devices on at least one occasion (American Cancer Society, 2009).

The mainstay of treatment is surgical excision with intention to cure (Prichard et al., 2002). However, the last decade has seen a paradigm shift in the surgical approach to this disease. The management of the primary tumour has become more conservative, with acceptance of narrower excision margins. Similarly, there has been a move away from the routine performance of an elective regional lymph node dissection, towards the utilization of sentinel lymph node biopsies to accurately stage the patient's disease. The purpose of this chapter is to highlight the appropriate surgical management of both the primary tumour and the associated regional lymph node basin. We also aim to distil current controversies in the management of the regional lymph node basin.

2. Diagnosis

Any suspicious naevi or skin lesions should be assessed, using either the ABCDE system or the 7-point checklist shown below.

Seven point checklist:	The ABCDE lesion system:
Major features are:	
Change in size	A Geometrical **A**symmetry in 2 axes
Irregular shape	B Irregular **B**order
Irregular colour	C At least 2 different **C**olours in lesion
Minor features are:	D Maximum **D**iameter >6 mm
Largest diameter 7 mm or more	E **E**levation of lesion
Inflammation	
Oozing	
Itch/change in sensation	

Table 1. Seven point checklist and ABCDE system for assessment of pigmented lesions
(Whited, JD et al. 1998)

2.1 Risk factors

Risk factors for the development of malignant melanoma are varied and include genetic
susceptibility, exposure to ultraviolet radiation, and immunologic deficits (Friedman et al.,
1991). The most important of these is intermittent ultraviolet exposure. Intermittent
unaccustomed sun exposure and sunburn history were found to have considerable roles as
risk factors for melanoma. Interestingly, they reported that high occupational exposure was
inversely associated to melanoma (Gandini et al., 2005).

Epidemiological studies have identified: blue, green or grey eyes, blonde or red hair, light
complexion, freckles, sun sensitivity, and the inability to tan, as risk factors for the
development of melanoma (Evans et al., 1988; Gellin et al., 1969). Countries with
predominantly fair-skinned populations have shown that increasing proximity to the
equator is associated with an increased risk of developing melanoma. Although it is not
possible to modify genetic factors, minimizing exposure to ultraviolet radiation, in particular
intermittent exposure to high intensity radiation, and the adoption of photoprotective
measures, can significantly reduce the risk of development of melanoma (Brozena, 1993;
Friedman, 1991). The most commonly practiced sun protection behaviours in a national
sample of US adults were the application of sunscreen and shade seeking. The use of
protective clothing (hats and long-sleeved shirts) was less frequently practiced (American
Cancer Society, 2009)

Other risk factors for the development of melanoma include: a positive family history
(Greene et al., 1985) personal history of melanoma or non-melanoma cancer or in-situ skin
carcinoma (Evans et al., 1988), large numbers of melanoctic naevi in childhood (Holman &
Armstrong, 1984), and xeroderma pigmentosum (Kraemer, 1984).

2.2 Biopsy

Suspicious lesions should undergo a full thickness excisional biopsy (Lees & Briggs, 1991).
This should include the full thickness of the lesion with a 1- 3 mm margin of clinically

normal skin and subcutaneous fat. The surgical incision should be planned with definitive treatment in mind. This should include longitudinal orientation in the extremities. In addition, narrow excision margins are recommended, in order to avoid interference with subsequent sentinel lymph node mapping (Royal College of Surgeons Guidelines, 2006).

As shave and punch biopsies make pathological staging of melanoma impossible, their routine use is not recommended (Royal College of Surgeons Guidelines, 2006). Incisional biopsies may also render lesions difficult to assess on histopathological criteria, but they may be acceptable in certain anatomic locations such as the palm or sole, digit, face, ear, subungal areas, or in very large lesions. Incisional biopsies have not been associated with a worse prognosis, in terms of local or regional recurrence rates or mortality (Ledeerman & Sober, 1985; Lees & Briggs, 1991; Austin et al., 1996; Royal College of Surgeons, 2006).

3. Surgical management of the primary tumour

The surgical management of the primary tumour has shifted from extensive surgical resection, which was not only debilitating but also disfiguring, to a more conservative approach. Patients with malignant melanoma should ideally be managed by a multidisciplinary team in a tertiary referral centre. This team should include: a dermatologist, surgeon, medical oncologist, pathologist, radiologist, counsellor, specialist nurse and palliative care specialist (Royal College of Surgeons, 2006).

Excision biopsy of histologically confirmed melanoma should be followed by excision of the melanoma scar with a macroscopic margin of normal skin (Royal College of Surgeons, 2006). Previously, wider excision margins have been used to prevent lymphatic spread to the draining lymph node basin. Numerous studies have, however, failed to show any statistically significant difference between wide excision margins ranging from 3 – 5 cm, and narrower margins of 1 – 2 cm, in terms of local recurrence, mortality and disease-free survival. In addition, wider excision margins are associated with greater morbidity. (Thomas et al., 2004). Excision margins around primary melanoma should not be less than 1 cm. Exception to this rule is made for in-situ melanoma, where confirmed histological excision is adequate (Haigh et al., 2003).

The risk of death from melanoma is dependent on a number of factors, including tumour thickness according to the Breslow classification (Breslow, 1980), the presence of ulceration in the primary tumour, micrometastases to sentinel nodes, tumour site and gender (Balch et al., 2001). As survival is directly dependent on tumour thickness, current guidelines recommend excision margins based on Breslow thickness of the initial excision biopsy (Royal College of Surgeons, 2006). For patients with T1 tumours, a margin of 1 cm is advised. In this group of patients, where melanoma are less than 1 mm thick, rates of local recurrence are not higher when an excision margin of 1 cm is used instead of wider margins (Veronesi et al., 1977). A 1 – 2 cm excision margin is recommended for T2 lesions. Long-term results of a randomised trial have shown that a melanoma greater than 0.8 mm and less than or equal to 2 mm thickness can be treated with excision margins of 2 cm, as safely as those with 5 cm margins. Rates of local recurrence are not higher in patients with the narrower 2 cm margin. Similarly, rates of overall survival and recurrence -free survival are not higher in patients with narrower resection margins (Cohn-Cedarmark et al., 2000). T3 and T4 lesions should have a 20 mm margin. Loco-regional recurrence rates have been shown to be higher in melanoma greater than or equal to 2 mm thickness that is excised with a 1 cm margin, instead of a 3 cm margin. However, overall survival rates are similar in both groups. There is insufficient data to support the preferred use of either a 2 cm or 3 cm margin, and consequently, it may be reasonable to allow the patient to decide, following an informed discussion of surgical options. The use of the larger 3 cm margin is however recommended in patients with deep tumours (> 4 mm depth), due to the higher risk of loco-regional recurrence (Thomas et al., 2004). In selected cases, however, margin size may be modified to accommodate individual anatomic or cosmetic considerations (Royal College of Surgeons, 2006). Table 2 shows a summary of recommended excision margins based on tumour size.

Margins	
Tis	Histologically clear margins are adequate
T1	1 cm margin recommended
T2	1-2 cm margin recommended
T3&T4	2 – 3 cm margin recommended

Table 2. Recommended excision margins based on tumour size

3.1 In-transit metastasis

In-transit metastases are defined as cutaneous or subcutaneous deposits of melanoma between the site of primary disease and regional lymph nodes (Hayes et al., 2004). Deposits may be localized around the primary tumour, may be widespread throughout the affected limb, or on the head, neck or trunk, depending on the primary site. The number of deposits generally increases over time (Hayes et al., 2004). They are thought to arise from dissemination of melanoma cells via lymphatics to tissues located primarily between the primary tumour and the regional lymph node basin. Other theories include that of drift metastases within tissue fluid of the limb (McCarthy, 2002) or the local implantation of circulating haematogenous melanoma cells (Heenan & Ghaznawie, 1999).

The presence of small in-transit metastatic melanoma presents specific surgical problems. Unlike nodal disease, which can be managed by regional lymph node dissection (with local recurrences being uncommon), in-transit disease is often widespread and may necessitate multiple surgeries as the disease progresses and new deposits become apparent. This may cause a great deal of distress for patients. In its most severe form, in-transit metastasis may become severely disabling and may be refractory to treatment. Treatment is therefore, palliative, even if staging investigations fail to show evidence of distant metastatic disease (Hayes et al., 2004). Recent studies have recommended that treatment should be tailored to the extent of the disease, with treatments associated with significant morbidity being reserved for bulky advanced metastases (Hayes et al., 2004).

In-transit metastases are sharply circumscribed with a clear line demarcating them from normal dermis and epidermis. This line does not contain any in-situ component. Therefore, wide excision margins are not recommended for these lesions, and, therefore, a complete macroscopic excision and primary closure is sufficient. If lesions are grouped closely together, an en bloc excision is acceptable (Hayes et al., 2004).

There are numerous treatments available for management of in-transit metastases that are not amenable to surgical excision. Carbon dioxide laser therapy has been used in the management of multiple small in-transit metastases that are not suitable for surgical excision. This treatment may be performed under local anaesthetic or if a very large number of lesions are present, general anaesthetic. It is suitable for use as a day-case procedure. If the lesion is small -measuring less than 3 mm- it may be vapourized completely. Larger lesions, however, are first circumscribed with the laser followed by excision of the central core. Haemostasis is achieved with a pressure dressing, following treatment. This procedure is tolerated well by patients, as it is relatively pain free. Wound healing may take up to 6 weeks following treatment. The value of carbon dioxide laser therapy is highest in patients with multiple small lesions, but is it is less useful in patients with larger deposits. It has been recommended that this treatment be undertaken before isolated limb perfusion, as the latter is associated with significant morbidity (Hayes et al., 2004).

Isolated limb perfusion (ILP) was first described in the 1960s (Creech & Krementz, 1966). This process involves the application of a tourniquet to the affected limb, thereby isolating it from the systemic circulation, and administering cyctotoxic agents via an extracorporeal bypass circuit. This procedure is performed under general anaesthetic. The first step is to expose and cannulate the artery and vein supplying the affected limb. The chemotherapeutic agent is then perfused over a period of 1 hour. Agents used include melphalan and dacarbazine. TNF-α has been shown to increase response rates, when given with melphalan (Lienard et al., 1992). It is thought to work by targeting neo-vasculature instead of being directly cytotoxic to tumour cells, and is of use in larger deposits (Fraker, 1999). This is then followed by a washout period lasting 30 minutes (Hayes et al., 2004). Advantages of this procedure include the delivery of high doses (up to tenfold higher than the dose tolerated systemically) of chemotherapeutic agents to the affected limb, with a reduction in systemic toxicity (Briele et al., 1985). Disadvantages of this treatment are numerous: local toxicity may be in the form of mild erythema or even epidermolysis and deep tissue damage (Wieberdink et al., 1982). High pressures may lead to compartment syndrome requiring fasciotomy (Mubarak & Owen, 1977). Hypotension and myelosuppression may result from leakage of perfusate into the systemic circulation (Hayes et al., 2004). One study found that patients with stage III disease, who were treated with BCG and dimethyltriazeno imidazole carboxamide (DTIC), trended towards a delay in recurrence and increased survival, but this was not statistically significant (Can Med Assoc J. 1983). Similarly, the use of interferon alpha for isolated limb perfusion is not supported by strong scientific evidence (RCSI guidelines, 2006).

More recently, the role of isolated limb infusion in the management of in-transit metastasis is being investigated. This technique is minimally invasive, easy to perform and is more economical than isolated limb perfusion (Brady et al, 2006; Mian et al, 2001). The size of the area treated depends on disease severity and ranges from a small section of a limb to the entire limb. The first step in this process is to determine the volume of the limb in order to allow calculation of the appropriate dose of chemotherapeutic agents. A number of techniques have been described for calculation of limb volume. These include the use of programs which take into account serial limb measurements. Other centres use the formula $\pi r2h$ to calculate limb volume at measured intervals. The next step is the placement of arterial and venous catheters into the contralateral limb. The catheter tips must lie above the knee or elbow. A hot air blanket is placed over the affected limb with the intention in inducing a temperature of 38-40 degrees Celcius (limb hyperthermia). The patient is anaesthetised and 30ml of papaverine is administered followed by a heparin flush. A tourniquet is then applied. A mixture of dactinomycin and melphalan are circulated for 20

TNM Staging Categories for Cutaneous Melanoma		
Classification	Thickness (mm)	Ulceration Status/Mitoses
Tis	NA	NA
T1	≤ 1.00	a: Without ulceration and mitosis < 1/ mm^2 b: With ulceration or mitoses ≥1/ mm^2
T2	1.01-2.00	a: Without ulceration b: With ulceration
T3	2.01-4.00	a: Without ulceration b: With ulceration
T4	> 4.00	a: Without ulceration b: With ulceration
N	No. of Metastatic Nodes	Nodal Metastatic Burden
N0	0	NA
N1	1	a: Micrometastasis* b: Macrometastasis†
N2	2 -3	a: Micrometastasis* b: Macrometastasis† c: In transit metastases/satellites without metastatic nodes
N3	4+ metastatic nodes, or matted nodes, or in transit metastases/satellites with metastatic nodes	
M	Site	Serum LDH
M0	No distant metastases	NA
M1a	Distant skin, subcutaneous, or nodal metastases	Normal
M1b	Lung metastases	Normal
M1c	All other visceral metastases	Normal
	Any distant metastasis	Elevated
Abbreviations: NA, not applicable; LDH, lactate dehydrogenase. Micrometastases are diagnosed after sentinel lymph node biopsy. †Macrometastases are defined as clinically detectable nodal metastases confirmed pathologically.		

Table 3. TNM staging categories for cutaneous melanoma (Balch et al., 2009)

minutes by withdrawing through the venous circuit and infusion into the arterial circuit. One litre of Hartmann's solution is then infused to remove the chemotherapeutic agents. Following the infusion the tourniquet and catheters are removed, a pressure dressing is applied and the patient's leg is elevated (Al-Hilli et al, 2007).

Isolated limb infusion has a number of advantages over isolated limb perfusion. Firstly, it is associated with a lower rate of complications including erythema, skin loss, compartment syndrome, myopathy, neuropathy and limb loss (1%). In addition, catheters are placed percutaneously making it less invasive with no requirement for a bypass circuit. Operating time is shorter than for isolated limb perfusion (4 hours for isolated limb perfusion versus 1 hour for isolated limb infusion). Complete response rates of 45% and partial response rates of 42% have been reported for isolated limb infusion compared to complete response rates of 40% and partial response rates of 40% for isolated limb perfusion (Brady et al, 2006; Mian et al, 2001).

The presence of in-transit metastases indicates a poor prognosis. The development of in-transit disease is rapidly followed by distant metastases (Hayes et al., 2004). The American Committee on Cancer Staging (AJCC) classify it as stage IIIB or IIIC disease, along with regional lymph node metastases. Five year survival rates in patients with stage III disease ranges from 18% to 60%. However, patients with in-transit metastasis have the worst prognosis, with 5 year survival of approximately 25% (Hayes et al., 2004).

3.2 Reconstruction

The optimal treatment of patients is primary closure, following excision of the primary tumour with adequate margins. Unfortunately, this is not always possible, and the patient may require reconstructive surgery. The type of reconstruction employed depends on the location of the melanoma. Skin grafts are often used, following excision of melanoma on the limbs. Traditionally, these were harvested from the contralateral limb, as melanoma was thought to metastasize primarily via lymphatic routes (Cade, 1961, Roberts et al., 2002). A recent study has shown that there is no difference in rates of donor site recurrence whether the ipsilateral or contralateral limb is used. The authors recommended that to improve patients post-operative recovery, the skin graft be harvested from the same limb as the primary tumour (Schumacher et al., 2010).

The use of skin grafts on the head and neck, however, is not always ideal, and may give rise to significant deformity. Local rotational skin flaps, such as rhomboid flaps, are safe, versatile, and aesthetically pleasing when used in this area (Lent & Aryian, 1994). They may also be of use in very large areas where a skin graft alone would give a poor cosmetic result.

4. Management of the regional lymph node basin

The outcome in patients diagnosed with melanoma is dependent, not only on tumour thickness, but also on the presence of regional or distant metastasis (Lees & Briggs, 1991). In fact, regional lymph node status is thought to be the most powerful prognostic indictor in clinically localized melanoma (Morton et al., 2006). The presence of regional nodal metastasis is associated with a 50% reduction in survival (Royal College of Surgeons, 2006). The rate of nodal metastatic disease is largely dependant upon the initial tumour thickness. T1 melanoma has a favourable outlook, with a 10% risk of occult nodal metastasis. Approximately 25% of patients, with melanoma between 1.5 - 4.0 mm thick, have lymph node metastasis at presentation. 60% of patients with melanoma greater than 4 mm will show regional lymph node metastasis at diagnosis. These data form the basis for the current guidelines on which patients should be offered a sentinel lymph node biopsy (Royal College of Surgeons, 2006).

Patients diagnosed with stage III disease commonly have clinically negative lymph nodes but are found to have micro-metastatic disease on their sentinel lymph node biopsy. Such patients have a more favourable outcome than patients with clinically involved nodes at presentation (Balch et al., 2009). The major determinants of outcome for stage III disease are: number of metastatic lymph nodes and the presence of either microscopic or macroscopic disease. Five-year survival rates for patients with stage IIIA disease is 67%, and 10-year survival is 60%. Five-year survival rates for patients with stage IIIB disease is estimated at 53%. Stage IIIC disease has a poorer prognosis with 5-year survival of approximately 26% (Balch et al., 2001).

5. The sentinel lymph node biopsy

The sentinel lymph node is defined as any lymph node that receives lymphatic drainage directly from a primary tumor site (Thompson, 2001; Uren et al., 1994). The rationale for undertaking a sentinel lymph node biopsy in melanoma is to firstly to provide prognostic information and secondly to allow node negative patients avoid an unnecessary lymph node dissection. The current indications for sentinel lymph node biopsy include intermediate thickness melanoma, 1 – 4 mm (Morton et al., 2006). However, a study published this year also recommended that patients with thin melanoma, greater than 0.75 mm and or ulceration, should be considered for a sentinel lymph node dissection, although this has as yet not gained widespread acceptance (Yonick et al., 2011).

The use of sentinel lymph node biopsy allows surgeons to appropriately select patients for complete lymph node dissection, instead of undertaking lymph node dissection in all patients. This practice allows assessment of the regional lymph node basin with low rates of morbidity (Gershenwald et al., 1999). By managing occult nodal metastases early, through sentinel lymph node dissection, the patients risk of melanoma-related death is reduced (Faries et al., 2010).

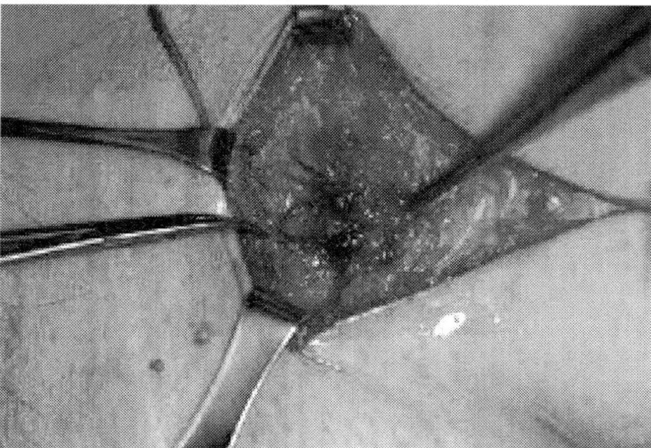

Fig. 1. The sentinel lymph node biopsy

The technical details of sentinel lymph node biopsy can be broken down into a number of steps. First, the patient undergoes preoperative lymphoscintigraphy which identifies the regional nodal basin and estimates the location of the sentinel node. Four intradermal injections of 0.1–0.2 ml of 10 mBq radiocolloid are performed around the melanoma or melanoma scar: the injection should raise a small wheal on the skin. The most commonly used radiotracers are 99mTc-labeled albumin (Europe), 99mTc-labeled sulfur colloid and 99mTc-antimony trisulfide colloid. Scintillation cameras are used to obtain dynamic images. These images allow identification of sentinel nodes within the regional nodal basin. They also allow discrimination of second-tier nodes, which may be falsely interpreted as sentinel nodes on delayed imaging. The surface location of the sentinel node may be marked on the skin preoperatively or, alternatively, a gamma probe can be use to locate the node intra-operatively. Intra-operative lymphatic mapping involves injection of vital blue dye (Isosulfan blue (Lymphazurin), Methylene Blue or Patent Blue V are used). A combination of radiotracers and blue dye has been shown to allow sentinel node identification in 99% of cases. The blue dye is injected intra-dermally (again to produce a wheal) in 2-4 locations at the site of the primary lesion, 10-15 minutes before skin incision. The dye is used to visualize the sentinel node intra-operatively. A gamma probe (covered in a sterile plastic sheath), which detects radiation, may be used to locate the sentinel node. Counts should be obtained over the skin before incision, to confirm the location of the sentinel node. A short skin incision is made, bearing in mind the potential need for complete lymph node dissection. The sentinel nodes are then identified using the blue dye and gamma probe as a guide, and they are removed with minimal dissection. An ex-vivo count should be obtained, by measuring the radioactivity of the sentinel node(s) after removal. A bed count is then also obtained following removal of the sentinel node(s), to ensure that no sentinel nodes remain (Bagaria et al., 2010).

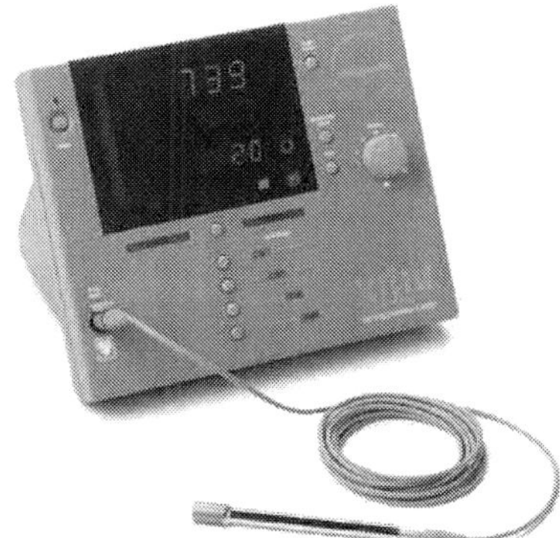

Fig. 2. Gamma probe used to locate sentinel lymph node

Significant controversy surrounds the use of sentinel lymph node biopsy in thin, early melanomas. There are a number of reasons for this. Firstly, patients with a low-risk of nodal metastases are exposed to the toxicity of a potentially unnecessary procedure. Secondly, the routine use of sentinel lymph node biopsy is expensive: global application of sentinel lymph node biopsy in all patients is estimated to cost between $700,000 and $1,000,000 for every sentinel node metastasis detected (Agnses et al., 2003).

Can we therefore use the sentinel lymph node technique selectively in patients with thin melanomas? Multiple studies have examined risk factors for poor prognosis in patient with thin melanoma. Age has been shown to be associated with a decreased overall and melanoma-specific survival (Faries et al., 2010). Paradoxically, age is associated with a lower risk of lymph node metastases. This paradox can be explained by decreased lymphatic function with advancing age (Conway et al., 2009). Other risk factors which have been put forward as predictors of lymph node metastasis include: sex, vertical growth phase, Breslow thickness, mitotic rate, Clark level, and tumour-infiltrating lymphocytes (Bedrosian et al., 2000; Bleicher et al., 2003; Cecchi et al., 2007; Gimotty et al., 2004; Kesmodel et al., 2005; Oliveira et al., 2003; Puleo et al., 2005; Vaquerano et al., 2006).

These specific factors remain controversial and several studies have questioned their importance (Stitzenberg et al., 2004; Wong et al., 2006). The use of vertical growth phase as a predictor of metastasis may be problematic as it is not reported in many centres and pathologists may not be experienced at distinguishing it from the radial growth phase. A similar problem is encountered when Clark level is used (Owen et al., 2001). Tumour-infiltrating lymphocytes are measured on a scale that is deemed to be subjective, and therefore may give rise to inter-observer variation. Mitotic rate, however, has been shown to be extremely important in melanoma risk assessment (Gimotty et al., 2005; Paek et al., 2007; Sondak et al., 2004) and is planned to be included in the updated American Joint Committee on Cancer Staging system. Ulceration has been associated with a worse prognosis and a higher rate of nodal metastasis, but this is an uncommon finding in thin lesions (McKinnion et al., 2003). A recent study by Faries et al, examining the rate of nodal recurrence in thin melanoma following wide local excision, only identified Breslow thickness, age, and sex as significant indicators of recurrence. Based on these findings, they developed a scoring system and nomogram for the risk of regional nodal metastasis. It has been recommended that this system may be used to reassure low-risk patients, who are anxious about metastasis, or to convince high-risk patients to proceed with a sentinel lymph node biopsy (Faries et al., 2010).

The role of sentinel lymph node biopsy for patients with thick melanomas (> 4 mm) also remains controversial. This specific group of patients have a high risk of nodal metastasis, with some studies showing rates as high as 60% (Balch et al., 2001; Gershenwald et al., 2000). However, as this group of patients are also at high risk of distant metastatic disease the role of either sentinel lymph node biopsy or regional lymph node clearance remain unclear, in terms of providing an improvement in overall survival. Recent studies, have however proposed an improvement in both disease free and overall survival with the presence of a negative sentinel lymph node (Scoggins et al., 2010). They therefore concluded that sentinel lymph node biopsy and complete lymph node dissection for sentinel node positive patients achieves good regional nodal disease control. Sentinel lymph node biopsy in this group of patients may, therefore important for prognosis as well as having therapeutic implications and should at least be considered in these patients (Scoggins et al., 2010).

6. Elective regional lymph node dissection

Complete lymph node dissection is performed with the intention of halting metastatic spread of melanoma in the early stages of the disease (Callery et al., 1982; Roses et al., 1985). Five-year survival rates in patients with negative complete lymph node dissection stands at 62.5%, compared with 20.3% in patients with positive non-sentinel nodes (Kunte et al.,

2009). Therefore, patients undergoing elective lymph node dissection should have improved survival, when compared with patients who are only treated following the appearance of metastases, a point that has been demonstrated in numerous retrospective studies (Balch et al., 1979, 1988; Callery et al., 1982; Milton et al., 1982; Roses et al., 1985). Before the advent of sentinel lymph node biopsy, a complete lymph node dissection was carried out for all patients with malignant melanoma irrespective of lymph node status. However, a number of randomized prospective trials have failed to show overall survival benefit to elective lymph node dissection, and propose that regional lymph nodal metastases represent markers of systemic disease (Balch et al., 1996; Sim et al., 1978; Veronesi et al., 1977, 1982).

It is unclear if an elective lymph node dissection is the appropriate next step in the management of patients with a positive sentinel lymph node biopsy. Currently, a complete lymph node dissection is carried out for all patients with a positive sentinel lymph node, irrespective of the type of metastases (micro-metastasis or macro-metastasis). The value of a complete lymph node dissection in this group of patients has not been extensively investigated (Garbe et al., 2008) and it must constantly be borne in mind that complete lymph node dissection is associated with significant patient morbidity (Guggenheim et al., 2008).

A significant survival benefit has been noted in patients with a positive sentinel lymph node biopsy, who undergo a complete lymph node dissection, when compared with patients undergoing complete lymph node dissection after nodal metastases become apparent (Kretschmer et al., 2004). In a study conducted by Morton et al. (2006), a 5-year survival rate of 72% was seen in patients with positive sentinel lymph nodes, followed by immediate lymph node dissection, whereas patients undergoing a delayed lymph node dissection had a 5-year survival rate of only 52%. However, further positive non-sentinel lymph nodes are found in a relatively small proportion of patients: previously quoted figures ranged from 17%-24% (Ghaferi et al., 2009; Lee et al., 2004; Rossi et al., 2008; Wright et al., 2010). However, a recent study has shown rates of further positive findings to be as low as 14.8% (Kunte et al., 2011).

Ideally, patients at high risk of non-sentinel nodal metastases could be identified and treated by regional lymph node dissection, and patients with a low risk of non-sentinel nodal metastases could be spared from further intervention (Wright et al., 2008). Recently, researchers have sought to identify factors, which increase a patient's likelihood of non-sentinel node metastases. Increasing Breslow depth has been associated with increased risk of non-sentinel node metastases, while a depth of less than 1 mm has no association with any further positive nodes on completion lymph node dissection (Kunte et al., 2011). Studies have failed to show an association between specific tumour and patient characteristics with an increased rate of non-sentinel nodal metastasis (Rossi et al., 2008). However, a number of histopathologic features have been shown to be associated with positive complete lymph node dissections. These include: nodular melanoma, ulceration, melanoma regression, naevus association, and no special tumour characteristics (Kunte et al., 2011). Using a size/ulceration score, Reeves et al. (2003) showed ulceration to be an independent predictor of non-sentinel node deposits.

Recent studies have examined the association between the size of sentinel lymph node deposits and the rate of positive complete lymph node dissection. Kunte et al. (2011) did not report any patients with micro-metastatic deposits on sentinel lymph node biopsy to have positive findings on complete lymph node dissection (Glumac et al., 2008). Another study showed a 3-year survival rate in patients with 1 mm sentinel lymph node metastasis to be

100%, while 3-year survival in patients with deposits greater than 1 mm was 80% (Van der Ploeg et al., 2009). Ollila et al. (2009), however, found a significantly higher rate of recurrence in patients with sub-micrometastatic disease (ie. sentinel lymph node deposits less than 0.1 mm), compared with node-negative patients. Unfortunately the role of complete lymph node dissection in patients with a positive sentinel lymph node biopsy remains unclear and further study is necessary to identify factors which may be incorporated into a model for assessing risk of identifying high risk patients.

7. Conclusion

The incidence of melanoma is rising steadily in the Western world. Increased awareness of the disease has not impacted on its poor prognosis. Surgery remains the mainstay of treatment for this difficult tumour. Indeed there is little in the way of adjuvant systemic therapy that improves overall survival. Adequate surgical margins with or without local reconstructive techniques can improve local recurrence rates. Utilization of the sentinel node biopsy technique allows accurate staging of disease and determination of prognosis. Positive sentinel lymph nodes should be treated with regional lymph node dissection to reduce loco-regional disease. The impact of this on overall survival has not yet been clearly elucidated. The future lies in the continued expansion of the molecular basis of melanoma and the hope of personalised targeted molecular therapies.

8. References

Agnese, DM; Abdessalam, SF; Burak, WE Jr; Magro, CM; Pozderac, RV & Walker, MJ. (2003). Cost-effectiveness of sentinel lymph node biopsy in thin melanomas. *Surgery*, Vol.134, No. 4, pp. 542-548.

Al-Hilli, Z; Khan, W; Hill, A. D. K. (2007). Isolated limb infusion for melanoma. *Surgeon*, Vol. 5, No. 5, pp. 310-2.

American Cancer Society. (1990). 1989 survey of physicians' attitudes and practices in early cancer detection. *CA*, Vol. 40, pp. 77-101.

Austin, JR; Byers, RM; Brown, WD; Wolf, P. (1996). Influence of biopsy on the prognosis of cutaneous melanoma of the head and neck. *Head Neck*, Vol. 18, pp. 107-117.

Bagaria, SP; Faries. MB; Morton. DL. (2010). Sentinel Node Biopsy in Melanoma: Technical Considerations of the Procedure as Performed at the John Wayne Cancer Institute. *J. Surg. Oncol.*, Vol. 101, pp. 669–676.

Balch, CM; Buzaid, AC; Soong, SJ; Atkins, MB ; Cascinelli, N; Coit, DG. et al. (2001). Final version of the American Joint Committee on Cancer staging system for cutaneous melanoma. *J Clin Oncol*, Vol. 19, pp 3635–3648.

Balch, CM; Gershenwald, JE; Soong, SJ. et al. (1996). Final Version of 2009 AJCC melanoma staging and classification. *J Clin Oncol*, Vol. 27, No. 36, pp. 6199–206.

Balch, CM; Soong, S-J; Bartolucci, AA. et al. (1996). Efficacy of an elective regional lymph node dissection of 1 to 4 mm thick melanomas for patients 60 years of age and younger. *Ann Surg*, Vol. 224, pp. 255–66.

Balch, CM; Soong. SJ; Gershenwald. JE. et al. (2001). Prognostic factors analysis of 17,600 melanoma patients: validation of the American Joint Committee on Cancer melanoma staging system. *J Clin Oncol*, Vol. 19, pp. 3622-34.

Balch, CM; Soong, SJ; Murad, TM; Ingalls, AL; Maddox, WA. (1979). A multifactorial analysis of melanoma. II. Prognostic factors in patients with stage I (localized) melanoma. *Surgery*, Vol.86, pp. 343–51.

Balch, CM. (1988). The role of elective lymph node dissection in melanoma: rationale, results, and controversies. *J Clin Oncol*, Vol. 6, pp. 163–72.

Bedrosian, I; Faries, MB; Guerry, DT. IV. et al. (2000). Incidence of sentinel node metastasis in patients with thin primary melanoma (_1 mm) with vertical growth phase. *Ann Surg Oncol.*, Vol. 7, No. 4, pp.262-267.

Bleicher , RJ; Essner, R; Foshag, LJ; Wanek, LA; Morton, DL. (2003). Role of sentinel lymphadenectomy in thin invasive cutaneous melanomas. *J Clin Oncol*, Vol. 21, No. 7, pp. 1326-1331.

Boring, CC; Squires, TS; Tong, T; Montgomery, S. (1994). Cancer Statistics 1994. *CA Cancer J Clin,* Vol. 44, No. 7.

Brady, MS; Brown, K; Patel, A; Fisher, C; Marx, A. (2006). Phase II trial of isolated limb infusion with melphalan and dactinomycin for regional melanoma and soft tissue sarcoma of the extremity. *Ann Surg Onc*, Vol. 13, No. 8, pp. 1123-9.

Breslow, A. (1980). Prognosis in cutaneous melanoma: tumor thickness as a guide to treatment. *Pathol Annu,* Vol. 15, pp. 1-22.

Briele, HA; Djuric, M; Jung, DT; Mortell, T; Patel, MK; Das Gupta, TK. (1985). Pharmacokinetics of melphalan in clinical isolation perfusion of the extremities. *Cancer Res*, Vol. 45, pp. 1885–1889.

Brozena, SJ; Fenske, NA; Perez, IR. (1993). Epidemiology of malignant melanoma, worldwide incidence, and etiologic factors. *Semin Surg Oncol,* Vol. 9, pp. 165–7.

Cade, S. (1961). Malignant melanoma. *Ann R Coll Surg Engl,* Vol. 28, pp. 331–366.

Callery, C; Cochran, AJ; Roe, DJ. et al. (1982). Factors prognostic for survival in patients with malignant melanoma spread to regional lymph nodes. *Ann Surg,* Vol. 196, pp. 69–75.

Cascinelli, N; Marchesini. R. (1989). Increasing incidence of cutaneous melanoma, ultraviolet radiation and the clinician. *Photochem Photobiol*, Vol. 50, pp. 497-505.

Cecchi, R; Buralli, L; Innocenti, S; De Gaudio, C. (2007). Sentinel lymph node biopsy in patients with thin melanomas. *J Dermatol,* Vol. 34, No. 8, pp. 512-515.

Clinical Guidelines Committee. (2006). Management of Cutaneous Melanoma Clinical Guidelines. *Dublin: Royal College of Surgeons in Ireland.*

Cohn-Cedarmark, G ; Rutqvist, LE ; Anderson, R. et al. (2000). Long-term results of a randomised study by the Swedish Melanoma Study Group on 2-cm versus 5-cm resection margins for patients with cutaneous melanoma with a tumour thickness of 0.8-2.0 mm. *Cancer,* Vol. 89, pp. 1495-1501.

Conway, WC; Faries, MB; Terando, AM. et al. (2009). Age-related lymphatic dysfunction in malignant melanoma patients. *Ann Srug Oncol,* Vol. 16, pp. 1548-1552.

Creech, O; Krementz, E. (1966). Techniques of regional perfusion. *Surgery ,*Vol. 60, pp. 938–947.

Evans, RD; Kopf, AW; Lew, RA .et al. (1988). Risk factors for the development of malignant melanoma: I. Review of case-control studies. *J Dermatol Surg Oncol*, Vol. 14, pp. 393-408.

Faries, MB; Wanek, LA; Elashoff, D; Wright, BE; Morton, DL. Predictors of Occult Nodal Metastasis in Patients With Thin Melanoma. (2010). *Arch Surg*, Vol. 145, No.2, pp. 137-142.

Fraker, DL. (1999). Hyperthermic regional perfusion for melanoma and sarcoma of the limbs. *Curr Probl Surg*, Vol. 36, pp. 841-907.

Friedman, RJ; Rigel. DS; Silverman, MK; Kopf, AW; Vossaert, KA . (1991). Malignant melanoma in the 1990s: the continued importance of early detection and the role of physician examination and self-examination of the skin. *CA Cancer J Clin, Vol.* 41, pp. 201-6.

Gandini, S; Sera, F; Cattaruzza, MS; Pasquini, P; Picconi, O; Boyle, P; Melchi, CF. Meta-analysis of risk factors for cutaneous melanoma : II. Sun exposure. *Eur J Cancer*, Vol. 41, pp. 45-60.

Garbe, C; Hauschild, A; Volkenandt, M; Schadendorf, D; Stolz, W; Reinhold, U. et al. (2008). Evidence and interdisciplinary consensusbased German guidelines: surgical treatment and radiotherapy of melanoma. *Melanoma Res,* Vol. 18, pp. 61-7.

Gellin, GA; Kopf, AW; Garfinkel, L. (1969). Malignant melanoma: A controlled study of possibly associated factors. *Arch Derm*, Vol. 99, pp. 43-48.

Gershenwald, JE; Mansfield, PF; Lee, JE; Ross, MI. (2000). Role of lymphatic mapping and sentinel lymph node biopsy in patients with thick ($\geq$4 mm) primary melanoma. *Ann Surg Oncol.*, Vol. 7, No. 2, pp. 160-165.

Gershenwald, JE; Thompson, W; Mansfield, PF. et al. (1999). Multi-institutional melanoma lymphatic mapping experience: the prognostic value of sentinel lymph node status in 612 stage I or II melanoma patients. *J Clin Oncol.* Vol. 17, No. 3, pp. 976-983.

Ghaferi, AA; Wong, SL; Johnson, TM; Lowe, L; Chang, AE; Cimmino, VM. et al. (2009). Prognostic significance of a positive nonsentinel lymph node in cutaneous melanoma. *Ann Surg Oncol*, Vol. 16, pp. 2978-84.

Gimotty, PA; Guerry, D; Ming, ME. et al. (2004). Thin primary cutaneous malignant melanoma: a prognostic tree for 10-year metastasis is more accurate than American Joint Committee on Cancer staging. *J Clin Oncol*, Vol. 22, No. 18, pp. 3668-3676.

Gimotty, PA; Van Belle, P; Elder, DE. et al. (2005). Biologic and prognostic significance of dermal Ki67 expression, mitoses, and tumorigenicity in thin invasive cutaneous melanoma. *J Clin Oncol,* Vol. 23, No. 31, pp. 8048-8056.

Glumac, N; Hocevar, M; Zadnik, V; Snoj, M. (2008). Sentinel lymph node micrometastasis may predict non-sentinel involvement in cutaneous melanoma patients. *J Surg Oncol*, Vol. 98, pp. 46-8.

Greene, MH; Clark, WH; Tucker, MA. et al. (1985). High risk of malignant melanoma in melanoma-prone families with dysplastic naevi. *Ann Intern Med*, Vol. 102, pp. 458-465.

Guggenheim, MM; Hug, U; Jung, FJ; Rousson, V; Aust, MC; Calcagni, M; Künzi, W; Giovanoli, P. (2008). Morbidity and recurrence after completion lymph node dissection following sentinel lymph node biopsy in cutaneous malignant melanoma. *Ann Surg,* Vol. 247, pp. 687-93.

Haigh, PI; DiFronzo, LA; McCready, DR. (2003). Optimal excision margins for primary cutaneous melanoma: a systematic review and meta-analysis. *Can J Surg*, Vol. 46, pp. 419-426.

Hayes, AJ; Clarke, MA; Harries, M; Thomas, JM. (2004). Management of in-transit metastases from cutaneous malignant melanoma. *Br J Surg*, Vol. 91, pp. 673-682.

Heenan, PJ; Ghaznawie, M. (1999). The pathogenesis of local recurrence of melanoma at the primary excision site. *Br J Plast Surg*, Vol.52, pp. 209–213.

Holman, CD; Armstrong, BK. (1984). Cutaneous melanoma and indicators of total accumulated exposure to the sun: An analysis separating histogenetic types. *J Natl Cancer Inst*, Vol. 73, pp. 75-82.

Jemal, A; Devesa, SS; Hartge, P; Tucker, MA. (2001). Recent trends in cutaneous melanoma incidence among whites in the United States. *J Natl Cancer Inst*, Vol. 93, No. 9, pp. 678-683.

Kesmodel, SB; Karakousis, GC; Botbyl, JD. et al. (2005). Mitotic rate as a predictor of sentinel lymph node positivity in patients with thin melanomas. *Ann Surg Oncol*, Vol. 12, No. 6, pp. 449-458.

Kopf, AW. (1988). Prevention and early detection of skin cancer/melanoma. *Cancer*, Vol. 62, No. 8, pp. 1791-1795.

Kraemer KH: Xeroderma Pigmentosum, in Dermis DJ, McGuire J (eds). (1984). *Clinical Dermatology*, vol 4, Philadelphia, Harper &Row Publishers, unit 19-7.

Kretschmer, L; Hilgers, R; Mohrle, M; Balda, BR; Breuninger, H; Konz ,B. et al. (2004). Patients with lymphatic metastasis of cutaneous malignant melanoma benefit from sentinel lymphonodectomy and early excision of their nodal disease. *Eur J Cancer*, Vol. 40, pp. 212-8.

Kunte, C; Geimer, T; Baumert, J; Konz, B; Volkenandt, M; Flaig, M; Ruzicka, T; Berking, C; Schmid-Wendtner, MH. (2011). Analysis of predictive factors for the outcome of complete lymph node dissection in melanoma patients with metastatic sentinel lymph nodes. *J Am Acad Dermatol.*, Vol. 64, No. 4, pp. 655-62.

Lederman, JS; Sober, AJ. (1985). Does biopsy type influence survival in clinical stage I cutaneous melanoma? *J Am Acad Dermatol*, Vol. 13, pp. 983-987.

Lee, JH; Essner, R; Torisu-Itakura, H; Wanek, L; Wang, H; Morton, DL. (2004). Factors predictive of tumor-positive nonsentinel lymph nodes after tumor-positive sentinel lymph node dissection for melanoma. *J Clin Oncol*, Vol. 22, pp. 3677-84.

Lees, VC; Briggs, JC. (1991). Effect of initial biopsy procedure on prognosis in Stage 1 invasive cutaneous malignant melanoma: review of 1086 patients. *Br J Surg*, Vol. 78, pp. 1108-1110.

Lent, WM ; Ariyan, S. (1994). Flap reconstruction following wide local excision for primary malignant melanoma of the head and neck region. *Ann Plast Surg*, Vol. 33, No. 1, pp. 23-7.

Lienard, D; Ewalenko, P; Delmotte, JJ; Renard, N; Lejeune, FJ. (1992). High-dose recombinant tumor necrosis factor alpha in combination with interferon gamma and melphalan in isolation perfusion of the limbs for melanoma and sarcoma. *J Clin Oncol*, Vol. 10, pp. 52–60.

Malignant tumors (melanomas and related lesions). In: Elder DE, Murphy GF. Melanocytic tumors of the skin. Atlas of tumor pathology. 3rd series. Fascicle 2. Washington, D.C.: Armed Forces Institute of Pathology, pp. 103-205.

McCarthy, WH. (2002). Melanoma: Margins for error—another view. *Aust NZ J Surg*, Vol. 72, pp. 304–306.

McKinnon, JG; Yu, XQ; McCarthy, WH; Thompson, JF. (2003). Prognosis for patients with thin cutaneous melanoma: long-term survival data from New South Wales Central Cancer Registry and the Sydney Melanoma Unit. *Cancer*, Vol. 98, No.6 , pp. 1223-1231.

Mian, R; Henderson, M; Speakman, D; Finkelde, D; Ainslie, J; McKenzie, A. (2001). Isolated limb infusion for melanoma: a simple alternative to isolated limb perfusion. *Can J Surg*, Vol. 44, No. 3, pp. 189-92

Milton, GW; Shaw, HM; McCarthy, WH. et al. (1982). Prophylactic lymph node dissection in clinical stage I cutaneous malignant melanoma: results of surgical treatment in 1319 patients. *Br J Surg*, Vol. 69, pp. 108-11.

Morton ,DL; Thompson , JF; Cochran, AJ; Mozzillo, N; Elashoff, R; Essner, R. et al. (2006). Sentinel-node biopsy or nodal observation in melanoma. *N Engl J Med*, Vol. 355, pp. 1307-17.

Mubarak, SJ; Owen, CA. (1977). Double-incision fasciotomy of the leg for decompression in compartment syndromes. *J Bone Joint Surg (US)*, Vol. 59A, pp. 184-187.

No authors listed. (1983). Randomized controlled trial of adjuvant chemoimmunotherapy with DTIC and BCG after complete excision of primary melanoma with a poor prognosis or melanoma metastases. *Can Med Assoc J.*, Vol. 128, No. 8, pp. 929-33.

Oliveira Filho, RS; Ferreira, LM; Bias, LJ; Enokihara, MM; Paiva, GR; Wagner ,J. (2003). Vertical growth phase and positive sentinel node in thin melanoma. *Braz J Med Biol Res*, Vol. 36, No. 3, pp. 347-350.

Ollila ,DW; Ashburn, JH; Amos, KD; Yeh, JJ; Frank, JS; Deal, AM. et al. (2009). Metastatic melanoma cells in the sentinel node cannot be ignored. *J Am Coll Surg*, Vol. 208, pp. 924-9.

Owen, SA; Sanders, LL; Edwards, LJ; Seigler, HF; Tyler, DS; Grichnik, JM. (2001). Identification of higher risk thin melanomas should be based on Breslow depth not Clark level IV. *Cancer*, Vol. 91, No.5, pp. 983-991.

Paek, SC; Griffith, KA; Johnson, TM. et al. (2007). The impact of factors beyond Breslow depth on predicting sentinel lymph node positivity in melanoma. *Cancer*, Vol. 109, No. 1, pp. 100-108.

Parker, SL; Tong, T; Bolden, S; Wingo, PA. (1996). Cancer statistics, 1996. *CA Cancer J Clin*, Vol. 47, pp. 5-27.

Prichard, RS; Hill, ADK; Skehan, SJ; O'Higgins, NJ. (2002). Positron emission tomography for staging and management of malignant melanoma. *Br J Surg*, Vol. 89, pp. 389-396.

Puleo, CA; Messina, JL; Riker ,AI. et al. (2005). Sentinel node biopsy for thin melanomas: which patients should be considered? *Cancer Control*, Vol. 12, No. 4, pp. 230-235.

Reeves, ME; Delgado, R; Busam, KJ; Brady, MS; Coit, DG. (2003). Prediction of nonsentinel lymph node status in melanoma. *Ann Surg Oncol*, 2003, Vol. 10, pp. 27-31.

Roberts, DL; Anstey, AV; Barlow, RJ. et al. (2002). U.K. guidelines for the management of cutaneous melanoma. *Br J Dermatol*, Vol. 146, pp. 7-17.

Roses, DF; Provet , JA; Harris, MN; Gumport, SL; Dubin, N. (1985). Prognosis of patients with pathologic stage II cutaneous malignant melanoma. *Ann Surg*, Vol. 201, pp. 103-7.

Rossi, CR; De Salvo, GL; Bonandini, E; Mocellin, S; Foletto, M; Pasquali, S. et al. (2008). Factors predictive of nonsentinel lymph node involvement and clinical outcome in melanoma patients with metastatic sentinel lymph node. *Ann Surg Oncol*, Vol. 15, pp. 1202-10.

Schumacher, HH;. Chia, HL. et al. (2010). Ipsilateral Skin Grafts for Lower Limb Melanoma Reconstruction Are Safe. *Plastic and Reconstructive Surgery*, Vol. 125, No. 2, pp. 89e-91e.

Scoggins, CR; Bowen, AL; Martin, RC; Edwards,MJ; Reintgen, DS; Ross, MI; Urist, MM; Stromberg ,AJ; Hagendoorn, L; McMasters, K. (2010). Prognostic Information From Sentinel Lymph Node Biopsy in Patients With Thick Melanoma. *Arch Surg*, Vol. 145, No. 7, pp. 622-627.

Sim, FH; Taylor, WF; Ivins, JC; Pritchard, DJ; Soule, EH. (1978). A prospective randomized study of the efficacy of routine elective lymphadenectomy in management of malignant melanoma: preliminary results. *Cancer*, Vol. 41, pp. 948–56.

Sondak, VK; Taylor, JM; Sabel, MS. et al. (2004). Mitotic rate and younger age are predictors of sentinel lymph node positivity: lessons learned from the generation of a probabilistic model. *Ann Surg Oncol*, Vol. 11, No. 3, pp. 247-258.

Stitzenberg, KB; Groben, PA; Stern, SL. et al. (2004). Indications for lymphatic mapping and sentinel lymphadenectomy in patients with thin melanoma (Breslow-thickness_1.0 mm). *Ann Surg Oncol*, Vol. 11, No. 10, pp. 900-906.

The American Cancer Society. (2010). What are the key statistics about Melanoma?, In : *The American Cancer Society*, 20.03.10, Available from http://www.cancer.org/Cancer/SkinCancer-Melanoma/DetailedGuide/melanoma-skin-cancer-key-statistics

Thomas, JM ; Newton-Bishop, J ; A'Hern, R. et al. (2004). Excision margins in high-risk malignant melanoma. New Engl J Med, Vol. 350, pp. 757-766.

Thompson, JF. (2001). The Sydney Melanoma Unit experience of sentinel lymphadenectomy for melanoma. *Ann Surg Oncol*, Vol. 8, pp. 44S–47S.

Uren, RF; Howman-Giles, R; Thompson, JF. et al.(1994). Lymphoscintigraphy to identify sentinel lymph nodes in patients with melanoma. *Melanoma Res*, Vol. 4, pp. 395–9.

Van der Ploeg, IM; Kroon, BB; Antonini, N; Valdes Olmos, RA; Nieweg, OE. (2009). Is completion lymph node dissection needed in case of minimal melanoma metastasis in the sentinel node? *Ann Surg*, Vol. 249, pp. 1003-7.

Vaquerano, J; Kraybill, WG; Driscoll, DL; Cheney, R; Kane, JM III. (2006). American Joint Committee on Cancer clinical stage as a selection criterion for sentinel lymph node biopsy in thin melanoma. *Ann Surg Oncol*, Vol. 13, No. 2, pp. 198-204.

Veronesi, U; Adamus, J; Bandiera, DC. et al. (1977). Inefficacy of immediate node dissection in stage I melanoma of the limbs. *New Engl J Med*, Vol. 297, pp. 627-630.

Veronesi, U; Adamus, J; Bandiera, DC. et al. (1982). Delayed regional lymph node dissection in stage I melanoma of the skin of the lower extremities. *Cancer*, Vol.49, pp.2420–30.

Whited, JD; Grichnik, JM. (1998) The rational clinical examination. Does the patient have a mole of a melanoma? JAMA,Vol. 279, pp. 696-701.

Wieberdink, J; Benckhuysen, C; Braat, RP; van Slooten, EA; Olthuis, GA. (1982). Dosimetry in isolation perfusion of the limbs by assessment of perfused tissue volume and grading of toxic tissue reactions. *Eur J Cancer Clin Oncol*, Vol. 18, pp. 905–910.

Wong, SL; Brady, MS; Busam, KJ; Coit, DG. (2006). Results of sentinel lymph node biopsy in patients with thin melanoma. *Ann Surg Oncol*, Vol. 13, No. 3, pp. 302-309.

Wright, BE; Scheri, RP; Ye, X. et al. (2008). Importance of sentinel lymph node biopsy in patients with thin melanoma. *Arch Surg*, Vol. 143, No. 9, pp. 892-900.

Wright, EH; Stanley, PR; Roy, A. (2010). Evaluation of sentinel lymph nodes positive for melanoma for features predictive of nonsentinel nodal disease and patient prognosis: a 49 patient series. *J Plast Reconstr Aesthet Surg*, Vol. 68, pp. 500-2.

Yonick, DV; Ballo, RM; Kahn, E; Dahiya, M; Yao, K; Godellas, C; Shoup, M; Aranha, GV. (2011). Predictors of positive sentinel lymph node in thin melanoma. *Am J Surg.*,Vol. 201, No. 3, pp. 324-8.

4

Challenging Problems in the Surgical Management of Melanoma

Asvin M. Ganapathi, Douglas S. Tyler and Paul J. Mosca
Department of Surgery, Duke University Medical Center
Durham, NC 27710
USA

1. Introduction

The surgical management of cutaneous melanoma can occasionally present serious challenges even to experienced surgeons. Management problems range from selecting the best surgical intervention at the time of initial diagnosis of a primary tumor to establishing whether surgery has a role in palliation of advanced disease. We will review the relevant literature and discuss recommended approaches to management in order to address several areas of debate or uncertainty in the surgical management of melanoma.

2. Surgical management of melanocytic lesions of uncertain malignant potential

The diagnosis of melanoma should be considered in the evaluation of all melanocytic skin lesions and all skin lesions with aggressive clinical behavior. Melanocytic lesions raising a suspicion of melanoma may be referred to using a variety of terms, such as "atypical Spitz nevus", "atypical melanocytic proliferation", "melanocytic tumor of uncertain malignant potential" ("MELTUMP"), "cellular blue nevus", and others. When referred a patient with such a lesion, it is critically important that the treating surgeon thoroughly review available histopathologic descriptions regarding the lesion, have outside slides reviewed by a qualified dermatopathologist, communicate with the pathologist to ensure that all information necessary to guide treatment is provided, and obtain outside dermatopathology consultation if indicated. Most importantly, the clinician must recognize that proper management of melanocytic lesions of uncertain malignant potential depends not only on the pathology report per se, but also on the clinical context of the lesion.

While melanoma is often a relatively straightforward diagnosis, there are many cases in which it is difficult or impossible to differentiate between melanoma and lesions of benign or uncertain biologic behavior [Barnhill et al., 1999; Scolyer et al., 2004]. One of the lesions that may be among the most difficult to differentiate from melanoma is the atypical Spitz tumor. This diagnosis not only carries important prognostic information for the patient, but also may be associated with significant anguish and can be a source of medicolegal liability if improperly managed. Consequently, it is important to convey the nature of uncertainty regarding the diagnosis, and when appropriate, advocate an aggressive approach to management.

One method that has been advocated as a strategy for differentiating between melanomas and similar lesions is the sentinel lymph node biopsy. The literature has shown that in cases of lesions with unknown malignant potential there is a 16-47% positive SLNB rate [Berk et al., 2010; Ghazi et al., 2010; Ludgate et al., 2009; Magro et al., 2010; Meyers et al., 2010]. Interestingly, atypical spitzoid lesions appear to have a high incidence of microscopic nodal involvement, but a more favorable prognosis than common melanomas [Ludgate et al, 2009]. In a study of 31 patients undergoing SLNB for atypical melanocytic neoplasms, younger median age (11 versus 23.5) and greater thickness (1.90 mm versus 1.09 mm) were associated with a nodal metastasis [Meyers et al, 2010]. Thus, a negative SLNB does not prove that a lesion is benign but does provide reassurance that it is localized. A positive SLNB result, on the other hand, is more valuable with respect to establishing the diagnosis, and it confirms the presence of regional nodal disease. Performance of SLNB should be considered in the management of atypical melanocytic neoplasms, particularly in a younger patient or a patient with a thicker lesion.

New and emerging technologies may provide additional tools to help differentiate these lesions from melanoma. One such technology is comparative genomic hybridization. It has been reported that approximately 95% of melanomas have chromosomal abnormalities [Scolyer et al., 2010], while melanocytic nevi rarely have such chromosomal aberrations [Bastian et al., 2000; Bastian et al., 2003; Carless & Griffiths, 2008; Casorzo et al., 2005; Pirker et al., 2003; Stark & Hayward, 2007]. One drawback to this technique is the availability and cost of this technology. Another method that may be helpful in distinguishing between nevi and melanoma is fluorescence in-situ hybridization (FISH) [Gerami et al., 2009; Morey et al., 2009; Newman et al., 2009; Pouryazdanparast et al., 2009]. Finally, it has also been shown that BRAF and NRAS mutations are commonly seen in melanomas but not in Spitz nevi, while HRAS mutations sometimes occur in Spitz nevi, but are not usually seen in melanomas [Scolyer et al, 2010].

Despite the availability of these sophisticated analyses, some lesions will remain difficult or impossible to definitively classify. In these cases, discussion in the context of a multidisciplinary melanoma/pigmented lesion clinic or conference is recommended. In cases in which a consensus is unable to be reached regarding the diagnosis, then appropriate wide excision, if possible, should be performed in order to treat, according to the "worst-case scenario". At times, melanoma may be confirmed upon re-excision, in which case it is reasonable to consider proceeding with SLNB if not already performed. As routine use of imaging or laboratory tests for staging is not recommended for localized, early stage primary melanomas, such extensive staging evaluation is rarely indicated prior to surgery for pigmented lesions of uncertain biologic potential. Certainly, if advanced melanoma is confirmed or strongly suspected, then appropriate staging is indicated. Finally, the foundation for management of diagnostically challenging pigmented skin lesions is effective two-way communication and careful attention to the patient's level of understanding, wishes, and expectations regarding management.

3. Indication for and appropriateness of sentinel lymph node biopsy

3.1 SLNB for thin and thick melanomas

While the value of sentinel lymphadenectomy in the nodal staging of malignant melanoma has been well documented in the literature, there remain questions regarding optimal application of the technique [Bagaria et al., 2010; Essner, 2010; Phan et al., 2009; van Akkooi et al., 2009]. In general, for a clinically node negative patient with a primary lesion that is thicker than 1 mm – particularly in the 1 – 4 mm range – consideration should be given to performing a sentinel lymph node biopsy (SLNB) [Garbe et al., 2010; Testori et al., 2009]. The value of SLNB in patients with melanomas less than 1 mm (T1; "thin") or greater than 4 mm (T4; "thick") in thickness remains less well defined.

Patients with primary tumors less than 1 mm in thickness generally do not have a high enough probability of harboring nodal micrometastasis to warrant SLNB for nodal staging. However, the need for SLNB is often considered in these T1 tumors, and it has even been suggested that this threshold should lowered to 0.75 mm [Wong et al., 2006b]. For tumors less than 1 mm in thickness, it is appropriate to factor in other clinical and histopathologic factors. Although it is tempting to recommend SLNB for *all* melanomas above 0.75 mm in thickness or less than 1 mm in thickness with adverse prognostic histopathologic features, this approach may be an overly liberal application of the technique. In fact, a number of studies have documented a very low incidence of positive SLNB in patients with T1 lesions, generally 5% or less [Berk et al., 2005; Cecchi et al., 2007; Karakousis et al., 2006; Kesmodel et al., 2005; Wong et al., 2006a]. In a Memorial Sloan Kettering study of patients with T1 melanomas undergoing SLNB, 8 (3.2%) of 223 patients had positive nodes [Wong et al, 2006a]. Interestingly, all those patients with positive nodes had melanomas between .75 and 1 mm in thickness *and* had a Clark level of IV (i.e., Breslow thickness-Clark level *discordance*). In this study, ulceration was not predictive of a positive SLN, but in several other studies, ulceration *was* found to be associated with regional nodal metastasis in patients with T1 melanomas undergoing SLNB [Karakousis et al, 2006; Sondak et al., 2004; Wagner et al., 2000].

It has become clear that mitotic activity is a significant histopathologic prognostic factor for survival in melanoma, and it has replaced Clark level in the 7th version of the AJCC staging system, upstaging the primary tumor from T1a to T1b [Balch et al., 2009]. Mitotic activity has also been shown to be predictive of nodal micrometastasis. A Michigan study found that not only does mitotic activity increase the probability of nodal metastasis in the setting of T1 primary tumors, but the relative impact of mitotic activity increases progressively with the number of mitoses observed [Paek et al., 2007]. Interestingly, the relationship between mitotic activity and nodal metastasis is most pronounced in younger patients, and this relationship diminishes markedly with advanced age. Younger age itself, angiolymphatic invasion, and trunk or lower extremity primary tumor have also been associated with a positive SLNB [Paek et al, 2007; Sondak et al, 2004]. Regression, however, has not been found to be a predictor of SLN metastasis [Cecchi et al., 2008; Socrier et al., 2010].

It is important to consider that sentinel lymphadenectomy is not without risk and adds significant expense to the care of melanoma patients. Potential complications include seroma, hematoma, usually transient and/or minor nerve palsies, lymphedema, and rarely anaphylaxis associated with isosulfan blue [Lucci et al., 2007; Roaten et al., 2005]. The overall complication rate of SLNB alone in the Sunbelt Melanoma Trial, which enrolled over 2100 patients, was 4.6% [Wrightson et al., 2003]. Given the overall low incidence of positive SLNB in patients with T1 lesions, it is inappropriate to perform SLNB routinely in this group of patients. Patients with thicker T1 lesions associated with histopathologic factors that increase the probability of nodal micrometastasis should prompt consideration of nodal staging, particularly in patients with a long life expectancy. In these appropriately selected patients with T1, clinically node negative primary tumors, a balanced discussion regarding the potential value, as well as the risks, of performing a sentinel lymph node biopsy is recommended.

A final issue regards nodal staging in patients who are clinically node-negative but have T4 (> 4 mm; "thick") primary tumors. It may be argued that there is little value associated with SLNB in patients with thick melanomas since there is a high rate of systemic and/or regional disease at the time of diagnosis, and that the prognostic utility of SLNB is lower in these patients [Perrott et al., 2003]. Other studies reinforced this belief by demonstrating no significant difference in overall survival in patients who undergo SLNB for thick melanomas relative to those who do not [Cherpelis et al., 2001; Essner et al., 2002; Jacobs et al., 2004]. However, a study done by Gajdos et al. demonstrated that patients with T4 tumors with a negative SLNB experienced a longer disease-free and overall survival than those with a positive SLNB [Gajdos et al., 2009]. In fact, some patients with T4 disease may be candidates for adjuvant therapy, and the status of the SLN may impact the decision regarding adjuvant treatment [Gajdos et al, 2009]. It has also been recommended that SLNB be performed for thick melanomas because of its strong independent prognostic value [Carlson et al., 2003; Ferrone et al., 2002; Gershenwald et al., 2000].

Thus, it appears that SLNB should be considered as an option in selected patients with T4 primary tumors. Certainly, the most elderly of patients and/or those patients with major medical comorbidities with a poor performance status would not typically be offered SLNB in this setting. In otherwise healthy candidates, SLNB may be especially helpful in patients with non-ulcerated primary tumors or patients in whom nodal staging is expected to impact management, including administration of adjuvant therapy.

3.2 SLNB for head and neck melanomas

Another group of patients for whom the value of performing a SLNB may be uncertain is that with head and neck primary tumors, and this topic has recently been reviewed in depth [De Rosa et al., 2011]. Since the frequency of positive SLNs is in the 7-26% range, SLNB may be a valuable staging tool for patients with head and neck melanomas [Alex et al., 1998; Carlson et al., 2000; Jansen et al., 2000; O'Brien et al., 1995; Rasgon, 2001; Wells et al., 1997]. One of the greatest concerns about performing SLNB for lesions in the head and neck is injury, particularly to nerve structures such as the facial nerve [Eicher et al., 2002]. Another concern is that the drainage pattern of the lymphatics of the head and neck is considerably more complex than those in other regions of the body. Detailed mapping of head and neck lymphatics has shown unexpected drainage patterns in 8-43% of patients. [Klop et al., 2011; O'Brien et al, 1995]. A study by Kelly et al. showed that, while the procedure was safe, there was a false negative rate of 9.5% and a failure to locate a lymph node in 32.5% of patients [Kelly et al., 2009]. This high failure rate was attributed to complex drainage patterns as well as surgeon experience.

Some surgeons have taken a liberal approach to application of SLNB in head and neck melanomas. Some recommend that SNLB be performed in all patients with head and neck tumors thicker than 0.75 mm [Patel et al., 2002], and indeed some studies have shown superior results. Gomez-Rivera and colleagues reported a success rate of SLNB in head and neck melanomas of 96% [Gomez-Rivera et al., 2008]. In another series of 106 patients, SLNs were identified in 89% of patients [Teltzrow et al., 2007]. The median follow-up was 47 months, and 8 additional patients developed recurrence within the regional nodes, which translated into a sensitivity of 68%. In another study, SLNs were identified in 41 of 44 patients (94%) and there were no regional nodal recurrences, but this study was limited by a short median follow-up of 22.4 months [MacNeill et al., 2005]. A large retrospective study of over a thousand patients who underwent SLNB for melanoma was performed, and head and neck location was associated with a higher false-negative SLN rate compared to primary tumors in other locations [Carlson et al., 2008].

Based on the literature, SLNB for head and neck melanomas is safe in the hands of experienced surgeon and when appropriate pre-operative planning is done. However, the risks should be fully discussed with the patient before proceeding with SLNB. In this region, there are more complex lymphatic drainage patterns involving multiple lymph node basins, and the success of identifying SLNs may be lower than in other regions, particularly when the surgeon has less experience with head and neck SLNB. It has been proposed that the higher-resolution, three-dimensional images achieved with SPECT/CT imaging may enhance detection of SLNs and decrease risks by limiting the dissection necessary for SLNB [Even-Sapir et al., 2003; Roarke et al., 2007; Vermeeren et al., 2010], but this remains to be determined. Patients should be informed that an attempted SLNB may be unsuccessful, in which case the risks, cost, and discomfort associated with the procedure are incurred without added benefit to wide excision alone. Nevertheless, sentinel lymphadenectomy is a reasonable, though not mandatory procedure and may provide valuable staging information as part of the surgical management of patients with head and neck melanomas.

3.3 Complex drainage patters or failure to localize sentinel lymph nodes by lymphoscintigraphy

In the previous section, the possibility that the surgeon may fail to identify SLNs was discussed. A specific manifestation of this problem that occasionally arises is the failure of radiocolloid lymphoscintigraphy to locate any SLNs whatsoever. A related problem regards the approach to sentinel lymph node biopsy when mapping has shown a complex drainage pattern, such as a diffuse chain of lymph nodes extending from the inguinofemoral nodal basin up into the pelvic nodal basin. There is little literature guiding management in these circumstances.

The first step in preparing for unexpected results or complexities of lymphoscintigraphy is planning, and this starts with properly informing patients about the potential implications of lymphoscintigraphy and the decision making process that might be anticipated as a consequence. The next critical element is good communication and a close collaborative relationship with the nuclear medicine staff. Third, there should be some thought about contingency plans prior to the procedure, and these may be individualized depending on the particular patient, anatomic considerations, and lymphoscintigraphy results.

Perhaps among the most common questions is how to manage a situation in which lymphoscintigraphy fails to localize any sentinel lymph nodes whatsoever. This problem may make it impossible to determine the draining nodal basins and therefore may lead to a lower rate of complete and accurate SLN identification [Rousseau et al., 2005]. Failure of scintigraphic localization may be due to technical issues, the radiocolloid agent itself, or anatomic factors such as anatomic site, node characteristics, or complexities of the lymphatic drainage pattern. The surgeon should probe into whether the nuclear medicine department has noted other instances in which there was a failure to localize SLNs with the same lot of radiotracer. Other relevant questions might concern the dose of tracer employed, whether any technical problems were noted, and the duration of time from injection to detection/scanning and surgery.

There are a variety of acceptable courses when lymphoscintigraphy fails to localize any SLNs. One successful approach used in the setting of breast surgery has been reported by Meretoja and colleagues [Meretoja et al., 2010]. 207 (15.8%) out of 1,309 patients undergoing lymphatic mapping were given a second injection of radiocolloid because of poor or no visualization of SLNs, and this was demonstrated to be an effective strategy for SLN identification with no apparent significant adverse effects. However, depending on the circumstances, a second injection may pose significant logistical problems for the patient, operating room, and surgeon. Alternatively, the procedure may be postponed in favor of repeating lymphoscintigraphy with SPECT/CT imaging, which provides a finer, three-dimensional image of lymphatic drainage and may enhance the ability to detect SLNs in the setting of complex drainage patterns [van der Ploeg et al., 2009; Vermeeren et al, 2010]. This is more resource-intensive, however, and SPECT/CT imaging is not available at all institutions that offer lymphoscintigraphy.

Another option is to perform the procedure using blue dye alone. In breast surgery, most surgeons restrict the dissection for SLNs to the axilla regardless of the small possibility that SLNs may be located in other nodal basins, and therefore employing blue dye alone in this setting is not problematic. Melanomas, on the other hand may be located anywhere, and lymphatic drainage patterns may be difficult to predict. While the draining nodal basin for most melanomas – particularly extremity lesions – can usually be predicted, there is inherent degree of guesswork associated with this approach; hence, it simply may be too unreliable for most lesions in locations such as the trunk, head and neck. In addition, there may be a lower success rate with the application of blue dye alone for SLNB if prior lymphoscintigraphy failed to localize a SLN [Rousseau et al, 2005].

Another option is to abort pathologic nodal staging altogether, which would seem to conflict with whatever the rationale was underlying the original decision to perform the procedure. However, this is a reasonable option if in the surgeon's judgment it is in the best interest of the patient. The opposite extreme is to perform an elective lymph node dissection, and this remains an acceptable alternative, as well. However, since there remains no proof that either SLNB or complete LND improves survival in melanoma, this may represent an overly aggressive approach for most patients. Furthermore, as with attempting SLNB with blue dye alone, particularly for non-extremity melanomas, this option may be limited because of uncertainty regarding which would be the appropriate (draining) lymph nodes basins to dissect.

Another scenario that may be encountered is diffuse uptake among a large number of nodes in multiple basins and/or along a diffuse chain such as the pelvic or even para-aortic nodes. In these cases, it is important to weigh the relative benefits and risks of performing a much more extensive nodal mapping procedure than may have been planned. Certainly, there are proponents of a very aggressive approach in this setting, a viewpoint that emphasizes the value of SLNB in properly staging patients. An alternative is to routinely biopsy Cloquet's node during inguinofemoral SLNB and to use the status of Cloquet's node as a surrogate for pelvic SLNB [Essner et al., 2006]. Another option is to use the presence or absence of "second-echelon" iliac/obturator SLNs identified by lymphscintigraphy to determine whether a deep pelvic LND should be added to superficial groin dissection in the setting of a positive inguinal SLN [van der Ploeg et al., 2008]. Unfortunately, there remains no consensus regarding the best approach to managing these patients.

In situations when the surgeon believes that the risks outweigh the benefits, it is reasonable to forego performing an extensive nodal staging procedure. For example, there may be a dominant appearing SLN in the inguinal region and multiple additional faint iliac nodes on lymphoscintigraphy. In this situation, the magnitude of the procedure would be much greater and might approach the degree of dissection associated with a pelvic LND. This scenario would sway the surgeon away from extending the SLNB to the pelvic nodal basin. On the other hand, a young patient with a single SLN mapping to the distal external iliac nodal chain would be a more reasonable candidate for a pelvic SLNB. The other proposed strategies are also reasonable alternatives to the management of patients with lymphatic mapping to iliac/obturator nodes.

In summary, there are a variety of unexpected results and complexities that may accompany lymphatic mapping and SLNB. It is of utmost importance to plan for potential issues that arise and to counsel patients proactively so that when they do arise, patients are prepared for the recommended contingency plans. Following lymphoscintigraphy and prior to surgery, an unexpected result that could alter the operative plan should be explained to the patient and any resulting questions should be addressed before finalizing the plan. In this manner, one can ensure that the recommended course is both rational given the circumstances of the case and acceptable to the individual patient.

4. Indication for and extent of lymph node dissection

The potential therapeutic value of regional node dissection remains a topic of significant debate for a number of solid tumors, including melanoma. While there have been clinical trials suggesting an improvement in survival in specific subgroups of patients undergoing prophylactic lymph node dissection, whether lymph node dissection itself actually improves overall survival in melanoma remains controversial.

Historically, prior to the advent of the sentinel lymph node biopsy, two alternative strategies were applied to lymph node dissection for primary cutaneous melanoma with clinically negative nodes. One approach was to perform a complete lymph node dissection (CLND) up-front at the time of definitive surgical excision of the primary tumor; this is referred to as "early" or "prophylactic" lymph node dissection. The other strategy involved performing only the definitive wide excision up front and then carrying out surveillance for the appearance of clinically enlarged nodes; this approach is called "delayed" or "therapeutic" LND (or simply "observation").

Several randomized, prospective trials have been performed in an effort to determine which approach is superior with respect to survival [Balch et al., 2000; Cascinelli et al., 1998; Sim et al., 1986; Veronesi et al., 1977]. While each of the studies had somewhat different methodologies and inclusion criteria, none of them showed an improvement in disease-free or overall survival without subgroup analysis. It should be noted, however, that the World Health Organization (WHO) study, which included only patients with truncal melanomas at least 1.5 mm in thickness, did show an approximately 21% *absolute* improvement in five-year survival favoring ELND over observation when only those patients in the ELND group with *positive* nodes were compared to those in the observation group (48.2% vs 26.6%, p = .04) [Cascinelli et al, 1998].

The Intergroup Melanoma Surgical Trial included clinically node-negative patients with 1-4 mm thick melanomas and again randomized them to ELND versus initial observation. In this trial, patients were *prospectively stratified* for tumor thickness, anatomic site, and the presence of ulceration. Overall 10-year survival was similar in the ELND and observation groups (77% vs 73%, p = .12). However, ELND was associated with a 30% *relative* reduction in 10-year mortality in *non*-ulcerated melanomas, 30% reduction for those with 1-2 mm thick melanomas, and 27% reduction for those with extremity melanomas (all statistically significant). Also significant was a 27% relative reduction in mortality in patients age 60 years or younger, though this was not a prospectively stratified subgroup [Balch et al, 2000]. These findings fueled the debate regarding the value of early LND for nodal metastasis and perhaps accelerated the interest in and acceptance of lymphatic mapping and sentinel lymphadenectomy for nodal staging in melanoma.

The sentinel lymph node biopsy technique was introduced as a nodal staging technique for melanoma by Don Morton and colleagues in the early 1990s [Morton et al., 1992]. Since then, numerous reports have verified its utility and reliability, have quantified its sensitivity and specificity, and have described the relative limitations and risks of the technique in the setting of melanoma and breast cancer, and an in-depth discussion of these topics is beyond the scope of this chapter. Nonetheless, while most melanoma experts agree that performance of a sentinel lymph node biopsy in appropriately selected, clinically node-negative patients provides important staging information, the question remains whether performing the technique improves survival. In the Multi-Center Selective Lymphadenectomy Trial I (MSLT-I), patients with 1-4 mm thick primary melanomas were randomized to SLNB versus observation [Morton et al., 2006]. This trial showed similar 5-year survival in both the SLNB and observation groups. However, subgroup analysis showed a 20% improvement in 5-year survival favoring patients who underwent SLNB followed by CLND for positive nodes in comparison with patients who underwent observation and eventually required CLND for clinically positive nodes (72.3% vs 52.4%, p = .004). In this study Morton et al. also demonstrated that there was a significant difference between nodal relapse in those who were SLNB negative (4.0%) and those who were SLNB positive but were assigned to the observation arm (15.6%), from which the authors concluded that micrometastases would progress within regional or distant nodes. Thus, data from the WHO trial and MSLT-I have been used in support of the viewpoint that early LND when metastases are clinically occult may serve not only to improve the accuracy of staging, but may improve survival.

However, this interpretation of the results of MSLT-I has been questioned by many authors, and it remains uncertain whether SLNB or CLND may be therapeutic in melanoma. It has been pointed out that MSLT-I was underpowered to correctly analyze the survival benefit of immediate v. delayed CLND. Additionally the argument has made that it was improper to draw conclusions about survival in immediate v. delayed CLND as this was a post-randomization sub-group analysis [Ross & Gershenwald, 2008]. The idea that *all* micrometastases (detected by SLNB) would ultimately develop into clinically relevant disease (i.e., palpable lymphadenopathy) has also been questioned, leading to skepticism that the subgroup comparison between SLN-positive patients and those eventually developing clinically positive nodes is a valid analysis [Hermanek et al., 1999; van Akkooi et al., 2006]. That is, perhaps some micrometastases have indolent biology and do not develop into clinically detectable nodal disease for many years. In fact, a study by Van Akkooi et al. demonstrated no overall survival benefit for immediate CLND [van Akkooi et al., 2007]. Complicating matters still further, recent studies have shown only a 50-69% rate of immediate CLND for patients with positive SLNs, which means that at least half of patients would not receive a survival benefit if indeed early CLND produced such a benefit [Bilimoria et al., 2008; Callender & McMasters; Cormier et al., 2005; McMasters]. In fact, for the majority of patients who have micrometases *only* in the SLN, whether CLND is even necessary to achieve the theoretical therapeutic benefit remains in question, as well. This is being addressed in MSLT-II, in which patients with *positive* SLNs are randomized to CLND versus close observation [Amersi & Morton, 2007]. Additionally, the EORTC is conducting the MINITUB trial as well to help determine the effect of timing of CLND on survival [van Akkooi et al.].

It is important to appreciate another level of complexity with regard to CLND following SLNB: if there is a survival benefit associated with CLND, based on the existing literature it would appear to be restricted to the subset of patients with positive SLNs. It is well documented that only about 20% of patients undergoing SLNB will have one or more SLNs with micrometastasis, and thus 80% of patients undergoing SLNB may be spared a CLND. Furthermore, among the 20% of patients with one or more "positive" SLNs, only about 20% of those patients will have additional nodes with detectable metastatic disease. Whether it is only this subgroup of node-positive patients that benefit from CLND and how to reliably predict this is unknown at the present time.

Clearly, not all "positive" SLNs are the same. SLN metastases range from isolated tumor cells identified by immunohistochemical staining alone to macroscopic metastases, and, importantly, disease burden is an important prognostic factor. Perhaps the most reliable predictor of both survival and the probability of non-SLN metastasis is the maximal diameter of the largest SLN metastasis [Francischetto et al., 2010; Guggenheim et al., 2008; Ranieri et al., 2002]. The Rotterdam Criteria for classifying SLN disease burden represents a prognostically relevant and useful strategy for stratifying patients and is based on the largest diameter of the largest metastasis in the SLN: less than 0.1 mm, 0.1 -1.0 mm, or greater than 1.0 mm [van der Ploeg et al., 2010]. Not only does the size of SLN metastases predict the presence of additional disease in non-SLNs, but the anatomic location of tumor deposits is predictive as well. Dewar and colleagues classified SLN metastases as subcapsular, combined subcapsular and parenchymal, parenchymal, multifocal, or extensive; subsequent CLND revealed no additional tumor-positive non-SLNS in the 26% of patients with only subcapsular SLN deposits among a total of 146 patients with positive SLNs [van der Ploeg et al, 2010]. Unfortunately, it remains a subject of controversy whether a specific size cutoff (such as 0.2 mm) or other characteristic of SLN metastases is a reliable enough indicator of non-SLN status to be used as a basis for determining whether to perform or to forego CLND [Francischetto et al, 2010; Guggenheim et al, 2008]. Ongoing studies investigating the need for CLND in the setting of a positive SLN, such as MSLT-II, should provide further insight to help address this important issue.

While questions regarding the need for CLND, ideal patient selection for CLND, and potential impact of CLND on survival in melanoma have not been resolved, one aspect that has been fairly well characterized is the morbidity associated with this procedure. Inguinal as opposed to axillary LND may be associated with particularly high morbidity. Sabel and colleagues reported on 212 patients who underwent inguinal LND and observed a rate of wound complications of 19% and lymphedema of 30%, both of which were significantly higher in patients with clinically positive nodes than those with microscopic nodal disease [Sabel et al., 2007]. Chang and colleagues recently reported the results of a prospective study of 53 patients undergoing inguinal LND, and they observed an overall 30-day wound complication rate of 77% [Chang et al., 2010]. Interestingly, addition of a pelvic lymph node dissection was not associated with a statistically significant increase in complication rate. Whether technical factors, such as preserving the greater saphenous vein, is associated with a lower complication rate remains uncertain [Sarnaik et al., 2009]. The leg endoscopic groin lymphadenectomy, a minimally invasive technique, is currently being evaluated as a potentially less morbid approach to inguinal lymph node dissection [Master et al., 2009].

In summary, nodal staging and the value of CLND in melanoma continue to be hotly debated topics, and important questions remain. What is known is that the SLN biopsy can provide valuable staging information that refines prognosis and may significantly impact clinical management. While it is unclear whether the SLNB itself and/or CLND (directly or indirectly) improve survival in patients with nodal metastasis, this remains a possibility. Therefore, although both SLNB and CLND have associated risks and costs, until the issue has been resolved, performing SLNB in appropriate candidates followed by CLND for positive nodes in acceptable-risk patients appears to be the default for most patients unless they are entered into a suitable clinical trial (such as MSLT-II). All patients should be counseled regarding the potential benefits and risks of these procedures as indicated and should be afforded the opportunity to make a proper informed decision regarding their management.

5. Surgical management of childhood melanoma

There is increasing appreciation that melanoma not only may arise in children and young adults, but it may be at least as aggressive as in older patients and may be increasing in incidence. A number of challenging clinical problems may arise in the management of pediatric melanomas, ranging from the diagnosis to the management of advanced disease. It is important to appreciate the potential lethality of this disease in younger patients and to ensure that fundamental principles of surgical management are applied to the pediatric population with the same degree of vigilance as they are to adults.

While the characteristics, diagnosis, and treatment of adult melanoma have been well studied, there are relatively few publications providing significant insight into the same disease in children. This section will describe some of the characteristics that are similar between childhood and adult melanoma, but also help to highlight the unique aspects of childhood melanoma, particularly in terms of diagnosis and treatment of this disease in this patient population.

5.1 Epidemiology

Melanoma has a current annual incidence the U.S. of over 68,000, and approximately 1-4% of affected individuals are 19 years or younger (pediatric or "childhood" melanomas) [Ceballos et al., 1995; NCI, 2011; Prosdocimo et al., 2002]. About 75% of these tumors occur in the 15-19 year age group [Hamre et al., 2002; Lange et al., 2007]. Males are more likely to be affected in younger age groups, and the incidence in females increases with age [Hamre et al, 2002; Lange et al, 2007]. Although head and neck melanoma is most common in ages 1-4, truncal melanomas are more common after age four [McMasters et al., 2001].

5.2 Classification of childhood melanomas

Childhood melanomas may be classified based on age and mechanism or route of occurence. One such system revolves around age and was reported by Jen and colleagues [Jen et al., 2009]:

- Congenital (in utero to birth)
- Infantile (birth to age 1 year)
- Childhood (1 year to puberty)
- Adolescent (Post Puberty)

The second such scheme is based on the origin or mode of development of melanoma [Downard et al., 2007]:

- Arising from transplacental spread
- Arising via transformation from a giant congenital melanocytic nevus

- Arising in association with predisposing conditions
- Arising from healthy skin
- Arising from a pre-existing nevus

5.3 Risk factors/diagnosis

Because of the low incidence of melanoma in children and the perception that it is an adult disease, it is not uncommon for a physician to overlook concerning findings that might otherwise have lead to a prompt diagnosis in an adult. Physicians should ensure that childhood melanoma is in the differential diagnosis of suspicious skin lesions, particularly when predisposing factors or conditions are present. As with adults, the size, shape and character of existing skin lesions should be noted, and a dermatologist should be consulted regarding the management of any concerning appearing pigmented lesions. Particularly at risk are children with a history of significant sun exposure or a predilection for sunburning, and those with freckles, fair skin, blue/green eyes, and/or blond/red hair [Elwood & Jopson, 1997; Roth et al., 1990].

One condition that has a known predisposition to transformation into melanoma is that of giant congenital melanocytic nevus (GCMN). GCMN is defined as a melanocytic nevus that is greater than 20 cm in diameter or, alternatively, that occupies more than 2% of the body's surface area [Chung et al., 2006; Tannous et al., 2005a]. The incidence of GCMN has an incidence of approximately 1 in 20,000 newborns. Approximately 30% of childhood melanomas arise from giant congenital melanocytic nevi, and it has been estimated that GCMN carries a 2-20% risk for malignant transformation [Fishman et al., 2002]. While prophylactic excision of GCMN remains a topic of some debate, in light of the potential life-threatening implications associated with transformation to malignant melanoma, counseling parents regarding the potential benefits and risks of excision, at a minimum, is warranted. Importantly, the cosmetic implications of excision may be significant, and large lesions may require skin grafting or more complex plastic surgical procedures. Patients who have undergone excision of a GCMN may still develop an extracutaneous melanoma on rare occasions and therefore should undergo long-term surveillance [Krengel et al., 2008]. In addition, congenital melanocytic nevi that are not considered "giant" still carry up to a 1-5% risk of malignant transformation, so these should also be carefully observed or, in some cases, prophylactically excised [Tannous et al., 2005b].

A rare condition that predisposes children to melanoma is xeroderma pigmentosum, which renders affected individuals 2,000 more times likely to develop melanoma than children without the condition [Pappo, 2003]. Mutation of the CDKN2A (p16) gene also dramatically increases the risk of melanoma. Although the precise incidence of childhood melanoma per se in kindreds with a CDKN2A germline mutation is unknown, there is as high as a 50-90% lifetime risk of melanoma in affected individuals [Bergenmar et al., 2009]. Finally, as is observed in adults, children who are immunosuppressed, either genetically or pharmacologically (e.g., following organ transplantation), are an estimated 3-6 times more likely to develop melanoma [Downard et al, 2007; Pappo, 2003]. As with all patients who are at elevated risk of developing melanoma, dermatology consultation and appropriate follow-up should be carried out for pediatric populations with these significant predispositions to melanoma and other skin cancers.

With regard to diagnosis, it should be noted that presentation of children with melanoma is often similar to that of adults, and a similar approach should be used to confirm the diagnosis of melanoma. However, the diagnosis may be difficult to establish, and delays in diagnosis may delay treatment in up to 40-60% of cases in children [Melnik et al., 1986; Ridha et al., 2007; Saenz et al., 1999]. Probably as a result of the diagnostic difficulty, childhood melanomas are often thicker at the time of diagnosis than melanomas occurring in adults [Ferrari et al., 2005; Rao et al., 1990; Schmid-Wendtner et al., 2002]. As noted above, one potentially valuable approach to differentiating between melanoma and a benign condition such as a Spitz nevus is to perform a sentinel lymph node biopsy [Downard et al, 2007]. Sometimes genetic testing may also be helpful, since this appears to be of potential value primarily in differentiating melanoma from Spitz nevi [Bauer & Bastian, 2006]. Ultimately, just as in adults, clinical suspicion should drive the work-up and management of suspected melanoma in the pediatric patient population [Jen et al, 2009].

5.4 Treatment

With regard to treatment, the same principles of wide local excision that are used in adults apply to children, as well. In pediatric patients, there should be a low threshold for involvement of a plastic surgeon in management, especially in cosmetically or functionally sensitive areas, such as the face, joints, or genitalia. As with adults, there is a role for SLNB, and in children this can also serve a dual role of nodal staging and helping to establish the diagnosis of melanoma. In fact, children may actually be more likely to have a positive SLN than adults – 44% for children versus 24% for adults in one study [Topar & Zelger, 2007]. Certainly, in the risk-benefit equation regarding surgical treatment, appropriate weight should be placed on the importance of early aggressive surgical extirpation and the implications of failing to do so when faced with a melanoma.

5.5 Prognosis

Overall the prognosis of melanoma in pediatric patients is similar to that in adults. It has been shown that there is no significant difference in the five and ten year survival rates between adults and children [Balch, 1992] or between adolescents and pre-pubescent children [Livestro et al., 2007]. One fairly large study demonstrated an overall five year disease free survival of 83.2% [Livestro et al, 2007]. In another study, the five year survival rate was 90% in 79 patients with a median Breslow thickness of 0.8mm [Karlsson et al., 1998]. Age less than 10 years, male sex, and metastasis have been shown to be negative prognostic factors for survival in pediatric melanomas [Strouse et al., 2005].

5.6 Summary

Melanoma may occur in the pediatric population as in adults and may have a similarly aggressive course. Furthermore, there is concern that the incidence of childhood melanoma is increasing. Consequently, there should be a high level of vigilance in the screening and detection of melanoma in this population. Xeroderma pigmentosum, GCMN, and other predisposing conditions should further heighten the awareness of pediatricians and lower their threshold for early referral to a dermatologist.

Once diagnosed, the management of melanoma in children is similar to that in adults, although there is limited literature available on the topic. Although the use of wide local excision is applicable in children, the size of their lesion must be taken into consideration as large lesions might require the involvement of other surgical subspecialties for reconstructive efforts. In addition, lymphatic mapping and SLNB may play a valuable role in the diagnosis and staging of childhood melanoma.

6. Surgical management of melanoma in pregnancy

Primary melanoma during pregnancy is frequently accompanied by significant emotional distress on the part of the patient and occasionally and uncertainty regarding the optimal approach to management on the part of the surgeon. In general, wide excision can be performed safely during pregnancy, and there is rarely a legitimate reason for undue delay. The dilemma usually surrounds the appropriateness and timing of sentinel lymph node evaluation and the technique of performing the procedure during pregnancy. The possibility that hormonal changes may influence the progression or management of melanoma is another topic of interest and debate.

6.1 Hormones and melanoma

Whether hormonal changes during pregnancy may impact the biological behavior of melanoma remains uncertain. Early studies dating back to the 1950s indicated that pregnant women with melanoma had a worse prognosis than women who were not pregnant [Driscoll & Grant-Kels, 2007]. The belief that hormones of pregnancy could negatively impact prognosis was reinforced by investigations demonstrating the presence of estrogen receptors on melanoma cells [Neifeld & Lippman, 1980]. However, later studies employing monoclonal antibodies refuted this finding and demonstrated that human melanoma cells do not express estrogen receptors [Flowers et al., 1987; Lecavalier et al., 1990]. However, a subsequent study showed that metastatic melanoma tissue specimens were positive for testosterone receptors, which, when activated, stimulate proliferation. These receptors also appeared to be activated by estrogen, and tamoxifen blunted the proliferative effect of estrogen on these receptors [Morvillo et al., 2002]. Importantly, the use of oral contraceptives (OCP) or hormone replacement therapy (HRT) did not appear to increase the risk of melanoma or worsen the prognosis of melanoma [Durvasula et al., 2002; MacKie, 1999; Pfahlberg et al., 1997]. While further research is warranted regarding this subject, it does not appear that exogenous hormones negatively impact prognosis in melanoma.

Although there is limited evidence because of the relative infrequency of melanoma in pregnancy, the survival of women who develop melanoma during pregnancy does not appear to be significantly different from that of women with melanoma who are not pregnant [Lens et al., 2004]. Another common concern is transplacental transmission of melanoma, but this phenomenon is extremely rare and occurs only in the setting of advanced, generally stage IV melanoma [Driscoll & Grant-Kels, 2008]. In a recent study of 22 gravid women with advanced melanoma (10 stage III and 12 stage IV), there were no cases of neonates born with melanoma and only one case of placental metastases among 18 evaluable patients [Pages et al., 2010]. Nonetheless, women are often advised to wait approximately 2-5 years after diagnosis before conceiving. Although melanoma may recur at any point, most recurrences will occur within this time frame. Thus, waiting several years before attempting conception may provide some reassurance that the melanoma is less likely to recur during pregnancy [Leachman et al., 2007]. Such a decision, of course, is a very personal and difficult one for any woman or couple, and should be supported with accurate information and appropriate counseling.

With regard to treatment of primary cutaneous melanoma occurring during pregnancy, the mainstay of treatment remains wide excision. This should be performed in a timely fashion following diagnosis as in the nonpregnant patient and often may be performed under local anesthetic [Veronesi et al., 1988]. Lidocaine has been shown to safe in pregnancy, but caution should be exercised when using epinephrine [Gormley, 1990; Lawrence, 1996]. Moderate sedation, monitored anesthesia care, and general anesthesia can all be administered safely in pregnancy, and hence more extensive procedures that are not readily amenable to local anesthesia should not deter the surgeon from appropriately aggressive surgical excision and, if needed, reconstructive surgery [Kuczkowski, 2004].

6.2 Sentinel lymph node biopsy

Performance of nodal staging with sentinel lymphadenectomy during pregnancy remains controversial because of uncertainty regarding the risk of blue dye administration and Technetium Tc 99m sulfur colloid (radiocolloid) lymphoscintigraphy to the fetus. The most commonly employed agents for SLNB – Technetium Tc 99m sulfur colloid, isosulfan blue, and methylene blue – are all pregnancy category C drugs. That is, there is no (or inadequate) evidence from human or animal studies regarding teratogenicity or effects on reproductive capacity to make conclusive recommendations regarding safety in pregnancy.

With radiocolloid lymphoscintigraphy, the fetus is generally exposed to less than 5 mGy of radiation. The Society of Nuclear Medicine recommends that a pregnancy test should be conducted if there will be exposure to greater than 50 mGy [Adelstein, 1999]. Despite this, a pregnancy test is typically performed prior to lymphoscintigraphy. While there remains uncertainty about the potential risks associated with the small amount of radioactivity used in radiocolloid lymphoscintigraphy, there is also concern regarding the use of blue dye during pregnancy. The most feared of these for all patients is a risk of anaphylaxis associated with the use of isosulfan blue, estimated to be as high as 1.1%, but closer to 0.1% in more recent and larger studies, and zero among the more than 2100 patients who underwent SLNB in the Sunbelt Melanoma Trial [Albo et al., 2001; Amr et al., 2005; Leong et al., 2000; Schwartz et al., 2003; Wilke et al., 2006; Wrightson et al, 2003]. Nonetheless, there is some hesitance about using the dye in patients who are pregnant based on this concern alone [Amersi & Hansen, 2006]. There are some centers that will only employ radiocolloid in SLNB due to the risk of anaphylaxis [Lederman & Sober, 1985]. Although anaphylaxis has been reported as a risk of methylene blue during SLNB, as well, this seems to be a very rare event [Jangjoo et al., 2010; Soni et al., 2009; Sutherland et al., 2009]. Another primary concern is the risk of teratogenicity, but as stated, this has not been precisely determined. Of note, a small study conducted by Mondi et al. where in which nine pregnant patients were exposed to the isosulfan blue dye and/or radiocolloid showed that there was no negative effect on the fetus at birth [Mondi et al., 2007].

In absence of guidance from quality scientific studies, the performance of SLNB with vital dyes and/or radiocolloid during pregnancy should be determined on an individual basis. Among the many considerations is location of the primary site; if the primary tumor is located on the abdomen, one must appreciate that, in concept, the direct local exposure of the fetus to radioactivity from a radiocolloid injection may be higher than the systemic exposure, though the precise level of exposure has not been established. If this is a concern, then using a smaller quantity of radiocolloid and performing the procedure as soon as is feasible following completion of lymphoscintigraphy are reasonable measures to minimize radiation exposure of the fetus. For patients in whom there is greater concern for lymph node metastasis, then performing a SLNB should receive a higher priority. While the use of isosulfan blue dye and radiocolloid should be considered, it is also reasonable to use only a single agent in order to decrease risk – generally radiocolloid for most melanomas, particularly when there is uncertainty regarding the location (and number) of draining lymph node basin(s).

Another option is to perform wide excision up-front and to postpone the SLNB until after delivery. While it is uncertain whether postponement of SLNB until the end of pregnancy may negatively impact prognosis, there are no published studies confirming this. There is evidence from a multicenter study of 76 patients that the performance of SLNB after definitive wide excision, when necessary, does not diminish the accuracy of the SLNB [Evans et al., 2003]. If radiocolloid is employed in SLNB during the postpartum period, breast-feeding mothers should have alternative plans for feeding for a few days after the procedure until the radioactivity has been cleared, as the half-life for radioactive decay of Technetium Tc 99m is approximately 6 hours. In all cases the potential risks of these therapies should be thoroughly discussed with the expecting mother or couple. In pointing out the potential benefits and risks, it should be stressed that, while a SLNB provides valuable staging information, it has not been shown to improve survival in patients undergoing the procedure. Clearly, further research and long-term data on the risks and benefits of SLNB in pregnancy would be needed before more definitive guidelines can be established.

7. The role of surgery in the management of advanced melanoma

Surgical procedures may be beneficial in the palliation and/or control of disease in advanced melanoma, including either locoregionally advanced or distant metastatic disease. There is ample literature justifying resection of stage IV disease when feasible, and this has recently been reviewed in depth [Mosca et al., 2008]. Selection of the appropriate clinical scenario and particular patient amenable to surgical intervention, however, can present challenging management problems. Regardless of the circumstances, in considering a role for surgery in the care of the advanced melanoma patient, it is vital to clearly establish the goal(s) of surgery and to carefully weigh surgery versus other alternatives.

Advanced melanoma may take a variety of forms, and the particular pattern of disease and biologic behavior, as well as standard patient factors, should drive the management strategy for each individual patient. Certainly, participation in clinical trials is encouraged for all eligible and interested patients. Some patients present with widespread and/or rapidly progressive distant metastases and typically are candidates only for palliative systemic therapy or supportive care alone, though surgery (or other treatment) is sometimes indicated for palliation of a specific symptom complex. Surgical intervention for the purpose of eradicating disease – which may also achieve symptom control – is generally contemplated in the context of relatively indolent locoregionally advanced and/or distant disease, typically involving only one or a limited number of sites (oligometastatic melanoma).

7.1 Resection of distant metastatic disease

Surgical resection for stage IV melanoma should be considered in appropriate patients. When complete resection is performed in the setting of distant disease, five-year survival rates in the range of 20-25%, and as high as 40%, may be achieved [Mosca et al, 2008]. Importantly, one study showed that, while patients who undergo complete resection of metastatic melanoma have a 5 year survival rate of 23%, the figure was 6% in patients who either do not undergo surgery or have gross residual disease remaining following surgery (R2 resection) [Agrawal et al., 1999; Essner et al., 2004; Ollila et al., 1996; Rose et al., 2001].

As with almost all major oncologic procedures, a key to achieving optimal outcomes is proper patient selection. For example, patients with a disease-free interval of greater than 36 months at the time of recurrence and those with a solitary metastasis have better outcomes a [Essner, 2003; Essner et al, 2004]. Tumor doubling time has also been correlated with prognosis; a tumor doubling time of greater than 60 days is associated with a more favorable prognosis relative to a shorter doubling time [Ollila et al., 1998].

Among the most important factors to consider with regard to resection of advanced stage melanoma is that of location. The locations of metastasis that confer the best chance of survival are skin, subcutaneous tissue, and/or lymph nodes, with resection of these metastases being associated with a median survival of 24 months [Ollila et al., 1999].

In contrast, visceral metastases are associated with a worse prognosis in comparison with that of skin/soft tissue/nodal metastases. Among visceral sites, metastasis to the lungs is associated with the longest survival. Factors that are positively associated with prognosis for resection of lung metastasis are ability to perform complete resection, a prolonged disease-free interval, one or two pulmonary nodules, prior response to chemotherapy, negative lymph nodes, and the absence of extrathoracic disease [Harpole et al., 1992; Petersen et al., 2007]. Metastasectomy is associated with a median survival of 20 months compared with only 7.2 months for patients who do not undergo surgical resection [Young et al., 2006].

When there is metastasis to the gastrointestinal tract, surgery is often limited to palliative measures for patients experiencing perforation, obstruction, or bleeding. A more aggressive approach should be taken to resection when there may be a potential survival benefit, such as when it appears that the metastasis can be completely excised (i.e. solitary metastasis) with acceptable risk [Schuchter et al., 2000; Wood et al., 2001]. The median survival for patients with gastrointestinal metastases is 5-11 months [Panagiotou et al., 2002], but there are reports of survival of many years in a minority of patients [Young et al, 2006]. Cholecystectomy, liver resection, pancreaticoduodenectomy, or other complex pancreaticobiliary surgical procedures may also be indicated for metastatic melanoma to those sites [Carboni et al., 2004; Cellerino et al., 2000; Rose et al, 2001]. Another site of metastasis for which complete resection may be associated with a significant survival benefit is that of the adrenal gland. In cases of complete resection, median survival is 25.7 months compared to only 9.2 months for palliative resection [Haigh et al., 1999]. Alternatively, stereotactic radiosurgery may provide significant benefit in terms of disease control or palliation of symptoms related to brain or spinal cord metastasis. However, the prognosis is poor with most studies demonstrating a median survival of 5-10 months [Gaudy-Marqueste et al., 2006; Mathieu et al., 2007; Powell et al., 2008; Samlowski et al., 2007; Tarhini & Agarwala, 2004].

7.2 Surgical management of advanced extremity melanoma

Advanced melanoma of the extremity may take the form of bulky and/or in transit disease. While this pattern may be amenable to surgical extirpation or palliation with intralesional injection of an immune modulator such as BCG [Storm et al., 1979], usually its pace rapidly advances beyond the ability to control it with local treatments. An effective approach to these cases is regional chemotherapy in the form of hyperthermic isolated limb perfusion (HILP) or a less invasive alternative called isolated limb infusion (ILI) [Ariyan & Brady, 2008; Padussis et al., 2008; Tyler & Ross, 2008].

Regional therapy for advanced melanoma (either HILP or ILI) can provide excellent disease control and may achieve long-term survival in a significant minority of patients with advanced extremity melanoma [Alexander et al., 2010; Grunhagen et al., 2006; Kroon et al., 2008; Lindner et al., 2002; Rossi et al., 2010; Sanki et al., 2007]. While a relatively wide range of response rates have been reported, these procedures, both of which usually employ a melphalan-based regimen, yield objective responses in the majority of patients. HILP has been reported to achieve overall and complete response rates of as high as 80-100% and 60-90%, respectively [Ariyan & Brady, 2008; Tyler & Ross, 2008]. In a randomized, prospective, multicenter U.S.-based cooperative group trial (ACOSOG Z0020) examining HILP with melphalan +/- TNF-α, the overall and complete response rates were more modest at 66% and 25% with no difference between the TNF-α and melphalan alone groups [Cornett et al., 2006].

ILI is a less invasive form of regional chemotherapy for the treatment of advanced extremity melanoma that has been reported to achieve overall and complete response rates as high as 85% and 41%, respectively [Lindner et al, 2002]. A recently reported multi-institutional U.S. study demonstrated a 64% overall and 31% complete response rates [Beasley et al., 2009a]. Unlike HILP, ILI does not require open surgical cannulation of vessels, but rather involves placement of catheters using a percutaneous interventional radiologic approach. Thus, while a lymph node dissection of the relevant basin, if not previously done, is typically performed as part of the exposure for HILP, it must be added as an additional procedure if necessary either under the same anesthetic as for ILI or in a staged fashion.

While rare systemic side effects may occur and mild to moderate skin/soft tissue toxicity are common, primary complications of concern are compartment syndrome, occurring in about 10% and limb loss occurring in up to 2% of patients. Regional chemotherapy may also be used to effectively palliate advanced extremity disease in the setting of stage IV melanoma [Kroon et al., 2009]. In ACOSOG Z0020, the incidence of grade 4 regional toxicity was 12% and was higher in the TNF-α group; and two out of 129 patients (1.6%), both in the TNF-α group, required amputation due to regional toxicity [Cornett et al, 2006]. While both HILP and ILI are effective therapies for controlling or eradicating extremity melanoma, ILI is a less invasive method that is associated with lower regional toxicity, but it is also a somewhat less effective alternative than HILP [Beasley et al., 2008].

Recently, novel approaches to enhancing the efficacy of regional chemotherapy have been investigated. One intriguing approach is to combine systemically administered targeted molecular therapies with conventional regional chemotherapy. Beasley and colleagues reported the results of a phase 1 dose-escalation trial of systemic ADH-1, an inhibitor of the adhesion molecule N-cadherin, in conjunction with ILI, and the treatment was well tolerated and yielded a robust complete response rate [Beasley et al., 2009b]. This was followed up with a phase II study, but no significant improvement in objective response rate was noted [Beasley et al., 2011]. However, this work introduced a new paradigm for the development of novel cytotoxic and targeted molcular therapeutics for the treatment of advanced melanoma. Another significant advancement is the emergence of gene expression profiling of tumor biopsies – usually readily accessible in this patient population – as a potential means of predicting treatment response and guiding selection of optimal therapeutics for regional chemotherapy [Augustine et al., 2010].

Invasive or minimally invasive surgical interventions may be indicated in a variety of settings for the treatment of advanced melanoma. The goal may be to achieve prolonged disease control or to palliate specific symptoms or some combination of the two. One should carefully select patients for major intervention so that the right patients receive the right treatment at the right time. Certainly, performing a major surgical procedure associated with significant risk and without clear benefit has the potential to shorten life and/or worsen the quality of life of a patient and therefore have the opposite consequences to those intended.

8. Conclusion

The surgical management of cutaneous melanoma can be challenging even in relatively straightforward cases because of its protean clinical presentations, variable location, and the wide range of demographic groups that it commonly affects. However, there are a number of recurring themes in surgery for melanoma that serve as a constant reminder that some clinical problems seem to have more questions than answers. Several of these complex areas of melanoma management have been reviewed in this chapter on challenging problems. Common threads that run through these areas of uncertainty are that optimal care first necessitates familiarity with current literature and guidelines on the topic, that patients should be properly educated and actively involved in the decision-making process, and that conscientious, multi-disciplinary cancer care serves as a foundation for proper clinical management. Despite this, in the case of each of the topics discussed, there remains a tension between taking an aggressive approach to a disease that in most cases may only be cured or effectively controlled with surgery, and trying to minimize the risk of sometimes debilitating morbidity that may accompany such treatment. A thoughtful, collaborative and patient-centered approach to these challenging cases helps to ensure that each patient receives the best possible surgical management for his or her melanoma.

9. References

Adelstein SJ. 1999. Administered radionuclides in pregnancy. *Teratology* 59:236-9

Agrawal S, Yao TJ, Coit DG. 1999. Surgery for melanoma metastatic to the gastrointestinal tract. *Annals of Surgical Oncology* 6:336-44

Albo D, Wayne JD, Hunt KK, Rahlfs TF, Singletary SE, et al. 2001. Anaphylactic reactions to isosulfan blue dye during sentinel lymph node biopsy for breast cancer. *American Journal of Surgery* 182:393-8

Alex JC, Krag DN, Harlow SP, Meijer S, Loggie BW, et al. 1998. Localization of regional lymph nodes in melanomas of the head and neck. *Arch Otolaryngol Head Neck Surg* 124:135-40

Alexander HR, Jr., Fraker DL, Bartlett DL, Libutti SK, Steinberg SM, et al. 2010. Analysis of factors influencing outcome in patients with in-transit malignant melanoma undergoing isolated limb perfusion using modern treatment parameters. *Journal of Clinical Oncology* 28:114-8

Amersi F, Hansen NM. 2006. The benefits and limitations of sentinel lymph node biopsy. *Curr Treat Options Oncol* 7:141-51

Amersi F, Morton DL. 2007. The role of sentinel lymph node biopsy in the management of melanoma. *Advances in Surgery* 41:241-56

Amr D, Broderick-Villa G, Haigh PI, Guenther JM, DiFronzo LA. 2005. Adverse drug reactions during lymphatic mapping and sentinel lymph node biopsy for solid neoplasms. *American Surgeon* 71:720-4

Ariyan CE, Brady MS. 2008. History of regional chemotherapy for cancer of the extremities. *International Journal of Hyperthermia* 24:185-92

Augustine CK, Jung S-H, Sohn I, Yoo JS, Yoshimoto Y, et al. 2010. Gene expression signatures as a guide to treatment strategies for in-transit metastatic melanoma. *Molecular Cancer Therapeutics* 9:779-90

Bagaria SP, Faries MB, Morton DL. 2010. Sentinel node biopsy in melanoma: technical considerations of the procedure as performed at the John Wayne Cancer Institute. *Journal of Surgical Oncology* 101:669-76

Balch CM. 1992. Cutaneous melanoma: prognosis and treatment results worldwide. *Semin Surg Oncol* 8:400-14

Balch CM, Gershenwald JE, Soong S-J, Thompson JF, Atkins MB, et al. 2009. Final version of 2009 AJCC melanoma staging and classification. *Journal of Clinical Oncology* 27:6199-206

Balch CM, Soong S, Ross MI, Urist MM, Karakousis CP, et al. 2000. Long-term results of a multi-institutional randomized trial comparing prognostic factors and surgical results for intermediate thickness melanomas (1.0 to 4.0 mm). Intergroup Melanoma Surgical Trial. *Annals of Surgical Oncology* 7:87-97

Barnhill RL, Argenyi ZB, From L, Glass LF, Maize JC, et al. 1999. Atypical Spitz nevi/tumors: lack of consensus for diagnosis, discrimination from melanoma, and prediction of outcome. *Hum Pathol* 30:513-20

Bastian BC, Kashani-Sabet M, Hamm H, Godfrey T, Moore DH, 2nd, et al. 2000. Gene amplifications characterize acral melanoma and permit the detection of occult tumor cells in the surrounding skin. *Cancer Res* 60:1968-73

Bastian BC, Olshen AB, LeBoit PE, Pinkel D. 2003. Classifying melanocytic tumors based on DNA copy number changes. *Am J Pathol* 163:1765-70

Bauer J, Bastian BC. 2006. Distinguishing melanocytic nevi from melanoma by DNA copy number changes: comparative genomic hybridization as a research and diagnostic tool. *Dermatol Ther* 19:40-9

Beasley GM, Caudle A, Petersen RP, McMahon NS, Padussis J, et al. 2009a. A multi-institutional experience of isolated limb infusion: defining response and toxicity in the US. *Journal of the American College of Surgeons* 208:706-15; discussion 15-7

Beasley GM, McMahon N, Sanders G, Augustine CK, Selim MA, et al. 2009b. A phase 1 study of systemic ADH-1 in combination with melphalan via isolated limb infusion in patients with locally advanced in-transit malignant melanoma. *Cancer* 115:4766-74

Beasley GM, Petersen RP, Yoo J, McMahon N, Aloia T, et al. 2008. Isolated limb infusion for in-transit malignant melanoma of the extremity: a well-tolerated but less effective alternative to hyperthermic isolated limb perfusion. *Annals of Surgical Oncology* 15:2195-205

Beasley GM, Riboh JC, Augustine CK, McMahon N, Grobmyer SR, et al. 2011. A multi-center phase II trial of systemic ADH-1 in combination with melphalan via isolated limb infusion (M-ILI) in patients with advanced extremity melanoma. *Journal of Clinical Oncology* 29:1210-5

Bergenmar M, Hansson J, Brandberg Y. 2009. Family members' perceptions of genetic testing for malignant melanoma--a prospective interview study. *European Journal of Oncology Nursing* 13:74-80

Berk DR, Johnson DL, Uzieblo A, Kiernan M, Swetter SM. 2005. Sentinel lymph node biopsy for cutaneous melanoma: the Stanford experience, 1997-2004. *Arch Dermatol* 141:1016-22

Berk DR, LaBuz E, Dadras SS, Johnson DL, Swetter SM. 2010. Melanoma and melanocytic tumors of uncertain malignant potential in children, adolescents and young adults--the Stanford experience 1995-2008. *Pediatric Dermatology* 27:244-54

Bilimoria KY, Balch CM, Bentrem DJ, Talamonti MS, Ko CY, et al. 2008. Complete lymph node dissection for sentinel node-positive melanoma: assessment of practice patterns in the United States. *Ann Surg Oncol* 15:1566-76

Callender GG, McMasters KM. Early versus delayed complete lymphadenectomy in melanoma: insight from MSLT I. *Ann Surg Oncol* 18:306-8

Carboni F, Graziano F, Lonardo MT, Lepiane P, Santoro R, et al. 2004. Pancreaticoduodenectomy for pancreatic metastatic melanoma. *Journal of Experimental & Clinical Cancer Research* 23:539-43

Carless MA, Griffiths LR. 2008. Cytogenetics of melanoma and nonmelanoma skin cancer. *Adv Exp Med Biol* 624:227-40

Carlson GW, Murray DR, Greenlee R, Alazraki N, Fry-Spray C, et al. 2000. Management of malignant melanoma of the head and neck using dynamic lymphoscintigraphy and gamma probe-guided sentinel lymph node biopsy. *Arch Otolaryngol Head Neck Surg* 126:433-7

Carlson GW, Murray DR, Hestley A, Staley CA, Lyles RH, Cohen C. 2003. Sentinel lymph node mapping for thick (>or=4-mm) melanoma: should we be doing it? *Annals of Surgical Oncology* 10:408-15

Carlson GW, Page AJ, Cohen C, Parker D, Yaar R, et al. 2008. Regional recurrence after negative sentinel lymph node biopsy for melanoma. *Annals of Surgery* 248:378-86

Cascinelli N, Morabito A, Santinami M, MacKie RM, Belli F. 1998. Immediate or delayed dissection of regional nodes in patients with melanoma of the trunk: a randomised trial. WHO Melanoma Programme. *Lancet* 351:793-6

Casorzo L, Luzzi C, Nardacchione A, Picciotto F, Pisacane A, Risio M. 2005. Fluorescence in situ hybridization (FISH) evaluation of chromosomes 6, 7, 9 and 10 throughout human melanocytic tumorigenesis. *Melanoma Res* 15:155-60

Ceballos PI, Ruiz-Maldonado R, Mihm MC, Jr. 1995. Melanoma in children. *N Engl J Med* 332:656-62

Cecchi R, Buralli L, Innocenti S, De Gaudio C. 2007. Sentinel lymph node biopsy in patients with thin melanomas. *Journal of Dermatology* 34:512-5

Cecchi R, Pavesi M, Buralli L, Innocenti S, De Gaudio C. 2008. Tumour regression does not increase the risk of sentinel node involvement in thin melanomas. *Chirurgia Italiana* 60:257-60

Cellerino P, Corsi F, Morandi E, Foschi D, Trabucchi E. 2000. Metastatic melanoma of the gallbladder. *European Journal of Surgical Oncology* 26:815-6

Chang SB, Askew RL, Xing Y, Weaver S, Gershenwald JE, et al. 2010. Prospective assessment of postoperative complications and associated costs following inguinal lymph node dissection (ILND) in melanoma patients. *Annals of Surgical Oncology* 17:2764-72

Cherpelis BS, Haddad F, Messina J, Cantor AB, Fitzmorris K, et al. 2001. Sentinel lymph node micrometastasis and other histologic factors that predict outcome in patients with thicker melanomas. *J Am Acad Dermatol* 44:762-6

Chung C, Forte AJV, Narayan D, Persing J. 2006. Giant nevi: a review. *Journal of Craniofacial Surgery* 17:1210-5

Cormier JN, Xing Y, Ding M, Lee JE, Mansfield PF, et al. 2005. Population-based assessment of surgical treatment trends for patients with melanoma in the era of sentinel lymph node biopsy. *J Clin Oncol* 23:6054-62

Cornett WR, McCall LM, Petersen RP, Ross MI, Briele HA, et al. 2006. Randomized multicenter trial of hyperthermic isolated limb perfusion with melphalan alone compared with melphalan plus tumor necrosis factor: American College of Surgeons Oncology Group Trial Z0020. *Journal of Clinical Oncology* 24:4196-201

De Rosa N, Lyman GH, Silbermins D, Valsecchi MD, Pruitt SK, et al. 2011. Sentinel node biopsy for head and neck melanoma: a systematic review. In press

Downard CD, Rapkin LB, Gow KW. 2007. Melanoma in children and adolescents. *Surg Oncol* 16:215-20

Driscoll MS, Grant-Kels JM. 2007. Hormones, nevi, and melanoma: an approach to the patient. *J Am Acad Dermatol* 57:919-31; quiz 32-6

Driscoll MS, Grant-Kels JM. 2008. Melanoma and pregnancy. *Giornale Italiano di Dermatologia e Venereologia* 143:251-7

Durvasula R, Ahmed SM, Vashisht A, Studd JW. 2002. Hormone replacement therapy and malignant melanoma: to prescribe or not to prescribe? *Climacteric* 5:197-200

Eicher SA, Clayman GL, Myers JN, Gillenwater AM. 2002. A prospective study of intraoperative lymphatic mapping for head and neck cutaneous melanoma. *Arch Otolaryngol Head Neck Surg* 128:241-6

Elwood JM, Jopson J. 1997. Melanoma and sun exposure: an overview of published studies. *Int J Cancer* 73:198-203

Essner R. 2003. Surgical treatment of malignant melanoma. *Surg Clin North Am* 83:109-56

Essner R. 2010. Lymphatic mapping and sentinel lymphadenectomy in primary cutaneous melanoma. *Expert Review of Anticancer Therapy* 10:723-8

Essner R, Chung MH, Bleicher R, Hsueh E, Wanek L, Morton DL. 2002. Prognostic implications of thick (>or=4-mm) melanoma in the era of intraoperative lymphatic mapping and sentinel lymphadenectomy. *Ann Surg Oncol* 9:754-61

Essner R, Lee JH, Wanek LA, Itakura H, Morton DL. 2004. Contemporary surgical treatment of advanced-stage melanoma. *Archives of Surgery* 139:961-6; discussion 6-7

Essner R, Scheri R, Kavanagh M, Torisu-Itakura H, Wanek LA, Morton DL. 2006. Surgical management of the groin lymph nodes in melanoma in the era of sentinel lymph node dissection. *Archives of Surgery* 141:877-82; discussion 82-4

Evans HL, Krag DN, Teates CD, Patterson JW, Meijer S, et al. 2003. Lymphoscintigraphy and sentinel node biopsy accurately stage melanoma in patients presenting after wide local excision. *Annals of Surgical Oncology* 10:416-25

Even-Sapir E, Lerman H, Lievshitz G, Khafif A, Fliss DM, et al. 2003. Lymphoscintigraphy for sentinel node mapping using a hybrid SPECT/CT system. *Journal of Nuclear Medicine* 44:1413-20

Ferrari A, Bono A, Baldi M, Collini P, Casanova M, et al. 2005. Does melanoma behave differently in younger children than in adults? A retrospective study of 33 cases of childhood melanoma from a single institution. *Pediatrics* 115:649-54

Ferrone CR, Panageas KS, Busam K, Brady MS, Coit DG. 2002. Multivariate prognostic model for patients with thick cutaneous melanoma: importance of sentinel lymph node status. *Ann Surg Oncol* 9:637-45

Fishman C, Mihm MC, Jr., Sober AJ. 2002. Diagnosis and management of nevi and cutaneous melanoma in infants and children. *Clin Dermatol* 20:44-50

Flowers JL, Seigler HF, McCarty KS, Sr., Konrath J, McCarty KS, Jr. 1987. Absence of estrogen receptor in human melanoma as evaluated by a monoclonal antiestrogen receptor antibody. *Arch Dermatol* 123:764-5

Francischetto T, Spector N, Neto Rezende JF, de Azevedo Antunes M, de Oliveira Romano S, et al. 2010. Influence of sentinel lymph node tumor burden on survival in melanoma. *Annals of Surgical Oncology* 17:1152-8

Gajdos C, Griffith KA, Wong SL, Johnson TM, Chang AE, et al. 2009. Is there a benefit to sentinel lymph node biopsy in patients with T4 melanoma? *Cancer* 115:5752-60

Garbe C, Peris K, Hauschild A, Saiag P, Middleton M, et al. 2010. Diagnosis and treatment of melanoma: European consensus-based interdisciplinary guideline. *European Journal of Cancer* 46:270-83

Gaudy-Marqueste C, Regis J-M, Muracciole X, Laurans R, Richard M-A, et al. 2006. Gamma-Knife radiosurgery in the management of melanoma patients with brain metastases: a series of 106 patients without whole-brain radiotherapy. *International Journal of Radiation Oncology, Biology, Physics* 65:809-16

Gerami P, Jewell SS, Morrison LE, Blondin B, Schulz J, et al. 2009. Fluorescence in situ hybridization (FISH) as an ancillary diagnostic tool in the diagnosis of melanoma. *Am J Surg Pathol* 33:1146-56

Gershenwald JE, Mansfield PF, Lee JE, Ross MI. 2000. Role for lymphatic mapping and sentinel lymph node biopsy in patients with thick (> or = 4 mm) primary melanoma. *Ann Surg Oncol* 7:160-5

Ghazi B, Carlson GW, Murray DR, Gow KW, Page A, et al. 2010. Utility of lymph node assessment for atypical spitzoid melanocytic neoplasms. *Annals of Surgical Oncology* 17:2471-5

Gomez-Rivera F, Santillan A, McMurphey AB, Paraskevopoulos G, Roberts DB, et al. 2008. Sentinel node biopsy in patients with cutaneous melanoma of the head and neck: recurrence and survival study. *Head & Neck* 30:1284-94

Gormley DE. 1990. Cutaneous surgery and the pregnant patient. *J Am Acad Dermatol* 23:269-79

Grunhagen DJ, de Wilt JHW, Graveland WJ, Verhoef C, van Geel AN, Eggermont AMM. 2006. Outcome and prognostic factor analysis of 217 consecutive isolated limb perfusions with tumor necrosis factor-alpha and melphalan for limb-threatening soft tissue sarcoma. *Cancer* 106:1776-84

Guggenheim M, Dummer R, Jung FJ, Mihic-Probst D, Steinert H, et al. 2008. The influence of sentinel lymph node tumour burden on additional lymph node involvement and disease-free survival in cutaneous melanoma--a retrospective analysis of 392 cases. *British Journal of Cancer* 98:1922-8

Haigh PI, Essner R, Wardlaw JC, Stern SL, Morton DL. 1999. Long-term survival after complete resection of melanoma metastatic to the adrenal gland. *Annals of Surgical Oncology* 6:633-9

Hamre MR, Chuba P, Bakhshi S, Thomas R, Severson RK. 2002. Cutaneous melanoma in childhood and adolescence. *Pediatr Hematol Oncol* 19:309-17

Harpole DH, Jr., Johnson CM, Wolfe WG, George SL, Seigler HF. 1992. Analysis of 945 cases of pulmonary metastatic melanoma. *J Thorac Cardiovasc Surg* 103:743-8; discussion 8-50

Hermanek P, Hutter RV, Sobin LH, Wittekind C. 1999. International Union Against Cancer. Classification of isolated tumor cells and micrometastasis. *Cancer* 86:2668-73

Jacobs IA, Chang CK, Salti GI. 2004. Role of sentinel lymph node biopsy in patients with thick (>4 mm) primary melanoma. *Am Surg* 70:59-62

Jangjoo A, Forghani MN, Mehrabibahar M, Sadeghi R. 2010. Anaphylaxis reaction of a breast cancer patient to methylene blue during breast surgery with sentinel node mapping. *Acta Oncologica* 49:877-8

Jansen L, Koops HS, Nieweg OE, Doting MH, Kapteijn BA, et al. 2000. Sentinel node biopsy for melanoma in the head and neck region. *Head Neck* 22:27-33

Jen M, Murphy M, Grant-Kels JM. 2009. Childhood melanoma. *Clin Dermatol* 27:529-36

Karakousis GC, Gimotty PA, Botbyl JD, Kesmodel SB, Elder DE, et al. 2006. Predictors of regional nodal disease in patients with thin melanomas. *Annals of Surgical Oncology* 13:533-41

Karlsson P, Boeryd B, Sander B, Westermark P, Rosdahl I. 1998. Increasing incidence of cutaneous malignant melanoma in children and adolescents 12-19 years of age in Sweden 1973-92. *Acta Dermato-Venereologica* 78:289-92

Kelly J, Fogarty K, Redmond HP. 2009. A definitive role for sentinel lymph node mapping with biopsy for cutaneous melanoma of the head and neck. *Surgeon* 7:336-9

Kesmodel SB, Karakousis GC, Botbyl JD, Canter RJ, Lewis RT, et al. 2005. Mitotic rate as a predictor of sentinel lymph node positivity in patients with thin melanomas. *Annals of Surgical Oncology* 12:449-58

Klop WM, Veenstra HJ, Vermeeren L, Nieweg OE, Balm AJ, Lohuis PJ. 2011. Assessment of lymphatic drainage patterns and implications for the extent of neck dissection in head and neck melanoma patients. *J Surg Oncol*

Krengel S, Breuninger H, Hauschild A, Hoger P, Merl V, Hamm H. 2008. Installation of a network for patients with congenital melanocytic nevi in German-speaking countries. *Journal der Deutschen Dermatologischen Gesellschaft* 6:204-8

Kroon HM, Lin DY, Kam PCA, Thompson JF. 2009. Isolated limb infusion as palliative treatment for advanced limb disease in patients with AJCC stage IV melanoma. *Annals of Surgical Oncology* 16:1193-201

Kroon HM, Moncrieff M, Kam PCA, Thompson JF. 2008. Outcomes following isolated limb infusion for melanoma. A 14-year experience. *Annals of Surgical Oncology* 15:3003-13

Kuczkowski KM. 2004. Nonobstetric surgery during pregnancy: what are the risks of anesthesia? *Obstetrical & Gynecological Survey* 59:52-6

Lange JR, Palis BE, Chang DC, Soong SJ, Balch CM. 2007. Melanoma in children and teenagers: an analysis of patients from the National Cancer Data Base. *J Clin Oncol* 25:1363-8

Lawrence C. 1996. Drug management in skin surgery. *Drugs* 52:805-17

Leachman SA, Jackson R, Eliason MJ, Larson AA, Bolognia JL. 2007. Management of melanoma during pregnancy. *Dermatol Nurs* 19:145-52, 61

Lecavalier MA, From L, Gaid N. 1990. Absence of estrogen receptors in dysplastic nevi and malignant melanoma. *J Am Acad Dermatol* 23:242-6

Lens MB, Rosdahl I, Ahlbom A, Farahmand BY, Synnerstad I, et al. 2004. Effect of pregnancy on survival in women with cutaneous malignant melanoma. *J Clin Oncol* 22:4369-75

Leong SP, Donegan E, Heffernon W, Dean S, Katz JA. 2000. Adverse reactions to isosulfan blue during selective sentinel lymph node dissection in melanoma. *Annals of Surgical Oncology* 7:361-6

Lindner P, Doubrovsky A, Kam PCA, Thompson JF. 2002. Prognostic factors after isolated limb infusion with cytotoxic agents for melanoma. *Annals of Surgical Oncology* 9:127-36

Livestro DP, Kaine EM, Michaelson JS, Mihm MC, Haluska FG, et al. 2007. Melanoma in the young: differences and similarities with adult melanoma: a case-matched controlled analysis. *Cancer* 110:614-24

Lucci A, McCall LM, Beitsch PD, Whitworth PW, Reintgen DS, et al. 2007. Surgical complications associated with sentinel lymph node dissection (SLND) plus axillary lymph node dissection compared with SLND alone in the American College of Surgeons Oncology Group Trial Z0011. *Journal of Clinical Oncology* 25:3657-63

Ludgate MW, Fullen DR, Lee J, Lowe L, Bradford C, et al. 2009. The atypical Spitz tumor of uncertain biologic potential: a series of 67 patients from a single institution. *Cancer* 115:631-41

MacKie RM. 1999. Pregnancy and exogenous hormones in patients with cutaneous malignant melanoma. *Curr Opin Oncol* 11:129-31

MacNeill KN, Ghazarian D, McCready D, Rotstein L. 2005. Sentinel lymph node biopsy for cutaneous melanoma of the head and neck. *Annals of Surgical Oncology* 12:726-32

Magro CM, Crowson AN, Mihm MC, Jr., Gupta K, Walker MJ, Solomon G. 2010. The dermal-based borderline melanocytic tumor: a categorical approach. *Journal of the American Academy of Dermatology* 62:469-79

Master V, Ogan K, Kooby D, Hsiao W, Delman K. 2009. Leg endoscopic groin lymphadenectomy (LEG procedure): step-by-step approach to a straightforward technique. *European Urology* 56:821-8

Mathieu D, Kondziolka D, Cooper PB, Flickinger JC, Niranjan A, et al. 2007. Gamma knife radiosurgery in the management of malignant melanoma brain metastases. *Neurosurgery* 60:471-81; discussion 81-2

McMasters KM. Why does no one want to perform lymph node dissection anymore? *Ann Surg Oncol* 17:358-61

McMasters KM, Reintgen DS, Ross MI, Gershenwald JE, Edwards MJ, et al. 2001. Sentinel lymph node biopsy for melanoma: controversy despite widespread agreement. *J Clin Oncol* 19:2851-5

Melnik MK, Urdaneta LF, Al-Jurf AS, Foucar E, Jochimsen PR, Soper RT. 1986. Malignant melanoma in childhood and adolescence. *American Surgeon* 52:142-7

Meretoja TJ, Joensuu H, Heikkila PS, Leidenius MH. 2010. Safety of sentinel node biopsy in breast cancer patients who receive a second radioisotope injection after visualization failure in lymphoscintigraphy. *Journal of Surgical Oncology* 102:649-55

Meyers MO, Yeh JJ, Deal AM, Byerly FL, Woosley JT, et al. 2010. Age and Breslow depth are associated with a positive sentinel lymph node in patients with cutaneous melanocytic tumors of uncertain malignant potential. *Journal of the American College of Surgeons* 211:744-8

Mondi MM, Cuenca RE, Ollila DW, Stewart JHt, Levine EA. 2007. Sentinel lymph node biopsy during pregnancy: initial clinical experience. *Ann Surg Oncol* 14:218-21

Morey AL, Murali R, McCarthy SW, Mann GJ, Scolyer RA. 2009. Diagnosis of cutaneous melanocytic tumours by four-colour fluorescence in situ hybridisation. *Pathology* 41:383-7

Morton DL, Thompson JF, Cochran AJ, Mozzillo N, Elashoff R, et al. 2006. Sentinel-node biopsy or nodal observation in melanoma. *N Engl J Med* 355:1307-17

Morton DL, Wen DR, Wong JH, Economou JS, Cagle LA, et al. 1992. Technical details of intraoperative lymphatic mapping for early stage melanoma. *Archives of Surgery* 127:392-9

Morvillo V, Luthy IA, Bravo AI, Capurro MI, Portela P, et al. 2002. Androgen receptors in human melanoma cell lines IIB-MEL-LES and IIB-MEL-IAN and in human melanoma metastases. *Melanoma Res* 12:529-38

Mosca PJ, Teicher E, Nair SP, Pockaj BA. 2008. Can surgeons improve survival in stage IV melanoma? *Journal of Surgical Oncology* 97:462-8

National Cancer Institute. 2011. *Cancer Topics: Melanoma.* http://www.cancer.gov/cancertopics/types/melanoma

Neifeld JP, Lippman ME. 1980. Steroid hormone receptors and melanoma. *J Invest Dermatol* 74:379-81

Newman MD, Lertsburapa T, Mirzabeigi M, Mafee M, Guitart J, Gerami P. 2009. Fluorescence in situ hybridization as a tool for microstaging in malignant melanoma. *Mod Pathol* 22:989-95

O'Brien CJ, Uren RF, Thompson JF, Howman-Giles RB, Petersen-Schaefer K, et al. 1995. Prediction of potential metastatic sites in cutaneous head and neck melanoma using lymphoscintigraphy. *American Journal of Surgery* 170:461-6

Ollila DW, Essner R, Wanek LA, Morton DL. 1996. Surgical resection for melanoma metastatic to the gastrointestinal tract. *Archives of Surgery* 131:975-9; 9-80

Ollila DW, Hsueh EC, Stern SL, Morton DL. 1999. Metastasectomy for recurrent stage IV melanoma. *Journal of Surgical Oncology* 71:209-13

Ollila DW, Stern SL, Morton DL. 1998. Tumor doubling time: a selection factor for pulmonary resection of metastatic melanoma. *Journal of Surgical Oncology* 69:206-11

Padussis JC, Steerman SN, Tyler DS, Mosca PJ. 2008. Pharmacokinetics & drug resistance of melphalan in regional chemotherapy: ILP versus ILI. *International Journal of Hyperthermia* 24:239-49

Paek SC, Griffith KA, Johnson TM, Sondak VK, Wong SL, et al. 2007. The impact of factors beyond Breslow depth on predicting sentinel lymph node positivity in melanoma. *Cancer* 109:100-8

Pages C, Robert C, Thomas L, Maubec E, Sassolas B, et al. 2010. Management and outcome of metastatic melanoma during pregnancy. *British Journal of Dermatology* 162:274-81

Panagiotou I, Brountzos EN, Bafaloukos D, Stoupis C, Brestas P, Kelekis DA. 2002. Malignant melanoma metastatic to the gastrointestinal tract. *Melanoma Res* 12:169-73

Pappo AS. 2003. Melanoma in children and adolescents. *Eur J Cancer* 39:2651-61

Patel SG, Coit DG, Shaha AR, Brady MS, Boyle JO, et al. 2002. Sentinel lymph node biopsy for cutaneous head and neck melanomas. *Arch Otolaryngol Head Neck Surg* 128:285-91

Perrott RE, Glass LF, Reintgen DS, Fenske NA. 2003. Reassessing the role of lymphatic mapping and sentinel lymphadenectomy in the management of cutaneous malignant melanoma. *J Am Acad Dermatol* 49:567-88; quiz 89-92

Petersen RP, Hanish SI, Haney JC, Miller CC, 3rd, Burfeind WR, Jr., et al. 2007. Improved survival with pulmonary metastasectomy: an analysis of 1720 patients with pulmonary metastatic melanoma. *Journal of Thoracic & Cardiovascular Surgery* 133:104-10

Pfahlberg A, Hassan K, Wille L, Lausen B, Gefeller O. 1997. Systematic review of case-control studies: oral contraceptives show no effect on melanoma risk. *Public Health Rev* 25:309-15

Phan GQ, Messina JL, Sondak VK, Zager JS. 2009. Sentinel lymph node biopsy for melanoma: indications and rationale. *Cancer Control* 16:234-9

Pirker C, Holzmann K, Spiegl-Kreinecker S, Elbling L, Thallinger C, et al. 2003. Chromosomal imbalances in primary and metastatic melanomas: over-representation of essential telomerase genes. *Melanoma Res* 13:483-92

Pouryazdanparast P, Newman M, Mafee M, Haghighat Z, Guitart J, Gerami P. 2009. Distinguishing epithelioid blue nevus from blue nevus-like cutaneous melanoma metastasis using fluorescence in situ hybridization. *Am J Surg Pathol* 33:1396-400

Powell JW, Chung CT, Shah HR, Canute GW, Hodge CJ, et al. 2008. Gamma Knife surgery in the management of radioresistant brain metastases in high-risk patients with melanoma, renal cell carcinoma, and sarcoma. *Journal of Neurosurgery* 109 Suppl:122-8

Prosdocimo T, Smith M, Polack EP. 2002. The diagnosis and treatment of childhood melanoma. *W V Med J* 98:149-51

Ranieri JM, Wagner JD, Azuaje R, Davidson D, Wenck S, et al. 2002. Prognostic importance of lymph node tumor burden in melanoma patients staged by sentinel node biopsy. *Annals of Surgical Oncology* 9:975-81

Rao BN, Hayes FA, Pratt CB, Fleming ID, Kumar AP, et al. 1990. Malignant melanoma in children: its management and prognosis. *Journal of Pediatric Surgery* 25:198-203

Rasgon BM. 2001. Use of low-dose technetium Tc 99m sulfur colloid to locate sentinel lymph nodes in melanoma of the head and neck: preliminary study. *Laryngoscope* 111:1366-72

Ridha H, Ahmed S, Theaker JM, Horlock N. 2007. Malignant melanoma and deep penetrating naevus--difficulties in diagnosis in children. *Journal of Plastic, Reconstructive & Aesthetic Surgery: JPRAS* 60:1252-5

Roarke MC, Ram P, Nguyen BD. 2007. Utility of SPECT/CT in preoperative planning for sentinel lymph node biopsy in melanoma and head/neck carcinoma: three illustrative cases. *Clinical Nuclear Medicine* 32:464-5

Roaten JB, Pearlman N, Gonzalez R, Gonzalez R, McCarter MD. 2005. Identifying risk factors for complications following sentinel lymph node biopsy for melanoma. *Archives of Surgery* 140:85-9

Rose DM, Essner R, Hughes TM, Tang PC, Bilchik A, et al. 2001. Surgical resection for metastatic melanoma to the liver: the John Wayne Cancer Institute and Sydney Melanoma Unit experience. *Archives of Surgery* 136:950-5

Ross MI, Gershenwald JE. 2008. How should we view the results of the Multicenter Selective Lymphadenectomy Trial-1 (MSLT-1)? *Ann Surg Oncol* 15:670-3

Rossi CR, Pasquali S, Mocellin S, Vecchiato A, Campana LG, et al. 2010. Long-term results of melphalan-based isolated limb perfusion with or without low-dose TNF for in-transit melanoma metastases. *Annals of Surgical Oncology* 17:3000-7

Roth ME, Grant-Kels JM, Kuhn MK, Greenberg RD, Hurwitz S. 1990. Melanoma in children. *J Am Acad Dermatol* 22:265-74

Rousseau C, Classe JM, Campion L, Curtet C, Dravet F, et al. 2005. The impact of nonvisualization of sentinel nodes on lymphoscintigraphy in breast cancer. *Annals of Surgical Oncology* 12:533-8

Sabel MS, Griffith KA, Arora A, Shargorodsky J, Blazer DG, 3rd, et al. 2007. Inguinal node dissection for melanoma in the era of sentinel lymph node biopsy. *Surgery* 141:728-35

Saenz NC, Saenz-Badillos J, Busam K, LaQuaglia MP, Corbally M, Brady MS. 1999. Childhood melanoma survival. *Cancer* 85:750-4

Samlowski WE, Watson GA, Wang M, Rao G, Klimo P, Jr., et al. 2007. Multimodality treatment of melanoma brain metastases incorporating stereotactic radiosurgery (SRS). *Cancer* 109:1855-62

Sanki A, Kam PCA, Thompson JF. 2007. Long-term results of hyperthermic, isolated limb perfusion for melanoma: a reflection of tumor biology. *Annals of Surgery* 245:591-6

Sarnaik AA, Puleo CA, Zager JS, Sondak VK. 2009. Limiting the morbidity of inguinal lymphadenectomy for metastatic melanoma. *Cancer Control* 16:240-7

Schmid-Wendtner MH, Berking C, Baumert J, Schmidt M, Sander CA, et al. 2002. Cutaneous melanoma in childhood and adolescence: an analysis of 36 patients. *Journal of the American Academy of Dermatology* 46:874-9

Schuchter LM, Green R, Fraker D. 2000. Primary and metastatic diseases in malignant melanoma of the gastrointestinal tract. *Curr Opin Oncol* 12:181-5

Schwartz JL, Mozurkewich EL, Johnson TM. 2003. Current management of patients with melanoma who are pregnant, want to get pregnant, or do not want to get pregnant. *Cancer* 97:2130-3

Scolyer RA, Murali R, McCarthy SW, Thompson JF. 2010. Histologically ambiguous ("borderline") primary cutaneous melanocytic tumors: approaches to patient management including the roles of molecular testing and sentinel lymph node biopsy. *Arch Pathol Lab Med* 134:1770-7

Scolyer RA, Thompson JF, Stretch JR, Sharma R, McCarthy SW. 2004. Pathology of melanocytic lesions: new, controversial, and clinically important issues. *J Surg Oncol* 86:200-11

Sim FH, Taylor WF, Pritchard DJ, Soule EH. 1986. Lymphadenectomy in the management of stage I malignant melanoma: a prospective randomized study. *Mayo Clinic Proceedings* 61:697-705

Socrier Y, Lauwers-Cances V, Lamant L, Garrido I, Lauwers F, et al. 2010. Histological regression in primary melanoma: not a predictor of sentinel lymph node metastasis in a cohort of 397 patients. *British Journal of Dermatology* 162:830-4

Sondak VK, Taylor JMG, Sabel MS, Wang Y, Lowe L, et al. 2004. Mitotic rate and younger age are predictors of sentinel lymph node positivity: lessons learned from the generation of a probabilistic model. *Annals of Surgical Oncology* 11:247-58

Soni M, Saha S, Korant A, Fritz P, Chakravarty B, et al. 2009. A prospective trial comparing 1% lymphazurin vs 1% methylene blue in sentinel lymph node mapping of gastrointestinal tumors. *Annals of Surgical Oncology* 16:2224-30

Stark M, Hayward N. 2007. Genome-wide loss of heterozygosity and copy number analysis in melanoma using high-density single-nucleotide polymorphism arrays. *Cancer Res* 67:2632-42

Storm FK, Sparks FC, Morton DL. 1979. Treatment for melanoma of the lower extremity with intralesional injection of bacille Calmette Guerin and hyperthermic perfusion. *Surgery, Gynecology & Obstetrics* 149:17-21

Strouse JJ, Fears TR, Tucker MA, Wayne AS. 2005. Pediatric melanoma: risk factor and survival analysis of the surveillance, epidemiology and end results database. *Journal of Clinical Oncology* 23:4735-41

Sutherland AD, Faragher IG, Frizelle FA. 2009. Intradermal injection of methylene blue for the treatment of refractory pruritus ani. *Colorectal Disease* 11:282-7

Tannous ZS, Mihm MC, Jr., Sober AJ, Duncan LM. 2005a. Congenital melanocytic nevi: clinical and histopathologic features, risk of melanoma, and clinical management. *Journal of the American Academy of Dermatology* 52:197-203

Tannous ZS, Mihm MC, Jr., Sober AJ, Duncan LM. 2005b. Congenital melanocytic nevi: clinical and histopathologic features, risk of melanoma, and clinical management. *J Am Acad Dermatol* 52:197-203

Tarhini AA, Agarwala SS. 2004. Management of brain metastases in patients with melanoma. *Curr Opin Oncol* 16:161-6

Teltzrow T, Osinga J, Schwipper V. 2007. Reliability of sentinel lymph-node extirpation as a diagnostic method for malignant melanoma of the head and neck region. *International Journal of Oral & Maxillofacial Surgery* 36:481-7

Testori A, Rutkowski P, Marsden J, Bastholt L, Chiarion-Sileni V, et al. 2009. Surgery and radiotherapy in the treatment of cutaneous melanoma. *Ann Oncol* 20 Suppl 6:vi22-9

Topar G, Zelger B. 2007. Assessment of value of the sentinel lymph node biopsy in melanoma in children and adolescents and applicability of subcutaneous infusion anesthesia. *Journal of Pediatric Surgery* 42:1716-20

Tyler D, Ross M. 2008. The role that regional therapy plays in the current day management of cancer that is confined to the extremities. Introduction. *International Journal of Hyperthermia* 24:183

van Akkooi AC, Bouwhuis MG, de Wilt JH, Kliffen M, Schmitz PI, Eggermont AM. 2007. Multivariable analysis comparing outcome after sentinel node biopsy or therapeutic lymph node dissection in patients with melanoma. *Br J Surg* 94:1293-9

van Akkooi AC, de Wilt JH, Verhoef C, Schmitz PI, van Geel AN, et al. 2006. Clinical relevance of melanoma micrometastases (<0.1 mm) in sentinel nodes: are these nodes to be considered negative? *Ann Oncol* 17:1578-85

van Akkooi AC, Voit CA, Verhoef C, Eggermont AM. New developments in sentinel node staging in melanoma: controversies and alternatives. *Curr Opin Oncol* 22:169-77

van Akkooi ACJ, Spatz A, Eggermont AMM, Mihm M, Cook MG. 2009. Expert opinion in melanoma: the sentinel node; EORTC Melanoma Group recommendations on practical methodology of the measurement of the microanatomic location of metastases and metastatic tumour burden. *European Journal of Cancer* 45:2736-42

van der Ploeg APT, van Akkooi ACJ, Schmitz PIM, Koljenovic S, Verhoef C, Eggermont AMM. 2010. EORTC Melanoma Group sentinel node protocol identifies high rate of submicrometastases according to Rotterdam Criteria. *European Journal of Cancer* 46:2414-21

van der Ploeg IMC, Valdes Olmos RA, Kroon BBR, Nieweg OE. 2008. Tumor-positive sentinel node biopsy of the groin in clinically node-negative melanoma patients: superficial or superficial and deep lymph node dissection? *Annals of Surgical Oncology* 15:1485-91

van der Ploeg IMC, Valdes Olmos RA, Kroon BBR, Wouters MWJM, van den Brekel MWM, et al. 2009. The yield of SPECT/CT for anatomical lymphatic mapping in patients with melanoma. *Annals of Surgical Oncology* 16:1537-42

Vermeeren L, van der Ploeg IMC, Olmos RAV, Meinhardt W, Klop WMC, et al. 2010. SPECT/CT for preoperative sentinel node localization. *Journal of Surgical Oncology* 101:184-90

Veronesi U, Adamus J, Bandiera DC, Brennhovd IO, Caceres E, et al. 1977. Inefficacy of immediate node dissection in stage 1 melanoma of the limbs. *New England Journal of Medicine* 297:627-30

Veronesi U, Cascinelli N, Adamus J, Balch C, Bandiera D, et al. 1988. Thin stage I primary cutaneous malignant melanoma. Comparison of excision with margins of 1 or 3 cm. *N Engl J Med* 318:1159-62

Wagner JD, Corbett L, Park HM, Davidson D, Coleman JJ, et al. 2000. Sentinel lymph node biopsy for melanoma: experience with 234 consecutive procedures. *Plastic & Reconstructive Surgery* 105:1956-66

Wells KE, Rapaport DP, Cruse CW, Payne W, Albertini J, et al. 1997. Sentinel lymph node biopsy in melanoma of the head and neck. *Plast Reconstr Surg* 100:591-4

Wilke LG, McCall LM, Posther KE, Whitworth PW, Reintgen DS, et al. 2006. Surgical complications associated with sentinel lymph node biopsy: results from a prospective international cooperative group trial. *Annals of Surgical Oncology* 13:491-500

Wong SL, Brady MS, Busam KJ, Coit DG. 2006a. Results of sentinel lymph node biopsy in patients with thin melanoma. *Annals of Surgical Oncology* 13:302-9

Wong SL, Brady MS, Busam KJ, Coit DG. 2006b. Results of sentinel lymph node biopsy in patients with thin melanoma. *Ann Surg Oncol* 13:302-9

Wood TF, DiFronzo LA, Rose DM, Haigh PI, Stern SL, et al. 2001. Does complete resection of melanoma metastatic to solid intra-abdominal organs improve survival? *Annals of Surgical Oncology* 8:658-62

Wrightson WR, Wong SL, Edwards MJ, Chao C, Reintgen DS, et al. 2003. Complications associated with sentinel lymph node biopsy for melanoma. *Annals of Surgical Oncology* 10:676-80

Young SE, Martinez SR, Essner R. 2006. The role of surgery in treatment of stage IV melanoma. *Journal of Surgical Oncology* 94:344-51

5

Immunotargeting of Melanoma

Jacek Mackiewicz[1] and Andrzej Mackiewicz[1,2]
*[1]Department of Cancer Immunology, Chair of Medical Biotechnology, Poznan University
of Medical Sciences and Greater Poland Cancer Center, Poznan,
[2]BioContract Sp. z o.o. Poznan,
Poland*

1. Introduction

The main task of the immune system is to defend the body against pathogens. The ability of the immune system to recognize and eliminate cancer cells is the basis for cancer immunotherapy. There is ample evidence of how important role plays the immune system to fight cancer: (i) spontaneous remission in patients with certain cancers; (ii) the presence of specific cytotoxic T lymphocytes in the environment of the tumor or regional lymph nodes, (iii) the presence of monocytes, lymphocytes and plasma cells infiltrating the tumor, (iv) increased incidence of some malignancies in immunosuppressed patients, (v) documented remissions of the disease after use of immunomodulators. Better understanding of the molecular and cellular mechanisms that control the immune system has enabled the development of many innovative and promising therapeutic strategies that modulate the immune response. It seems that in the next 5 to 10 years past surgery, radiotherapy and chemotherapy, immunotherapy will find a permanent position in the treatment of cancer modalities.

2. Anti-tumour immune response

Cancerogenesis is closely associated with non-lethal damage of genetic material. Such genetic damage (mutations) can stem from environmental factors, e.g. chemical, radioactive or viral, or can be hereditary. Neoplastic transformation occurs due to accumulation of mutations, predominantly in two gene classes: protooncogenes and suppressor genes. Mutated protooncogenes, termed oncogenes, promote autonomous cell proliferation. Proteins produced by the oncogenes transmit signals to cell nucleus and induce cell division. In contrast, mutated suppressor genes become inactivated and their protein products, deprived of their suppression properties, are not capable of controlling incorrect proliferation. Mutations in apoptosis-regulation genes via the synthesis of improper proteins develop mechanisms preventing programmed cell death.

Burnet's and Thomas' immune surveillance theory assumes that newly formed neoplastic cells are continually monitored by the human immune system which recognises and eliminates them. At some point, however, tumour cells escape immune surveillance, what may result in fully-fledged tumours. During the last twenty years, a number of mechanisms which enable tumour cells to evade effector immune mechanisms have been identified. They include:

- reduced expression/absence of expression of major histocompatibility complex antigens class I and II – (MHC I and II) (Resifo *et al.*, 1993; Garrido *et al.*, 1993; Ward *et al.*, 1990)
- loss of tumour antigens (Knurth *et al.*, 1989; Uyttenhove *et al.*, 1983; Ward *et al.*, 1989)
- improper intracellular antigen processing to prepare antigens for presentation (defects in proteosome function or adenosine-tri-phosphatate (ATP) dependent proteins transporting TAP peptides (Selinger *et al.*, 1998)
- reduction/loss of costimulatory signals of e.g. B7 molecules on the surface of tumour cells
- suppressed expression of adhesion molecules
- inhibited expression of the Fas receptor and/or Fas ligand resulting in the apoptosis of cytotoxic T lymphocytes (CTL) and/or natural killer (NK) cells (Strand *et al.*, 1996; Hahne *et al.*, 1996; Walker *et al.*, 1997)
- synthesis and secretion of immunosuppressive factors, e.g. interleukin (IL)10, TGF-beta, prostaglandine E_2 suppressing immune response (Boon *et al.*, 1995; Schmidt-Wolf *et al.*, 1995)
- expression of TRIAL (TNF-related apoptosis inducing ligand) on the tumour cell surface leading to T lymphocyte apoptosis (Baker *et al.*, 1998)
- prolonged stimulation of specific T cells resulting in clonal exhaustion or AICD (activation-induced cell death) (Overwijk *et al.*, 2001)

The term "cancer immunosurveillance" is no longer sufficient to precisely describe the difficult interactions that arise among a developing tumor and the immune system of the host. It was believed that cancer immunosurveillance was protecting the host by the adaptive immune system in the early phase of cell transformation. Dunn and coworkers described that not only the adaptive but also innate immune system plays a role in the process and serve not only to defend the host from tumor development but also to sculpt, or edit, the immunogenicity of tumors that may finally form. The authors use a wider term - "cancer immunoediting" to more suitably stress the double roles of immunity in not only preventing but also shaping neoplastic disease. According to this theory cancer immunoediting comprises of three phases: elimination, equilibrium and escape.

Elimination phase is based on the original concept of cancer immunosurveillance. If during this phase the developing tumor can be successfully eliminated the immunoediting process is completed without progression to the subsequent phases.

If the neoplasm circumvents the immune surveillance system, it may enter the next sub-clinical stage, termed the *equilibrium phase,* in which tumour tries to establish itself and withstand the growing pressure exerted by the immune system. Although lymphocytes and the secreted IFN-gamma attack the tumour cell, its genetic instability and multiple mutations protect it against destruction. The equilibrium phase is a long-term process and may last for years. The next stage is the *escape phase* which can stem from the exhaustion or suppression of the immune system, reduced expression of type I MHC on neoplastic cells or decreased sensitivity to interferon (IFN) gamma. The equilibrium phase does not occur in non-immunogenic tumours and the modified cell automatically enters the escape phase. This clinical stage is associated with fast growth and progression of the tumour (Dunn *et al.*, 2002 & 2006).

In tumours induced by viruses and chemical substances it has been found that tumour-related antigens are immunogenic and trigger specific cellular and humoral responses. Cytotoxic cells, including CD8+ CTL, NK cells and CD4+ T helper cells, are presumed to play a decisive role in the process. Cellular immune response also involves neutrophil granulocytes (Cavallo *et al.*, 1992) and macrophages. Humoral response is executed by antibodies which are directed against tumour antigens produced by activated B lymphocytes – plasmocytes. The process leading to the lysis of tumour cells in this mechanism may comprise activation of the complement system or induction of ADCC (Antibody Dependent Cell-mediated Cytotoxicity).

The role of different subpopulations of helper T lymphocytes (Th cells) has not been fully explored yet (Nishimura *et al.*, 1999). Cytokines secreted by helper T cells activate humoral or cellular anti-tumour immune response. Depending on the profile of secreted cytokines, Th cells are divided into two sub-groups: Th1 producing IL-2, IFN-gamma and IL-12 inducing cellular immune response; and Th2 secreting IL-4, IL-5, IL-6 and IL-10 which stimulate the humoral response and suppresses the cellular response (Swain *et al.*, 1995). Moreover, the subpopulation of regulatory T cells CD4+/CD25+[hihg]Foxp3 may inhibit immune response by paracrinous secretion of immunosuppressive cytokines IL-10 and TGF-beta. Th17 lymphocytes belong to the most recently described CD4+Th . A characteristic feature of these cells is the secretion of interleukin-17 but also IL-22, IL-26, IL-6, TNF-alfa. So far, no unequivocal influence of Th17 lymphocytes for the development of cancer has been described. It was shown that IL-17 may promote tumor cell growth by inducing tumor vascularization or enhancing inflammation. Meanwhile, a lot of data suggests the antitumor activity of Th17 cells. It therefore appears that Th17 cells may have different effects on tumor growth depending on its immunogenicity, clinical stage (different role in the early and late stages), as well as the origin of cancer and the influence of inflammation and angiogenesis in tumor microenvironment (Hus et al., 2010).

Effective anti-tumour response elicited by the immune system consists of two phases, induction and effector. The induction phase is marked by stimulation of specific anti-tumour response, while the effector phase involves a selective elimination of tumour cells. The following mechanisms are sequentially activated in the induction phase:

1. Presentation of tumour antigens in the context of HLA (Human Leukocyte Antigens) class I to CD8+ lymphocytes, or HLA class II to CD4+ lymphocytes;
2. Providing the costimulatory signal for T lymphocytes, e.g. binding of B7.1 molecules (CD80, CD86) with the CD28 receptor on the surface of T lymphocytes (Janeway *et al.*, 1994)
3. Providing the proliferation signal for immune cells in the area of tumour antigen presentation (typically cytokines or growth factors) (Pardoll *et al.*, 1995)

Induction of immune response is initiated by antigen presentation by dendritic cells (DCs) (Banchereau *et al.*, 1998). DCs phagocyte antigens from necrotic or apoptotic tumour cells and then migrate into regional lymph nodes, where they undergo maturation. In the lymph nodes, they present the antigen on their surface to T lymphocytes CD8+ (in the context of HLA I) and to T lymphocytes CD4+ (in the context of HLA II). This is where CD8+ and CD4+ CTLs are formed together with antibodies directed against specific tumour antigens.

The stimulation of humoral response requires a presentation of tumour antigen by a B lymphocyte to the specific CD4+T lymphocyte. Direct lymphocyte interaction, as well as production of cytokines by CD4+, triggers transformation of the B lymphocyte into a plasma cell and secretion of antibodies.

The effector phase of anti-tumour response may include the following cell destruction mechanisms by:

1. Specific activated CD8+ and CD4+ CTLs
2. Activated NK cells
3. Tumour-infiltrating granulocytes and macrophages
4. Specific antibodies determining activation of the complement system or ADCC
5. Inhibition of tumour neoangiogenesis by cytokines, such as IFN-gamma secreted by activated T lymphocytes (CD8+ and CD4+) into the tumour microenvironment.

Absence of one or several components listed above makes it possible for tumour cells to escape immune surveillance, which leads to tumour progression. Mechanisms involved in the induction and effector phases of anti-tumour response which have been identified so far makes it possible to apply immunotherapy to restore the capacity to recognise and eliminate tumour cells in immune defence mechanisms (Nanda *et al.,* 1995).

3. Tumour immunotherapy

Tumour immunotherapy is a treatment strategy based on intentional interference with the human immune system in order to enhance or modify the body's defence mechanisms against the developing tumour. Immune therapy can be divided into two major categories: passive and active. Within each category the therapy might be either specific or non-specific.

3.1 Passive non-specific immunotherapy

Passive non-specific immunotherapy involves transfer of factors or activated effector cells to elicit a non-specific activation of the immune system provoking anti-tumour response. Immunotherapeutic approaches may use e.g. cytokines or LAK (Lymphokine Activated Killers) cells.

Cytokines are low molecular weight proteins which play a vital role in all phases of immune response, both humoral and cellular. In order to display biological activity, cytokine must target a specific receptor on imune cells (T and B lymphocytes, NK cells, monocytes/macrophages and granulocytes). Various cytokines may demonstrate an antagonistic, agonistic, additive or synergistic effects in biological processes. Known anti-tumour effects of cytokines include (i) direct cytotoxic effect (TNF-sensitivity of cancer cells to cytotoxic effects of various biological or chemical factors (IFN-gamma, TNF-alpha), (ii) inhibition of tumour cells proliferation (IFN-alpha, IFN-gamma) and (iii) activation of NK cells (Granulocyte-Macrophate Colony-Stimulating Factor – GM-CSF, IL-2, IL-6).

The first recombinant cytokine registered for clinical application was IFN-alpha which has been used in the treatment of hairy-cell leukaemia, chronic myeloid leukaemia, melanoma, Kaposi's sarcoma, metastatic renal cell cancer and malignant lymphoma.

Several randomised phase III trials evaluating IFN-alfa-2a and IFN-2b in low, medium and high dose have been conducted. Only in two of them statistically significant improvement of OS (*overall survival*) was observed. High dose IFN-alfa-2b (Intron®) has been approved by the U.S. FDA (*Food and Drug Administration*) based on the results of ECOG 1684 trial. Intron is indicated in patients after resection of high-risk melanoma (stage IIB and stage III). In the registration trial 287 patients after surgical removal of melanoma were randomised into two study arms: INF-alfa-2b vs observation. At a median follow-up of 6.9 years, a statistically significant improvement in survival was demonstrated for the patients treated with IFN-alfa-2b. However at 12,6 years of follow-up, OS was not significantly different between the two study groups, even though there was a significant benefit for relapse free survival (RFS). About 80% of patients developed grade 3 and 4 toxicity (Kirkwood *et al.,* 1996). In another phase III study (ECOG 1694) efficacy of high-dose IFN-alfa-2b was compared with an experimental vaccine GM2-KLH21. After 2 years of median follow-up the median RFS and OS were significantly longer in patients treated with IFN-alfa-2b (Kirkwood *et al.*, 2000). Concerns raising the vaccine control group used in ECOG 1694 lead to initiation of another randomized phase III trial (EORTC 18961). The study which enrolled 1314 patients with stage II melanoma evaluated efficacy of GM2-KLH21 compared with observation. The trial was closed early by the data monitoring committee because of longer survival in the observation arm (Eggermont *et al.*, 2008a). Recently (March 2011) pegylated-IFN-alfa-2b (Sylatron®) has been approved for the treatment of patients with melanoma with microscopic or gross nodal involvement after definitive surgical resection including complete lymphadenectomy. The approval was based on the results of EORTC 18991 trial published in Lancet in the year 2008. The study enrolled 1256 patients with resected stage III melanoma to either observation or pegylated-IFN-alfa-2b. The estimated median RFS was 34.8 months (95% confidence interval (CI): 26.1, 47.4) and 25.5 months (95% CI: 19.6, 30.8) in the Sylatron and observation arms, respectively [hazard ratio (HR) 0.82 (95% CI: 0.71, 0.96); unstratified log-rank p = 0.011]. Unfortuntly, there was no difference in OS between the Sylatron and the observation arms [HR 0.98 (95% CI: 0.82, 1.16)]. The grade 3 and 4 adverse events were less frequent in patients treated with pegylated-IFN-alfa-2b than observed in subjects receiving IFN-alfa-2b in earlier trials (Eggermont *et al.*, 2008b).

Another cytokine registered in the USA for palliative treatment of renal cancer and melanoma is IL-2, however, it has recently been demonstrated that high doses of IL-2 stimulate Treg lymphocytes, what in fact suppresses immune response (Ahmadzadeh *et al.*, 2006).

IL-2 was approved by FDA in 1998 for the treatment of patients with metastatic melanoma. Overall objective response rates in patients treated with high dose IL-2 was 17% (Rosenberg *et al.*, 1994a). In a highly selected patient population with metastatic melanoma (270 patients) complete response (CR) was observed in 6% with median duration of response over 59 months. Partial response (PR) was seen in 10% of IL-2 treated patients. Disease did not progress in any patient responding for more than 30 months. Grade 3 and 4 toxicity was very frequent (Atkins *et al.*, 1993 & 1994). In another trial 684 patients with metastatic melanoma received high-dose IL-2 either alone or in combination with a variety of melanoma vaccines. The overall objective response rates were highest in patients treated with gp100:209-217(210M) peptide vaccine (22%) compared to IL-2 (13%) alone (P=0.01) (Smith *et al.*, 2008). Number of clinical trials evaluating the efficacy of biochemotherapy (combination of chemotherapy and biological agents) have been conducted. In a small phase III trial the investigators compared sequential CVD (dacarbazine, cisplatin, vinblastine) chemotherapy with IL-2 and interferon alfa with CVD alone. Patients treated with biochemotherapy responsed more frequently (48%) to the treatment than receiving chemotherapy alone (25%). The median OS was 11,9 months vs. 9,2 months for biochemotherapy and CVD alone respectively (Eton *et al.*, 2002). In another similar phase III randomized trial (E3695) the observation seen in the previous study was not confirmed – no improvement in OS between both study arms (CVD + IL-2 + IFN-alfa-2b vs CVD) (Atkins *et al.*, 2008). A recent meta-analysis of 18 trials involving 2621 patients with metastatic melanoma showed that biochemotherapy improves overall response rate without benefit of survival (Ives *et al.*, 2007).

At the American Society of Clinical Oncology (ASCO) 2010 annual meeting Lawson *et al.* presented results of a phase III trial (E4697) evaluating efficacy of GM-SCF in the adjuvant treatment in patients with resected high risk melanoma (stage III and IV). Patients were injected with 250 µg of GM-CSF or placebo s.c. daily for 14 consecutive days in a 4 week intervals. The treatment duration was 1 year. Median disease free survival (DFS) of patients treated with GM-CSF was significantly longer than of patients receiving placebo – 11,8 vs. 8,8 months (p=0,034). Median OS was 72,1 vs. 59,8 months respectively in the study arm evaluating GM-CSF and placebo, but the difference was not statistically significant (P=0,551). Toxicity was consistent with known effects of GM-CSF (Lawson *et al.*, 2010).

Another type of passive non-specific immunotherapy is the transfer of LAK cells. In this method, mononuclear cells are isolated from the blood of a patient, stimulated with IL-2 *ex vivo* and injected back with a simultaneous administration of high doses of IL-2 for continuous lymphocyte stimulation. LAK-based therapy was used by Rosenberg in a clinical trial of renal cancer and melanoma. It was found, however, that the therapeutic effect was rather achieved by IL-2, but not LAK cells, which is why further trials were discontinued (Rosenberg *et al.*, 1985 & 1993).

3.2 Passive specific immunotherapy

Passive specific immunotherapy is a treatment method based on the administration of factors or effector cells targeting specific tumour cells. Examples include application of antibodies directed against antigens present on tumour cells or cell therapies using tumour-infiltrating lymphocytes (TIL) which are isolated, cultured, activated and then transferred back into the patient. High expectations are currently held for the recently developed therapy based on modification of autologous lymphocytes isolated from PBLs (Peripheral Blood Lymphocytes) (Morgan *et al.*, 2006).

Passive immunotherapy employing antibodies was first described as far back as 100 years ago. However, it was not until the development of a viable technique of generating monoclonal antibodies (mAb) (Kohler *et al.*, 1975) that the method found more extensive applications in tumour therapy. The dynamic development of genetic engineering techniques has enabled generation of humanised and human mAb (technology using transgenic mice – Xenomouse®) (Green, 1999) deprived to the maximum extent possible of toxic effects associated with the induction of HAMA (Human Anti Murine Antibody) reaction.

Modified specific mAb used in immunotherapy act by binding directly to the tumour antigen, activate ADCC and CDC (Complement Dependent Cytotoxicity). Monoclonal antibodies can also block receptors on tumour cells, e.g. growth factor receptors. Antibodies conjugated with radioisotopes, cytostatics, enzymes, cytokines or toxins immediately destroy cells which they target.

The first mAb registered by the FDA in 1997 was Rituximab (MabThera®) used in the treatment of patients with low malignancy B-cell non-Hodgkin lymphomas. To date there are several mAb (trastuzumab, cetuximab, panitumumab, bevacizumab, ibritumomab, tiuxetan, tositumomab, gemtuzumab, ozogamicin, alemtuzumab) approved for the treatment of various malignancies. Ipilimumab, anti-CTLA4 (Cytotoxic T-lymphocyte-associated antigen 4) mAb has been recently registered for the treatment of metastatic melanoma (described in section: active non-specific immunotherapy).

Angiogenesis is of profound importance in melanoma development (Streit *et al.*, 2003). Malignant melanocytes excrete vascular endothelial growth factor (VEGF) and fibroblast growth factor (FGF) (Kurzen *et al.*, 2003, Lacal et *al.*, 2000, Lev *et al.*, 2003 & 2004). The VEGF is the fundamental regulator of new vessels formation in the tumour and its expression is related to poorer prognosis in melanoma patients (Ugurel *et al.*, 2001). Bewacizumab is a mAb directed against VEGF. Its effectiveness has been proven in the treatment of colon and kidney cancer (Saltz *et al.*, 2008, Melichar *et al.*, 2008). In the treatment of advanced melanoma its efficacy was evaluated in combination with low dose interferon-alfa-2b in a phase II trial which did not show extension of survival in studied patients (Varker *et al.*, 2007). In another phase II trial enrolling 62 metastatic melanoma patients, the effectiveness of bewacizumab in combination with temozolomide was tested. Objective clinical responses were observed in 26% of patients, while 30% of the patients developed SD (*stabilization disease*) lasting for 1.5-7.5 months (median of 3 months) (Von Mos R *et al.*, 2007). In a subsequent phase II trial with 214 randomized patients, the therapy with bevacizumab in combination with carboplatin and paklitaxel (first line treatment) improved effectiveness as the median OS was significantly longer (12.3 months) than in the control group (8.6 months) treated with chemotherapy alone. The toxicity of treatment was similar in both study arms (the number of grade 3-5 adverse events was 2% greater in the group treated with bevacizumab) (O'Day *et al.*, 2009). At the ASCO 2009 annual meeting, preliminary results were presented on the effectiveness of treatment with bevacizumab in combination with nab-paklitaxel in 41 patients with non-resectable III and IV stage melanoma (50% in M1c stage). Nab-paklitaxel is composed of paklitaxel and albumin. This combination alleviates the adverse events caused by administration of paklitaxel alone. The percent of 6 and 12-months survival was 91 and 83%, while the median OS was not reached (Boasberg *et al.*, 2009). The preliminary results of a phase II trial evaluating the efficacy of bevacizumab in combination with everolimus in first line treatment of advanced melanoma were presented at ASCO 2009 conference. Fifty six patients were qualified to the study, but the preliminary analysis included 31 subjects. PR was observed in 1 patient, SD in 19 patients and the median PFS was 3.5 months. The most frequent adverse event was mucositis. Grade 3 toxicity was observed in 13% of patients, other grade 3 adverse events were noted in less than 10% of subjects (Peyton *et al.*, 2009).

α_v integrin family such as α_vb3 and α_vb5 are related to the promotion of angiogenesis in the tumor and contribute to its growth. Human mAb CNTO 95 (intetumumab) directed against integrin has been found to show anticancer and antiangiogenic activity in animal models (Trikha *et al.*, 2004). At the ASCO 2009 annual meeting results of the phase II trial with 129 metastatic melanoma patients enrolled, were reported. The patients were randomised into four study arms: (i) intetumumab 5 mg/kg; (ii) intetumumab 10 mg/kg; (iii) intetumumab 10 mg/kg + DTIC; (iv) *placebo* + DTIC. Median OS of patients respectively in the above-mentioned groups was 9.8; 14; 10.9 and 7.6 months. The treatment was well tolerated and the percent of patients with serious adverse events was the highest in the arm treated with dacarbazine (DTIC) plus *placebo* (Loquai *et al.*, 2009). Volociximab is a chimeric monoclonal antibody that combines with $\alpha 5\beta 1$ integrin, inhibiting angiogenesis in tumors by damaging the bonds between endothelial cells and fibronectin in the intracellular cytoplasm. Effectiveness of volociksimab was evaluated in a phase II trial which enrolled 19 patients diagnosed with advanced melanoma after progression during the first line treatment. Objective clinical responses were observed only in 5% of the patients. Responses to the treatment were associated with the expression of integrin $\alpha 5\beta 1$ in patients tumor samples.The treatment was relatively well tolerated. Grade 1 and 2 toxicity (nausea, vomiting, diarrhoea) occurred in 68% of patients (Linette *et al.*, 2008).

Overexpression of glycoprotein NMB (GPNMB) was observed in many malignancies including melanoma. CRO11-vcMMAE is a human mAb targeting extracellular domain of

GPNMB, combined with the tubulin destabilising factor – monomethyl auristatin E (MMAE). The whole complex is stable in the blood, while MMAE is released within the tumour (Tse *et al.*, 2006). CRO11-vcMMAE was evaluated in phase I/II clinical trials. At ASCO 2009 the phase II study results were reported (MTD 1.88 mg/kg); this trial enrolled 36 patients with metastatic melanoma treated earlier with systemic therapy. 4 PR and 19 SD were observed, while the median PFS was 4 months. The most often noted grade 3 and 4 included neutropenia (22% patients) and rash (19%). Rash grade 2 and higher correlated with longer PFS (Hwu *et al.*, 2009).

Another therapeutic strategy of specific immunotherapy is the use of TIL cells which are extracted from patients tumors and incubated *ex vivo* in the presence of IL-2. Next they are transferred back into corresponding patients with a simultaneous administration of IL-2. In 1994, *et al.* observed objective clinical responses in 34% of patients with metastatic melanoma (Rosenberg *et al.*, 1994b). However, therapeutic benefit was assigned to i.v. injected IL-2 which stimulated lymphocytes.

To increase the efficacy of adoptive cell therapy, prior to TIL infusion, chemotherapy and/or total body irradiation (in order to obtain limfodepletion – elimination of suppressor T-cells) followed by administration of IL-2 was applied. Although effectiveness of this strategy was limited in the treatment of leukemia (Curti *et al.*, 1998; Schultze *et al.*, 2001) some activity in the therapy of melanoma was observed (Oble *et al.*, 2009). Patients with metastatic melanoma prior to TIL and IL-2 infusion received a limphodepleting dose of cyclophosphamide and fludarabine (Dudley *et al.*, 2005). In 51% (n=35) of treated patients objective response rate was observed. A very high overall response rate (70%) was seen in another trial where in melanoma patients prior to TIL transfusion a total body irradiation with a dose of 1200 cGy (in 3 fractionated doses) was obtained (Rosenberg *et al.*, 2008). Clinical trials, which tested peripheral blood lymphocytes stimulated with cytokines did not produce the desired result due to low numbers of antigen-specific lymphocytes. In order to increase the number of antigen-specific lymphocytes an *in vitro* stimulation with DC loaded with particular antigen can be obtained. In a phase I study patients with metastatic melanoma were treated with CD8+ T cell isolated from peripheral blood and incubated *ex vivo* with mature autologous DC pulsed with melanoma antigen Melan-A. Objective responses were seen in 3 out of all 11 patients. (Mackensen *et al.*, 2006). It has been proven that administration of CD4+ T-cells instead of CD8+ lymphocytes may turn out to be more effective in adoptive cell therapy (Perez-Diez *et al.*, 2002). Remission was observed in a patient with metastatic melanoma who received autologous CD4 + T cells specific for the melanoma antigen NY-ESO-1 (Hunder *et al.*, 2008).

Morgan *et al.* isolated PBLs which were then modified *ex vivo* with genes coding for TCR specific for a number of tumour-associated antigens (MART-1, gp100, NY-ESO-1 or p53). They demonstrated that modified PBLs recognise, in the context of HLA-A2, the above-mentioned tumour antigens present on melanoma, lung and breast cancer cells. The interaction of TCR and tumour peptides was associated with the production of a large quantity of IFN-gamma. In the clinical trial, Morgan *et al.* enrolled 31 patients with advanced melanoma resistant to IL-2 therapy. All subjects received autologous PBLs engineered with the anti-MART-1 TCR gene. Two patients showed a prolonged remission lasting more than 20 months. Patients who achieved a clinical response also exhibited high levels of modified circulating lymphocytes after 1 year from the injection of transduced PBLs. No toxicity was found to be associated with this type of therapy (Morgan *et al.*, 2006).

3.3 Active non-specific immunotherapy

Active non-specific immunotherapy is a therapeutic method based on stimulation of the immune system, cell-mediated immune response in particular, with antigens that are not present in tumour cells. Historically, the therapy has involved microorganisms, microbial fragments, enzymes and hormones. In recent years, due to the development of advanced genetic engineering technology and growing understanding of immune mechanisms involved in tumour growth, immune response-modulating mAbs were constructed.

Substances which contribute to the stimulation of immune processes include non-specific immunostimulators and immunomodulators. Immunostimulators include (i) intact microorganisms (living BCG – *Bacillus Calmette-Guérin*, killed *Corynebacterium parvum*), (ii) cell wall elements (BCG, *Nocardia*), (iii) microbial glycoproteins derived from *Klebsiella*, (iv) synthetic components, e.g. endotoxins (lipopolysaccharides). Immunomodulators include (i) thymus extracts (TPI, THF, TFX), (ii) synthetic thymus hormones (thymosin alpha-1, thymopoietin), (iii) tuftsin, (iv) enkephalins and endorphins (v) lymphocyte extracts (transfer factor, immunogenic RNA) (Hersh *et al.*, 1991).

Some of the substances listed above, when injected directly into the tumour, have triggered local inflammatory reaction associated with the infiltration of APCs, neutrophils, and T and B lymphocytes. Regression of injected tumours was often accomplished, however, the method was not capable of producing a specific systemic anti-tumour responses.

No active non-specific immunotherapy modality has entered routine clinical practice as yet.

Passive non-specific immunotherapy includes also monoclonal antibodies modulating the immune system. CTLA-4 is an immune checkpoint molecule that is up-regulated on activated T-cells, which suppresses further activation of specific CD4+ and CD8+ T-cells by interaction with DC or directly as a result of a contact between suppressor and effector T lymphocytes. The anti-CTLA4 monoclonal antibody by blocking the interaction of CTLA-4 with CD80/86 switches off the mechanism of immune suppression and enables continous, unrestrained stimulation of T-cells by DC (J. Mackiewicz & Kwinta, 2010). Two IgG monoclonal antibodies directed against CTLA-4 – ipilimumab and tremelimumab have been tested in number of clinical trials in patients with melanoma. In 2011 (March) ipilimumab (Yervoy®) has been approved by FDA for the treatment of metastatic melanoma patients that failed previous systemic therapy. The approval was based on the results of a randomized phase III trial which included 676 HLA-A*0201–positive patients with unresectable stage III or IV melanoma. Patients enrolled were treated previously with IL-2 or chemotherapy and were randomly assigned for administration of ipilimumab plus glycoprotein (gp)100 vaccine (403 patients), ipilimumab alone (137), or gp100 alone (136). Ipilimumab, at a dose of 3 mg per kilogram of body weight, was administered with or without gp100 every 3 weeks for up to four treatments. Patients receiving ipilimumab plus a peptide vaccine had a median survival of 10 months, compared with 6.4 months of patients receiving the gp100 alone (P<0.001). Subjects treated with ipilimumab alone had a nearly identical median survival — 10.1 months — in the 3-group clinical trial ($P < 0.003$). Immune related adverse events (grade 3 and 4) occurred in 10-15% of patients treated with ipilimumab and in 3% treated with gp100 alone (Hodi *et al.*, 2010)

Another monoclonal antibody targeting CTLA-4 is tremelimumab (administered in the dose of 15 mg/kg every 3 months), which effectiveness has been evaluated in a phase II trial in previously treated patients. From among 256 patients with metastatic melanoma enrolled into the study, objective clinical responses were observed in 8.3% patients, while the median OS was 10.2 months (Kirkwood *et al.*, 2008). The above results inclined the next phase III trial in which 643 patients were treated with tremelimumab in monotherapy or in combination with DTIC/TMZ in the first line setting. Analysis of preliminary results did not show the advantage of tremelimumab over the standard therapy (OS 11.8 *vs* 10.7) and the trial was terminated (Ribas *et al.*, 2008). The effectiveness of treatment with tremelimumab in combination with high doses interferon-alfa-2b was evaluated in phase II trial in which from among 16 patients with inoperable stage III and IV melanoma, clinical response was observed in 19%. The most frequent grade 3 and 4 adverse events included: neutropenia (3 patients, 19%), elevated level of the liver enzymes (2, 13%), fatigue (6, 38%), anxiety (2, 13%) (Tarhini *et al.*, 2008).

Another human mAb modulating the immune system is MDX-1106 (Medarex) directed against PD-1 (a molecule close to that of CTLA-4), which undergoes expression on activated T lymphocytes. Results of the phase I trial have shown regression of the tumours in patients with advanced melanoma and low toxicity of the treatment (Brahmer *et al.*, 2008).

The monoclonal antibody BMS-663513 targeting co-stimulating molecule CD137 (4-1BB) acts according to a different mechanism. Binding of the ligand or anti-CD137 antibody with 4-1BB receptor on the surface of T lymphocytes provides a co-stimulating signal enhancing the cell's activation and triggering its proliferation. The phase I trial enrolling 54 patients with solid tumors has shown acceptable toxicity level and a certain clinical activity of BMS-663513 (Sznol *et al.*, 2008). We look forward to the results of large randomised phase II study which has just been completed (US National Institutes of Health [NIH], 2008a). CP-870.893 is a human agonistic mAb against co-stimulating molecule CD40 that is up-regulated on the surface of the APC. Phase I trial has shown PR in 4 (27%) out of 15 patients with advanced melanoma and 1 CR lasting 18 months after single administration of the drug (Vonderheide *et al.*, 2006). Currently, the trial evaluating the efficacy of CP-870,893 in combination with carboplatin and paclitaxel has been completed and the results probably will be disclosed soon (US National Institutes of Health [NIH], 2008b).

3.4 Active specific immunotherapy

Active specific immunotherapy is a method of treatment which stimulates immune response to antigens specific for a given tumour type.

Active specific immunotherapy includes therapeutic cancer vaccines which encompass cell and non-cell based products. Cell based vaccines comprise: cancer cell lysates, whole cancer cells with adjuvants, gene modified whole cancer cells, DCs pulsed with DNA, RNA, peptides, proteins or cell lysates, pulsed DCs modified with immune stimulators, fused cancer cells with DCs cells or B-lymphocytes. Non-cell based vaccines include DNA vaccines (naked, plasmid), peptide vaccines, protein vaccines, viral-vector vaccines, anti-idiotypic antibody vaccines, particle based vaccines (Table 1) (J. Mackiewicz & A. Mackiewicz, 2009).

3.4.1 Therapeutic cancer vaccines

As early as in 1883, a New York surgeon William Colley was the first to make an attempt at administering a cancer vaccine. Colley injected bacterial toxins into sarcoma patients and observed disease remission.

First-generation cancer vaccines were created from irradiated autologous or allogeneic tumour cells. Cell lysates or natural cell-surface tumour antigens (such as gangliosides GD-2 and GM-2) were also used. In first-generation vaccines, injected cells or antigens were phagocytosed and degraded by mononuclear cells which are then presented to T and B lymphocytes in the context of MHC molecules class I and II. Second generation vaccines include gene-modified tumour vaccines (GMTV) which use (autologous, allogeneic or mixed) tumour cells modified with genes encoding tumour antigens, immunostimulating factors, e.g. cytokines. Their functions include supply and presentation of tumour antigens together with providing co-stimulatory signal for the stimulation of specific anti-tumour mechanisms.

Vaccine type	Vaccine	Reference
Peptide	Glycoprotein 100 (gp100)/tyrosinase complex with Incomplete Freund Adjuvant (IFA) and granulocyte macrophage colony-stimulating factor (GM-SCF)	Weber et al., 2003
	Melanoma specific peptide (MART-1) + Incomplete Freund Adjuvant (IFA)	Wang et al., 2003
	Melanoma specific peptide MAGE-A3	Goldman & DeFrancesco 2009
Heat Shock Protein (HSP)	Autologous, tumor-derived heat-shock protein peptide complex glicoprotein96 + granulocyte macrophage colony-stimulating factor (GM-CSF)+ineterferon-alfa	Pilla et al., 2006
DNA	DNA coding epitopes of melanoma antigens: MELAN-A/MART-1	Weber et al., 2008
	DNA coding co-stimulating molecule – B7	Fynan et al., 1993
Viral vector	Vaccinia virus expressing three costimulatory molecules, B7.1, ICAM-1, and LFA-3 (rV-TRICOM)	Kaufman et al., 2006
Anti-idiotipic antibody	BEC2 anti-idiotypic monoclonal antibody vaccine that mimics GD3 ganglioside	Chapman et al., 2004

Table 1. Selected clinical non-cellular based vaccine studies in patients with melanoma

The strategy of immunisation with genetically unmodified autologous DCs is based on *ex vivo* preincubation of DCs with tumour antigens, followed by administration to patients. This type of immunotherapy activates an antigen-specific cell-mediated response.

3.4.1.1 Non-modified cell vaccines

Vaccines based on whole tumour cells and stimulating factors (adjuvants) were one of the first and fundamental specific tumour immunotherapy strategies. Berd *et al.* (1990) evaluated the effects of immunisation of forty late-stage melanoma patients with a vaccine consisting of irradiated autologous melanoma cells mixed with BCG. Objective clinical response was observed in 5 patients, whereas median survival time was 10 months. The next stage was the use of established cell lines (allogeneic vaccines) which present antigens specific for a given tumour type. Their immunogenicity was enhanced by response to alloantigens present on vaccine cells. Allogeneic vaccines have superseded autologous vaccines due to the difficulties in obtaining the sufficient number of cells for repeated vaccinations. A vaccine consisting of three established allogeneic melanoma lines (Cancervax®) and BCG as an adjuvant was developed by Morton *et al.* (1992). The ensuing phase II trial involved 157 advanced melanoma patients. Objective clinical response was observed in 15-20% of trial subjects (Chan *et al.*, 1998). On the other hand, the outcome of randomised phase III clinical trials of patients treated with Cancervax failed to confirm prolonged survival of patients in comparison with the control group which received only BCG (Morton *et al.*, 2007).

Melacine is a melanoma tumor cell lysate vaccine consisting of two allogeneic melanoma cell lines (MSM-M-1 and MSM-M-2) combined with Detox® adjuvant (Vaishampayan *et al.*, 2002). After encouraging early phase studies the vaccine failed the phase III trial. Though, retrospective analysis showed that patients receiving Melacine and expressing at least two of five HLA antigens present on the vaccine cells developed longer RFS and OS (p =.0.0002 and p = 0.0001, respectively). For that reason, the HLA pattern of the patient served here as a biomarker and allowed stratification of patients who would respond to the treatment. The Melacine may serve as an example of personalized therapeutic vaccine (J. Mackiewicz & A. Mackiewicz, 2010).

Wallach et al in a multicenter randomized phase III trial assessed the efficacy of VMO – Vaccinia Melanoma Oncolysate. This preparation is a melanoma cell lysate (four cell lines) derived by infection of these lines by the vaccinia virus. The study enrolled 217 patients after resection of metastases to the lymph nodes. Test results showed no significant differences in RFS and OS (Wallack *et al.*, 1998).

3.4.1.2 Intracellular gene transfer

Systems of intracellular gene transfer can be broadly divided into non-viral (physical) and viral. The former category includes (i) electroporation (mechanical introduction of DNA in the electric field), (ii) "gene gun" (injection of DNA-coated gold beads into cells by means of pressurised helium). Non-viral chemical strategies are based on modifications of cell membrane permeability for macromolecules under the influence of cationic compounds or enabling penetration of liposome-encapsulated genes marked by high affinity to cell membranes. The most common gene transfer systems used in genetic therapy of human cancer nowadays are based on viral vectors: retroviral, adenoviral, adeno-associated viruses (AAV)) and lentiviral.

Recombinant retroviruses are predominantly based on Moloney murine leukaemia virus (MoMLV). They are used to transduce cells both in vitro and in vivo. Retroviruses transfer genetic material to dividing cells, with viral DNA becoming permanently incorporated into the host's genome, thus producing constant expression of the therapeutic gene in target cells and their descendants. Retroviruses are vectors of choice for constructing cellular cancer vaccines. When administered *in vivo* to humans, murine-enveloped retroviruses are quickly eliminated via complement activation. Consequently, human vectors or human-enveloped vectors were constructed.

Adenoviral vectors are used to modify tumour cells *in vivo*. A typical feature of adenoviral vectors is highly efficient transduction of target cells. On the other hand, as there is no interaction of genetic material with the host's genome, gene expression is trasient. In the case of serial administration of adenoviral vectors, they are eliminated from the human body due to the presence of specific adenoviral antibodies in the human serum. The main feature distinguishing adenoviral carriers from retroviral vectors is the ability to deliver genes into non-dividing cells. Adeno-associated vectors (AAV) have a low capacity and an ability of episomal (extrachromosomal) replication of genetic material and simultaneous integration of inserted genetic material with the host cell's DNA. Initially, AAV vectors contained "contaminants" in the form of immunogenic adenoviral particles necessary for AAV packaging, however new techniques have recently been developed to purify AAV vectors.

Lentiviral vectors are based on the human immunodeficiency virus type 1 (HIV-1). They have a capacity of permanent integration of genetic material with dividing and non-dividing cell genomes and are thus an efficient tools used to transduce early CD34+ stem cells (approximately 40%).

3.4.1.3 Genetically modified cell vaccines

Rapid development of genetic engineering and gene transfer systems, combined with increasing knowledge of tumour immunology, have triggered a dynamic development of

Immunostimulating factor	Dominant type of anti-tumour effect
IL-2	Direct anti-tumour effect Stimulation and proliferation of CD8+ lymphocytes and NK cells
IFN-gamma	Direct anti-tumour effect Stimulation of macrophages, induction of immune response, stimulation of expression of MHC and B7 cells Induction of chemokines which suppress neo-angiogenesis: IP-10, MIG
IL-12	Secreted by DCs, powerfully stimulates CD4+, CD8+ and NK cells. Secondary secretion of IFN-gamma and polarisation towards Th1-type response
IL-18	Secondary secretion of IFN-gamma and polarisation towards Th1-type response Suppressed secretion of IL-10 by stimulated T lymphocytes Stimulation of cytotoxic activity of NK cells by the Fas ligand
GM-CSF	Differentiation and maturation of DCs Stimulation of expression of MHC proteins, tumour antigens and co-stimulatory cells in antigen-presenting cells
IL-4	Tumour infiltration by macrophages and eosinophils Differentiation and maturation of DCs Stimulation of CD4+ cells
TNF	Direct anti-tumour effect (cytotoxic effect) Stimulation of specific and non-specific cell-mediated and humoral response
IL-7	Stimulation of CD4+ and CD8+ cells
IL-6+sIL6R	Stimulation of CD4+, CD8+ and NK cells, DCs maturation, presentation of cryptic antigens by DCs, inhibition of Treg formation, induction of GM-CSF secretion by lymphocytes
B7	Co-stimulatory signal for T cells
HLA-B7	As an allogeneic HLA molecule – stimulation of local production of interferons and cytokines in the tumour microenvironment

Table 2. Factors stimulating anti-tumour immune response used in genetic cancer therapy

gene-modified tumour cell vaccines (GMTV). GMTV vaccines are based on whole tumour cells that can be modified with genes encoding (i) immunostimulatory cytokines (such as IL-2, IL-4, IL-6, IL-7, IL-12, IFN-gamma, TNF) (Table 2), (ii) costimulatory molecules (CD80, CD86), (iii) adhesion molecules, (iv) histocompatibility (MHC) antigens. The aim of genetic modification of cancer cells is to augment their immunogenicity, e.g. via phenotype modifications (increased expression of MHC I and II) or activation of effector mechanisms of the immune system via the delivery of costimulatory signals (J. Mackiewicz & A. Mackiewicz, 2010). GMTV have been tested in many early phase clinical trials in the adjuvant and therapeutic settings (Table 3).

Type of modified cells	Vector	Gene	Trial phase	Number of patients	Clinical response (stable disease) [mixed disease]	Author and publication
Autologous	Liposomes	HLA-B7	I	5	1	Nabel GJ *et al.*, 1993
Autologous	Retrovirus	IL-7	I	10	0 (4) [2]	Moller *et al.*, 1998
Autologous	Gene gun	IL-12	I	6	0 (3)	Sun Y *et al.*, 1998
Autologous	Retrovirus	GM-CSF	I	29	0	Soiffer *et al.*, 1998
Autologous	Retrovirus	GM-CSF	I	35		Soiffer *et al.*, 2003
Autologous	Retrovirus	IL-2	II	12	(3)	Palmer *et al.*, 1999
Allogeneic	?	IL-2	I	12	[3]	Arienti *et al.*, 1996
Allogeneic	?	IL-4	I	12	[2]	Arienti *et al.*, 1999
Allogeneic	?	IL-2	I/II	33	2 (7)	Osanto *et al.*, 2000

Table 3. Results of gene therapy in metastatic melanoma – phase I/II trials

Mackiewicz et al. at the European Society of Medical Oncology (ESMO) meeting 2010 presented results of two phase II clinical trials conducted in almost 200 patients after resection of stage III and IV melanoma. In both studies patients were vaccinated with AGI-101 composed of two irradiated melanoma cell lines modified to express Hyper-IL-6 – a fusion protein composed of interleukin 6 (IL-6) and soluble IL-6 receptor . AGI-101 (5 x 10^7 cells per dose) was administered 8 times at 2-week intervals (induction phase) and then monthly (maintenance phase). At disease progression the induction phase (+/- surgery) was restarted, followed by a second maintenance phase. At progression 43 (Trial 3) and 39 (Trial 5) patients were re-induced +/- surgery followed by a second maintenance phase; of those 11 and 16 patients respectively are alive following re-induction. The 5-year survival in Trial 3 was 66,7%, 43,8% and 26,1% respectively in stage IIIB, IIIC and IV. In Trial 5 the 5-year survival was as follows 56,3%, 39,8% and 41,2% correspondingly in stage IIIA/B, IIIC and IV. The OS observed in trial 3 was 4,4 years and 3,1 year in trial 5 (A. Mackiewicz *et al.*, 2010). The vaccine was well tolerated as no vaccine related toxicity of CTC>2 was detected. Intensive research of melanoma vaccines is currently curried out in a number of countries worldwide. However, no vaccine, has been approved by regulatory authorities so far.

3.4.1.4 Vaccines based on dendritic cells

Extensive research of DCs has shown that they are the most efficient APCs (Banchereau *et al.*, 1998; Hart *et al.*, 1997). DCs play a vital role in inducing immune response. They are the only representatives of APCs that are capable of inducing primary response of virgin T lymphocytes. The use of DCs for antigen presentation offers an opportunity to trigger immune response even to weakly immunogenic tumour antigens and break immune tolerance.

Human DCs are generated by isolation of immature DCs from blood (Fong *et al.*, 2000) and differentiation *ex vivo* in the presence of IL-4 and GM-CSF, myeloid progenitor cells (CD34 +) or monocytes (CD14 +) (Sallusto *et al.*, 1994). Obtained immature DCs can be pulsed with tumor cell lysates (Nair SK et al. 1997) or synthetic peptides (Gitlitz *et al.*, 2003), modified with genes encoding tumor antigens or tumor cells RNA (Ashley *et al.*, 1997). For immunization are also used hybrids of DCs with tumor cells (Avigan *et al.*, 2004).

In a small trial, a group of 11 patients with advanced-stage melanoma were immunised with autologous DCs previously incubated with the MAGE-3 peptide presented by HLA-A1. Regression of cancerous lesions in the skin, lungs and the liver was achieved in 6 cases (Thurner *et al.*, 1999). In one of the few randomized phase III studies, Schadendorf *et al* injected metastatic melanoma patients with autologous DC pulsed with peptides presented in the context of HLA class I and II. However, preliminary analysis has not demonstrated superiority of vaccine over dacarbazine (control arm) and the study was terminated (Schadendorf *et al.*, 2006). Nevertheless, only 53 patients in the vaccine group and 55 in the control arm were participating in the trial and the vaccine was administered depending on the amount of DC cells, usually only from two to several times. Though, subsequent analysis showed that immunized patients with HLA-A2 +/HLA-B44 haplotyp lived longer than those treated with dacarbazine (Engel-Noerregaard *et al.*, 2009).

Peptide-pulsed DCs have certain limitations as well, including (i) short period of antigen presentation, dependent on the half-life of the MHC-peptide complex, (ii) the fact that using a given peptide is only limited to patients with an appropriate MHC haplotype (Amoscato *et al.*, 1998). It is believed that the strategy of modified DCs can be both more efficient and more universal. DCs can also be loaded with genes encoding tumour antigens, immunostimulatory factors or cytokines. Furthermore, DCs derived from different patients can be modified with the same genetic sequence (no need to match appropriate MHC haplotypes), while expression of a given introduced sequence is long-term.

Metharom *et al.* immunised mice with dendritic cells transduced with the mTRP-2 gene (tumour antigen of B16 murine melanoma cells). Tumour regression was observed in 4 out of 7 mice (Metharom *et al.*, 2001).

In a phase I/II trial, melanoma patients were immunised with autologous DCs transduced with tumour-derived mRNA, which enables lymphocytes to present – beside shared melanoma antigens – a wide range of tumour antigens that are unique for a given patient, as well as previously unknown antigens. The trial showed that the vaccine is completely safe. Response of T lymphocytes against tumour antigens encoded by tumour-derived mRNA in vivo was observed in the majority of cases (Kyte et al., 2006).

Melanoma DC vaccines tested to date, despite encouraging results noted in phase I and II trials, have not proven effective in phase III randomised trials.

4. Cancer immunotherapy clinical trial design

Results of many promising early-phase clinical studies evaluating the effectiveness of immunotherapy have not been confirmed in phase III trials. It is becoming clear that these failures could be related to the design of clinical trials (Finke *et al.*, 2007). At present, clinical trials design of new therapeutic strategies including immunotherapy are based on criteria developed for cytotoxic drugs. However immunotheraputics, especially of active immunotherapy have very different clinical characteristics, mechanism of action and toxicity prifile than chemotherapeutic agents. Accordingly, new clinical immunotherapy trial design paradigm was developed (Hoos, *et al.*, 2007). Here we outline some aspects which should be considered while designing clinical trials for the assessment of the effectiveness of immunotherapy.

Patients qualified to earlier clinical trials evaluating the efficacy of immunotheraputics were in late stage of the disease often treated previously with chemo- or radiotherapy. However, the highest clinical benefit was observed in patients with minimal residual disease and such patient population should be considered as candidates for immunotherapy trials (mainly cancer vaccine trials).

Clinical trial end points evaluating chemotherapeutic agents drugs may not be adequate for immunotherapy trials. The Response Evaluation Criteria in Solid Tumors (RECIST) in the assessment of objective clinical response to chemotherapy may not reflect the benefit from immunotherapy. The time points between tumor assessments in trials evaluating immunotherapeutics should be longer (in contrast to chemotherapy trials) giving time for the immune system to mount response to the treatment. In a recent phase II metastatic melanoma study, patients treated with AGI-101H (genetically modified melanoma vaccine secreting Hyper-IL-6) developed clinical response usually after 3-4 months of treatment. However, in many patients tumor shrinkage was observed after several months or even years following SD (Nawrocki & A. Mackiewicz, 2007, Nawrocki *et al.*, 2000). Nevertheless, in many studies assessed tumors tend to enlarge first due to infiltration of inflammatory cells and then shrink. Furthermore immunotherapy may fall to induce tumor decrease, but yet still be effective in slowing the rate of progression giving the patient benefit in OS. The cancer Vaccine Clinical Trial Working Group (CVCTWG) propose that patients after initial clinically not significant progression should not be excluded from the treatment and following tumor regression their response rate could be scored based on the largest tumor volume measured after the start of treatment, not necessarily from baseline tumor volume (Hoos *et al.*, 2007). Based on the observations from phase II clinical trial evaluating earlier described ipilimumab in metastatic melanoma patients' new guidelines for evaluation of immune-related response criteria (irRC) have been developed. In some patients treated with ipilimumab responses after initial increase in total tumor burden in the presence of new lesions were observed. Those patterns were associated with favorable survival. According to irRC: (i) new, nonmeasurable lesions do not define progression; (ii) new measurable lesions are not defined as progression but are incorporated into tumor burden; (iii) progression of the disease has to be confirmed by a repeat consecutive assessment no less than 4 weeks from the first documented date (Wolchok, 2009).

OS is a "gold standard" used for efficacy evaluation of new drugs and is a primary end point of choice in phase III clinical studies. OS is a very good end point, but might be affected by subsequent therapies, is time consuming, and requires large samples of patients. In efficacy randomized phase II trials using adoptive component might be required.

DFS and PFS used respectively in adjuvant and metastatic disease setting are acceptable surrogate primary end points which can shorten the time of randomized efficacy trials. However, definitions of DFS and PFS might not be consistent for immunotherapy trials. While as mentioned before patient's immune system needs time to develop clinical activity and even patients after progression of disease still may benefit from treatment. In terms of classical DFS/PFS description patients with relapse or progression of the disease could be excluded from the trial to early. Modifications of these definitions have been proposed:

confirmation of progression after at least second tumor assessments; not taking into account early progression within a defined time-interval (eg, three month from the beginning of the treatment). In patients who developed early progression with subsequent response to study treatment, the time of DFS and PFS should be calculation from the first day of drug administration (Hoos *et al.*, 2007). Moreover, in some malignancies like melanoma where there is no optional effective second line treatment, immunotherapy should be continued.

In patients developing progression, changes in immunotherapy schedule (induction phase) or metastasectomy may need to be performed. In our own melanoma study patients treated with AGI-101H vaccine received induction phase (8 doses in 2 week interval), with subsequent maintenance phase (1 dose monthly). After developing progression induction phase schedule followed by maintenance was performed. We observed that patients undergoing re-induction benefit from the treatment (Nawrocki & A. Mackiewicz, 2007, A. Mackiewicz *et al.*, 2010). Similar observation was seen in the ipilimumab phase III study conducted in metastatic melanoma patients. Ipilimumab was administered four times in 3 week intervals (induction phase). Patients with SD for 3 months duration after week 12 or a confirmed PR or CR were offered reinduction after developing progression. Among 31 patients given reinduction therapy with ipilimumab, a CR, PR or SD was achieved by 21 patients.

A properly designed immunotherapy clinical trial is very important, while these agents in contrast to chemical agents or small molecules like tyrosine kinases inhibitors might cure patients with immunogenic malignancies (eg. melanoma, renal cell carcinoma) even when the disease is disseminated. In a highly selected patient population with metastatic melanoma (270 patients) treated with IL-2, CR was observed in 6% with median duration of response over 59 months. PR was seen in 10% of IL-2 treated patients. Disease did not progress in any patient responding for more than 30 months (Atkins *et al.*, 1993 & 1994). Another example is a study evaluating ipiliumumab in metastatic melanoma patients, where best overall response (CR+PR) rate of only 10.9% was observed. However 60.0% of patients developed an objective response for at least 2 years (26.5 to 44.2 months[ongoing]) (Hodi *et al.*, 2010).

5. Conclusions and further directions of the development

Recent approval of DC based prostate cancer vaccine – Stipuleucel-T or immunostimultory antibody – Yervoy prove the potential of active immunotherapeutic approaches to treat cancer. Recent better understanding of immune tolerance mechanisms and their braking, development of vaccine design and the paradigm of immunotherapy clinical trials design will lead to the boosting of progress in the field of active cancer immunotherapy. Since examples already include melanoma, certainly immune targeting especially specific active immunotherapy approaches such as melanoma therapeutic vaccine will continue to be tested and finally successful. Most likely immunotherapy will need to be combined with other modalities such as for ex. small molecules, but certainly without support of the immune system elimination of cancer may not be possible.

6. References

Ahmadzadeh, M. & Rosenberg, S.A. (2006). Blood. *IL-2 administration increases CD4+ CD25(hi) Foxp3+ regulatory T cells in cancer patients*. Vol. 107, No. 6, (March 2006), pp. 2409-2414.

Amoscato, A.A., Prenovitz, D.A.& Lotze, M.T. (1998). J Immunol *Rapid extracellular degradation of synthetic class I peptides by human dendritic cells.* Vol. 161, No. 8, (October 1998), pp. 149-157.

Arienti, F., Sulé-Suso, J. & Belli, F. et al. (1996). Hum Gene Ther. *Limited antitumor T cell response in melanoma patients vaccinated with interleukin-2 gene-transduced allogeneic melanoma cells.* Vol. 7, No. 16, (October 1996), pp. 1955-1963.

Arienti, F., Belli, F. & Napolitano, F. et al. (1999). Hum Gene Ther. *Vaccination of melanoma patients with interleukin 4 gene-transduced allogeneic melanoma cells.* Vol. 10, No. 18, (1999 December), pp. 2907-2916.

Ashley, D.M., Faiola, B., Nair, S., Hale, L.P., Bigner, D.D. & Gilboa, E. (1997). J Exp Med. *Bone marrow-generated dendritic cells pulsed with tumor extracts or tumor RNA induce antitumor immunity against central nervous system tumors.* Vol. 186, No. 7, (October 199) pp. 1177-1182.

Atkins, M.B, Robertson, M.J. & Gordon, M. (1997). Clin Cancer Res. *Phase I evaluation of intravenous recombinant human interleukin 12 in patients with advanced malignancies.* (March 1997), Vol. 3, No. 3, pp. 409-417.

Atkins, M.B., Lotze, M.T. & Dutcher, J.P. et al. (1999). J Clin Oncol. *High-dose recombinant interleukin 2 therapy for patients with metastatic melanoma: analysis of 270 patients treated with 1985 and 1993.* (July 1999), Vol. 17, No 7, pp. 2105-2116.

Atkins, M.B., Kunkel, L., Sznol, M. & Rosenberg, S.A. (2000.) Cancer J Sci Am. *High-dose recombinant interleukin 2 therapy in patients with metastatic melanoma: long-term survival update.* (February 2000), 6 Suppl. 1, pp. 11-14.

Atkins, M.B., Hsu. J. & Lee, S. et al. (2008). J Clin Oncol. *Phase III trial comparing concurrent biochemotherapy with cisplatin, vinblastin, dacarbazine, interleukin-2, and interferon alfa-2b with cisplatin, vinblastin and dacarbazine alone (E3695): A trial coordinated by* eastern cooperative oncology group. (December 2008), Vol. 26, No. 35, pp. 5748-5754.

Avigan, D., Vasir, B. & Gong, J., et al. (2004). Clin Cancer Res. *Fusion cell vaccination of patients with metastatic breast and renal cancer induces immunological and clinical responses.* (July 2004), Vol. 10, No. 14, pp. 4699-4708.

Baker, A.B., Philips, J.H. & Figer, C.G. et al. (1998). J Immunol. *Killer cell inhibitory receptors for MHC class I molecules regulate lysis of melanoma cells mediated by NK cells, gamma-delta T cells and antigen specific CTL.* (Jun 1998), Vol. 160, No. 11, pp. 5239-5245.

Banchereau, J. & Steinman, R.M. (1998). Nature. *Dendritic cells and the control of immunity.* (March 1998), Vol. 392, No. 6673, pp. 245-252.

Berd, D., Maguire, H.C. Jr & McCue, P., et al. (1990). J Clin Oncol. *Treatment of metastatic melanoma with an autologus tumor-cell vaccine. Clinical and immunologic results in 64 patients.* (November 1990), Vol. 8, No. 11, pp. 1858-67.

Boasberg, P., Cruickshank, S., Hamid, O., O'Day, S., Weber, R. & Spitler, L. (2009). J Clin Oncol. *Nab-paclitaxel (Abraxane) and bevacizumab as first line therapy in patients with unresectable stage III nad IV melanoma;* Suppl. 27. Abstr 9061.

Boon, T., Gajewski, T.F. & Coulie, P.G. (1995). Immunol Today. *From defined human tumor antigens of effective immunization?* (July 1995),Vol. 16, No. 7, pp. 334-345.

Brahmer, J.R., Topalian, S. & Wollner, I. et al. (2008) J. Clin. Oncol. *Safety and activity of MDX-1106 (ONO-4538), an anti-PD-1 monoclonal antibody, in patients with selected refractory or relapsed malignancies.* Suppl. 26, Abstract. 3006.

Bristol Myers Squibb, (January 2008). A Randomized, Multi-Dose, Open-Label, Phase II Study of BMS-663513 as a Second-Line Monotherapy in Subjects With Previously Treated Unresectable Stage III or IV Melanoma. *US National Institutes of Health (NIH).* 24.01.2011, Available from http://clinicaltrial.gov/ct2/show/NCT00612664?term=4-1BB&rank=1

Cavallo, F., Giovarelli, M., Gulino, A., Vacca, A., Stoppacciaro, A., Modesti, A. & Forni, G. (1992). J Immunol . *Role of the neutrofils and CD4+ T lymphocytes in the primary and memory response to nonimmunogenic murine mammary adenocarcinoma made immunogenic by IL-2 gene.* (December 1992), Vol. 149, No. 11, pp.3627-3635.

Chan, A.D. & Morton, D.L. (1998). Semin Oncol. *Active immunotherapy with allogeneic tumor cell vaccines. Present status.* (December 1998), Vol. 25, No. 6, pp. 611-622.

Chapman, P.B., Wu, D., Ragupathi, G., Lu, S., Williams, L., Hwu, W.J., Johnson, D. & Livingston, P.O. (2004) Clin. Cancer. Res. *Sequential immunization of melanoma patients with GD3 ganglioside vaccine and antiidiotypic monoclonal antibody that mimics GD3 ganglioside.* (July 2004), Vol. 10, No. 14, pp. 4717-4723.

Curti, B.D., Ochoa, A.C. & Powers, G.C. et al. (1998) J. Clin. Oncol. *Phase I trial of anti-CD3-stimulated CD4+ T cells, infusional interleukin-2, and cyclophosphamide in patients with advanced cancer.* (August 1998), Vol. 16, No. 8, pp. 2752–2760.

Dudley, M.E., Wunderlich, J.R. & Yang, J.C. et al. (2005). J Clin Oncol. *Adoptive cell transfer therapy following non myeloablative but lymphodepleting chemotherapy for the treatment of patients with refractory metastatic melanoma.* (April 2005), Vol. 23, No. 10, pp.2346-2357.

Dunn, G.P., Bruce, A.T., Ikeda, H. & Old, L.J. Schreiber RD. (2002). *Nat Immunol Cancer immunoediting: from immunosurveillance to tumor escape.* (November 2002), Vol. 3, No. 11, pp. 991-998.

Dunn, G.P., Koebel, C.M. & Schreiber, R.D. (2006). Nat Rev *Immunol Interferons, immunity and cancer immunoediting.* (November 2006), Vol. 6, No. 11, pp. 836-848.

Eggermnont, A.M., Suciu, S. & Ruka, W. et al. EOTRC 18961: (2008a). J Clin Oncol *Post-operative adjuvant ganglioside GM2-KLH21 vaccination treatment vs observation in stage II (T3-T4N0M0) melanoma: 2nd interm analysis led to an early disclosure of the results.;* Suppl. 15, Abstract. 9004.

Eggermont, A.M., Suciu, S. & Santinami, M et al. (2008b). Lancet. *Adjuvant therapy with pegylated interferon alfa-2b versus observation alone in resected stage III melanoma: final results of EORTC 18991, a randomised phase III trial.* (July 2008), Vol. 372, No. 9633, pp. 117-126.

Engel-Noerregaard, L., Hansen, T.H, Andersen, M.H., Straten PT & Svane IM. (2009) Cancer Immunol. Immunother. *Review of clinical studies on dendritic cell-based vaccination of patients with malignant melanoma: assessment of correlation between clinical response and vaccine parameters.* (January 2009), Vol. 58, No. 1, pp. 1-14.

Eton, O., Legha, S.S. & Bedikian, A.Y. et al. (2002). J Clin Oncol. *Sequentional biochemiotheapy versus chemotherapy for metastatic melanoma: results* from a phase III randomized trial. (April 2002), Vol. 20, No. 8, pp. 2045-2052.

Finke, L.H., Wentworth, K., Blumenstein, B., Rudolph, N.S., Levitsky, H. & Hoos, A. et al. (2007). Vaccine. *Lessons from randomized phase III studies with active cancer immunotherapies – Outcomes from the 2006 Meeting of the Cancer Vaccine Consortium (CVC).* (September 2007), Suppl. 25, pp. 97-109.

Fong, L. & Engleman, E.G. (2000). AnnuRev Immunol. *Dendritic cells in cancer immunotherapy.* (April 2000), Vol. 18, pp. 245-273.

Fynan, E.F., Webster, R.G., Fuller, D.H., Haynes, J.R., Santoro, J.C. & Robinson, H.L. Proc. Natl. Acad. Sci. USA *(1993). DNA vaccines: protective immunizations by parenteral, mucosal, and gene-gun inoculations.* (April 1993), Vol. 90, No. 24, pp. 11478-11482.

Garrido, F., Cabrera, T. & Concha, A. et al. (1993). Immunol Today. *Natural history of HLA expression during tumor development.* (October 1993), Vol. 14, No. 10, pp. 491-499.

Gitlitz, B.J., Belldegrun, A.S. & Zisman, A., et al. (2003). J Immunother. *A pilot* trial of tumor *lysate-loaded dendritic cells for the treatment of metastatic renal cell carcinoma.* (October 2003), Vol. 26, No. 5, pp. 412-9.

Goldman, B. & DeFrancesco, L. (2009). Nature Biotech. *The cancer vaccine roller coaster.* (November 2009), Vol. 27, No. 2, pp. 129-140.

Green, L.L. (1999). J Immunol Methods. *Antibody engineering via genetic engineering of the mouse: XenoMouse strains are a vehicle for the facile generation of therapeutic human monoclonal antibodies.* (December 1999), Vol. 231, No 1-2, pp. 11-23.

Hart, D.N. (1997). Blood. *Dendritic cells: unique leukocyte populatons which control the primary immune response.* (November 1997), Vol. 90, No. 9, pp. 3245-87.

Hahne, M., Rimoldi, D. & Schroter, M. et al. (1996). Science. *Melanoma cell expression of Fas ligand: implications for tumor immune escape.* (November 1996), Vol. 274, No. 5291, pp. 1363-1366.

Hodi, F.S., O'Day, S.J. & McDermott, D.F. et al. (2010). N Engl J Med. *Improved survival with ipilimumab in patients with metastatic melanoma.* (August 2010), Vol. 363, No. 8, pp. 711-723.

Hoos, A., Parmiani, G. & Hege, K. (2007) J. Immunother. *A clinical development paradigm for cancer vaccines and related biologics.* (January 2007), Vol. 30, No.1, pp. 1-15.

Hunder, N.W., Wallen, H. & Cao, J. et al. (2008). N Engl J Med. *Treatment of metastatic melanoma with autologous CD4+ T cells against NY-ESO-1.* (Jun 2008), Vol. 358, No. 25, pp. 2698-2703.

Hus, I., Maciąg, E. & Rolinski, J. (2010). Postepy Hig Med Dosw. *The role of Th17 cells in anti-cancer immunity.* (July 2010), Vol. 64, pp. 244-250 e-ISSN 1732-2693.

Hwu, P., Sznol, M. & Pavlick., A. (2009). J Clin Oncol. *A phase I/II study of CR011-vcMMAE, an antibody-drug conjugate (DC) targeting glycoprotein NMB (GPNMB) in patients (pts) with advanced melanoma.* Suppl. 27. Abstr 9032.

Ives, N.J., Stowe, R.L. & Lorigan, R. et al. (2007). J Clin Oncol. *Chemotherapy compared with biochemotherapy form the treatment of metastatic melanoma: a meta-analysis of 18 trials involving 2,621 patients.;* (December 2007), Vol. 25, No. 34, pp. 5426-5434.

Janeway, C.A. Jr. & Bottomly, K.: (1994). Cell. *Signals and signs for lymphocyte responses.* (January 1994), vol. 76, No. 2, pp. 275-285.Kaufman, H.L., Cohen, S., Cheung, K., DeRaffele, G., Mitcham, J., Moroziewicz, D., Schlom, J. & Hesdorffer, C. (2006). Hum. Gene Ther. *Local delivery of vaccinia virus expressing multiple costimulatory molecules for the treatment of established tumors.* (February 2006), Vol. 17, No. 2, pp. 239-244.

Kirkwood, .JM., Strawderman, M.H. & Ernstoff, M.S. et al. (1996). J Clin Oncol. *Interferon alfa-2b adjuvant therapy of high-risk resected cutaneous melanoma: the Estern Cooperative Oncology Group Trial EST 1684.* (January 1996), Vol. 14, No. 1, pp. 7-17.

Kirkwood, J.M., Ibrahim, J.G. & Sondak VK et al. (2000). J Clin Oncol. *High- and low-dose interferon alfa-2b in high-risk melanoma: first analysis of intergroup trial E1690/S911/C9190.* ; (Jun 2000), Vol. 18, No. 12, pp. 2444-2458.

Kirkwod, J.M., Lorigan, P. & Hersey, P. et al. . (2008). J Clin Oncol. *A phase II trial of tremelimumab (CP-675,206) in patients with advanced refractory or relapsed melanoma.* (July 2008), Suppl. 26: Abstr 9023.

Knurth, I., Horsten, U. & Pflanz, S. et al. (1999). J Immunol. *Activation of the signal transducer glycoprotein 130 by both IL-6 and IL-11 requires two distinct binding epitopes.* (January 1999), Vol. 162, No. 3, pp. 1480-1487.

Kohler, G. & Milstein, C. (1975). Nature. *Continuous cultures of fussed cells secreting antibody of predefined specificity.* (August 1975), Vol. 256, No. 5517, pp. 256-475.

Kurzen, H., Schmitt, S., Naher H, Mohler T. Anticancer Drugs. (2003). *Inhibition of angiogenesis by non-toxic doses of temozolomide.* (August 2003), Vol. 14, No. 7, pp. 515-522.

Kyte, J.A., Mu, L. & Aamdal, S. et al. (2006). Cancer Gene Ther. *Phase I/II trial of melanoma therapy with dendritic cells transfected with autologous tumor m-RNA.*(October 2006), Vol. 13, No. 10, pp. 905-18.

Lacal, P.M., Failla, C.M. & Pagani, E. et al. (2000) J. Invest. Dermatol. *Human melanoma cells secrete and respond to placenta growth factor and vascular endothelial growth factor.* (December 2000, Vol. 115, No. 6, pp. 1000-1007.

Lawson, D.H., Lee, .S.J. & Tarhini, A.A. et al. (2010). J Clin Oncol. *E4697: Phase III cooperative group study of yeast-derived granulocyte macrophage colony-stimulating factor (GM-CSF) versus placebo as adjuvant treatment of patients with completely resected stage III-IV melanoma.* Suppl. 15, Abstract 8504.

Lev, D.C., Ruiz, M. & Mills, L. et al. (2003). Mol. Cancer Ther. *Dacarbazine causes transcriptional up-regulation of interleukin 8 and vascular endothelial growth factor in melanoma cells: a possible escape mechanism from chemotherapy.* (August 2003), Vol. 2, No. 8, pp. 753-763.

Lev, D.C., Onn, A. & Melinkova, V.O. et al. (2004) J. Clin. Oncol. *Exposure of melanoma cells to dacarbazine results in enhanced tumor growth and metastasis in vivo.* (Jun 2004), Vol. 22, No. 11, pp. 2092-2100.

Linette, G., Cranmer, L. & Hodi, S. et al. (2008). J Clin Oncol. *A multicenter phase II study of volociximab in patients with relapsed metastatic melanoma.* (July 2008), Suppl. 26. Abstract 3505.

Loquai, C., Pavlick & A. Lawson, D. et al. (2009). J Clin Oncol. *Randomised phase 2 study of the safety and efficacy of a human anyi- α_v integrin monoclonal antibody Intetumumab (CNTO 95) alone and in combination with dacarbazin in patients with stage IV melanoma: 12 month results.* (July 2009), Suppl. 27. Abstract 9029.

Mackensen, A., Meidenbauer, N. & Vogl S et al. (2006). J Clin Oncol. *Phase I study of adoptive T-cell therapy using antigen specific CD8+ T cells for the treatment of patients with metastatic melanoma.* (November 2006), Vol. 24, No. 31, pp. 5060-5069.

Mackiewicz, A., Wysocki, P. & Mackiewicz, J.et al. (2010). Ann of Oncology. *Long term survival of high risk melanoma patients immunized with an allogeneic whole cell genetically modified vaccine (AGI-101) after complete resection.* (October 2010), Vol. 21, Suppl. 8.

Mackiewicz, J. & Mackiewicz, A. (2009) Eur J Pharmacol. *Design of clinical trials for therapeutic cancer vaccines development.* (December 2009), Vol. 625, No. 1-3, pp. 84-89.

Mackiewicz, J. & Mackiewicz, A. (2010). Contemporary Oncology. *Immunotherapy of cancer and perspectives of its development.* (February 2010), Vol. 14, No. 2:59-71.

Mackiewicz, J. & Kwinta, L. (2010). Contemporary Oncology. *New targeted therapies in the treatment of patients with metastatic melanoma.* (January 2010), Vol. 14, No. 1, pp. 15-22.

Mackiewicz, J. & Mackiewicz, A. (2010). Transplant Proc. *Gene-modified cellular vaccines: technologic aspects and clinical problems;* (October 2010), Vol. 42, No. 8, pp. 3287-3292.

Melichar, B., Koralewski, B. & Ravaud, A. et al. (2008). Ann Oncol. *First-line bevacizumab combined with reduced dose interferon-alpha2a is active in patients with metastatic renal cell carcinoma.* (August 2008), Vol. 19, No. 8, pp. 1470-1476.

Metharom, P., Ellem, K.A., Schmidt, C. & wie, M.Q. (2001). Hum Gene Ther. *Lentiviral vetor-mediated tyrosone-related protein 2 gene transfer to dendritic cells for the therapy of melanoma.* (December 2001), Vol. 18, No. 12, pp. 2203-2213.

Möller, P., Sun, Y. & Dorbic, T. et al. (1998). Br J Cancer. *Vaccination with IL-7 gene-modified autologous melanoma cells can enhance the anti-melanoma lytic activity in peripheral blood of patients with a good clinical performance status: a clinical phase I study.* (November 1998), Vol. 77, No. 11, pp. 1907-1916.

Morgan, R.A., Dudley, M.E. & Wunderlich, JR. et al. (2006). Science. *Cancer Regression in Patients After Transfer of Genetically Engineered Lymphocytes.* (October 2006), Vol. 314, No. 5796, pp. 126-129.

Morton, D.L., Foshag, L.J. & Hoon, D.S. et al. (1992). Ann Surg. *Prolongation of survival in metastatic melanoma after active specific immunotherapy with a new polyvalent melanoma vaccine.* (October 1992), Vol. 216, No. 4, pp. 463-482.

Morton, D.L., Mozzillo, N. & Thompson, J.F. et al. (2007). J Clin Oncol. *An international, randomized, phase III trial of bacillus Calmette-Guerin (BCG) plus allogeneic melanoma vaccine (MCV) or placebo after complete resection of melanoma metastatic or regional or distant sites.* Suppl. 25:Abstr 8508.

Nabel, G.J., Nabel, E.G. & Yang, Z.Y. et al. (1993). Proc Natl Acad Sci U S A. *Direct gene transfer with DNA-liposome complexes in melanoma: expression, biologic activity, and lack of toxicity in humans.* (January 1993), Vol. 90, No. 23, pp. 11307-11311.

Nair, S.K., Snyder, D., Rouse, B.T. & Gilboa, E. (1997). Int J Cancer. *Regression of tumors in mice vaccinated with professional antigen-presenting cells pulsed with tumor extracts.* (March 1997), Vol. 70, No. 6, pp. 706-715.

Nanda, N.K. & Sercarz, E.E. (1995). Cell *Induction of anti-self-immunity to cure cancer.* (July 1995), Vol. 82, No. 1, pp. 13-17.

Nawrocki, S. & Mackiewicz A. (2007). Expert. Opin. Investig. Drugs. *Clinical trials of active cancer immunotherapy.* (August 2007), Vol. 16, No. 8, pp. 1137-1141.

Nawrocki, S., Murawa, P. & Malicki, J. et al. (2000). Immunol. Lett. *Genetically modified tumour vaccines (GMTV) in melanoma clinical trials.* (September 2000), Vol. 74, No. 1, pp. 81-86.

Nishimura, T., Iwakabe, K. & Sekimoto, M. et al. (1999). J Exp Med. *Distinct role of antigen-specific T helper type 1 (Th1) and Th2 cells in tumor eradication in vivo.* (September 1999), Vol. 190, No. 5, pp. 617-627.

Oble, D.A., Loewe, R., Yu, P. & Mihm. Jr. M.C. (2009). Cancer Immunol. *Focus on TILs: prognostic significance of tumor infiltrating lymphocytes in human melanoma.* (April 2009), Vol. 9, p. 3.

O'Day, S.J., Kim, G.P. & Sosman, J.A. et al. BEAM: (2009). Ann Oncol. *A randomized phase II study evaluating the activity of bevacizumab In combination with carboplatin plus paklitaxel In patients with previously untreated Advanced Melanoma.* Suppl. 8. Abstract 23LBA.

Osanto, S., Schiphorst, P.P., Weijl, N.I. et al. (2000). *Hum Gene Ther. Vaccination of melanoma patients with an allogeneic, genetically modified* interleukin 2-producing melanoma cell line. (May 2000), Vol. 11, No. 5, pp. 739-50.

Overwijk, W.W. & Restifo, N. (2001).Trends in Immunology. *Creating therapeutic cancer vaccines: notes from the battlefield.* (January 2001), Vol. 22, No. 1, pp. 5-7.

Palmer, K., Moore, J. &Everard, M. et al. (1999). Hum Gene Ther. *Gene therapy with autologous, interleukin 2-secreting tumor cells in patients with malignant melanoma.* (August 1999), Vol. 10, No. 8, pp. 1261-1268.

Pardoll DM. Paracrine cytokine adjuvants in cancer immunotherapy. (1995). Annu Rev Immunol. Vol. 13, pp. 399-415.

Perez-Diez, A., Joncker, N.T., Choi, K., Chan, W.F., Anderson, C.C., Lantz, O. & Matzinger, P. (2007). Blood. *CD4 cells can be more efficient at tumor rejection than CD8 cells.* (Jun 2007), Vol. 109, No. 12, pp. 5346–5354.

Peyton, J.D., Spigel, D.R., Burris, H.A., Lane, C., Rubin, M., Browning, M., Trent, D. & Hainsworth, J.D. (2009). J Clin Oncol. *Phase II trial of bevacizumab and everolimus in the treatment of patients with metastatic melanoma: Preliminary results.* Suppl. 27. Abstract 9027.

Pfizer, (January 2008). A Phase 1 Study Of CP- 870,893 In Combination With Paclitaxel And Carboplatin In Patients With Metastatic Solid Tumors. *US National Institutes of Health (NIH).* 17.11.2009, Available from
http://clinicaltrials.gov/ct2/show/NCT00607048?term=CP-870%2C893&rank=1NIH

Pilla, L., Patuzzo, R. & Rivoltini, L. et al. (2006). Cancer Immunol. Immunother. *A Phase II trial of vaccination with autologous, tumor-derived heat-shock protein peptide complex Gp96, in combination with GM-SCF and interferon-alfa in metastatic melanoma patients.* (August 2006), Vol. 55, No. 8, pp. 958-968.

Restifo, N.P., Kawakami, Y. & Marincola, F.et al. (1993). J Immunother. *Molecular mechanisms used by tumors to escape immune recognition: immunogenetherapy and the cell biology of major histocompatibility complex class I.* (October 1993), Vol. 14, No. 3, pp. 182-190.

Ribas, A., Hauschild, A. & Kefford, R. et al. (2008). J Clin Oncol. *Phase III, open-label, randomized, comparative study of tremelimumab (CP-675,206) and chemotherapy (temozolomide [TMZ] or dacarbazine [DTIC]) in patients with advanced melanoma.* Suppl. 26, Abstr LBA9011.

Rosenberg, S.A., Lotze, M.T. & Muul, L.M. et al. (1985). N Engl J Med. *Observation on the systemic administration of autologous lymphokine-activated-killer cells and recombinant interleukin-2 t patients with metastatic cancer.* (December 1985), Vol. 313, No. 23, pp. 1485-1892.

Rosenberg, S.A., Lotze, M.T. & Yang, J.C. et al. (1993). J Natl Cancer Inst. *Porspective randomized trial of high-dose interleukin 2 alone or in conjugation with lymphokine-activated-killer cells for the treatment of patients with advanced cancer.* (April 1993), Vol. 85, No. 8, pp. 622-632.

Rosenberg, S.A., Yang, J.C. & Topalian, S.L. et al. (1994a). JAMA. *Treatment of 283 consecutive patients with metastatic melanoma or renal cell cancer using high dose bolus interleukin 2.* (March 1994), Vol. 271, No. 12, pp. 907-913.

Rosenberg, S.A. Yannelli, J.R., Yang, J.C. et al. (1994b). J Natl Cancer Inst. *Treatment of patients with metastatic melanoma with autologous tumor-infiltrating lymphocytes and interleukin-2.* (August 1994), Vol. 86,1 No. 15, pp. 1159-1566.

Rosenberg, S.A., Restifo, N.P. & Yang, J.C. et al. (2008). Nat Rev Cancer. *Adoptive cell transfer: a clinical path to effective cancer immunotherapy.* (April 2008), Vol. 8, No. 4, pp. 299-308.

Sallusto, F. & Lanzavecchia, A. (1994). J Exp Med. *Efficient presentation of soluble antigen by cultured human den*dritic cells is maintained by granulocyte/macrophage colony-stimulating factor plus interleukin 4 and downregulated by tumor necrosis factor alpha. (April 1994), Vol. 179, No. 4, pp. 1109-1118.

Saltz, L.B., Clarke, S. & Díaz-Rubio, E. (2008). J Clin Oncol. et al. *Bevacizumab in combination with oxaliplatin-based chemotherapy as first-line therapy in metastatic colorectal cancer: a randomized phase III study.* (April 2008), Vol. 26, No. 12, pp. 2013-2019.

Schadendorf, D., Ugurel, S., Schuler-Thurner, B. et al. (2006). Ann Oncol. *Dacarbazine (DTIC) versus vaccination with autologous peptide-pulsed dendritic cells (DC) in first-line treatment of patients with metastatic melanoma: a randomized phase III trial of the DC study group of the DeCOG.* (April 2006), Vol. 17, No. 4, pp. 563–570.

Schmidt-Wolf, G. & Schmidt-Wolf, I.G.H. (1995). Immunol Today. *Cytokines and gene therapy.* (April 1995), Vol. 16, No. 4, p173-175.

Schultze, J.L., Anderson, K.C., Gilleece, M.H., Gribben, J.G. & Nadler, L.M. (2001). Br. J. Haematol. *A pilot study of combined immunotherapy with autologous adoptive tumour-specific T-cell transfer, vaccination with CD40-activated malignant B cells and interleukin 2.* (May 2001), Vol. 113, No. 2, pp. 455–460.

Selinger, B., Hardes, C., Lohmann, S., Momburg, F., Tampe, R. & Huber, C. (1998). Eur J Immunol. *Down regulation of the MHC class I antigen-processing machinery after oncogenic transformation of murine fibroblasts.* (January 1998), Vol. 28, No. 1, pp. 122-132.

Smith, F.O., Downey, S.G. & Klapper, J.A. et al. (2008). Clin Cancer Res. *Treatment of metastatic melanoma using interleukin-2 alone or in conjunction with vaccines.* (September 2008), Vol. 14, No. 17, pp. 5610-5618.

Soiffer, R., Lynch, T. & Mihm, M. et al. (1998). Proc Natl Acad Sci U S A. *Vaccination with irradiated autologous melanoma cells engineered to secrete human granulocyte-macrophage* colony-stimulating factor generates potent antitumor immunity in patients with metastatic melanoma. (October 1998), Vol. 95, No. 22, pp. 13141-13146.

Soiffer, R., Hodi, F.S. & Haluska, F. et al.(2003). J Clin Oncol. *Vaccination with irradiated, autologous melanoma cells engineered to secrete granulocyte-macrophage colony-stimulating factor by adenoviral-mediated gene transfer augments antitumor immunity in patients with metastatic melanoma.* (May 2003), Vol. 21, No. 17, pp. 3343-3350.

Strand, S., Hofmann, W.J. & Hug, H. et al. (1996). Nature Med. *Lymphocyte apoptosis induced by CD 95 (APO-1/CD95) ligand – expressing tumor cells – a mechanism of immune evasion.* (December 1996), Vol. 2, No. 12, pp. 1361-1366.

Streit, M. & Detmar, M. (2003). Oncogene. *Angiogenesis, lymphangiogenesis, and melanoma metastasis.* (May 2003), Vol. 22, No. 20, pp. 3172-3179.

Sun, Y., Jurgovsky, K., Möller, P., Alijagic, S., Dorbic, T., Georgieva, J., Wittig, B. & Schadendorf, D. (1998). Gene Ther. *Vaccination with IL-12 gene-modified autologous melanoma cells: preclinical results and a first clinical phase I study.* (April 1998), Vol. 5, No. 4, pp. 481-490.

Swain, S.L. (1995). J Leukoc Biol. *CD4 T cell development and cytokine polarization: an overview.* (May 1995), Vol. 57, No. 5, pp. 797-819.

Sznol, M., Hodi, F.S. & Margolin, K. (2008). J Clin Oncol. *Phase I study of BMS-663513, a fully human anti-CD137 agonist monoclonal antibody, in patients (pts) with advanced cancer (CA).* Suppl. 26. Abstract 3007.

Tarhini, A.A., Moschos, S.S., Schlesselman, J.J. et al. (2008). J Clin Oncol. *Phase II trial combination biotherapy of high-dose interferon alfa-2b and tremelimumab for recurrent inoperable stage III or IV melanoma.* Suppl. 26, Abstract 9009.

Thurner, B., Haendle, I. & Roder, C. et al. (1999). J Exp Med. *Vaccination with Mage-3A1 peptide-pulsed mature, monocyte-derived dendritic cells expands specific cytotoxic T cells and induces regression of some metastases in advanced stage IV melanoma.* (December 1999), Vol. 190, No. 11, pp. 1669-1678.

Trikha, M., Zhou, Z., Nemeth, J.A. et al. (2004). Int. J. Cancer. *CNTO 95, a fully human monoclonal antibody that inhibits αv integrins, has antitumor and antiangiogenic activity in vivo.* (Jun 2004), Vol. 110, No. 3, pp. 326-335.

Tse, K.F., Jeffers, M., Pollack, V.A. et al. (2006). Clin. Cancer Res. *CR011, a fully human monoclonal antibody-auristatin E conjugate, for the treatment of melanoma.* (February 2006), Vol. 12, No. 4, pp. 1373-1382.

Ugurel, S., Rappl, G., Tilgen, W. & Reinhold, U. (2001). J Clin Oncol. *Increased serum concentration of angiogenic factors in malignant melanoma patients correlates with tumor progression and survival.* (January 2001), Vol. 19, No.2, pp. 577-583.

Uyyttenhove, C., Maryanski, J. & Boon, T. (1983). J Exp Med. *Escape of mouse mastocytoma P815 after nearly complete rejection is due to antigen-loss variants rather then immunosupression.* (March 1983), Vol. 157, No. 3, pp. 1040-1052.

Vaishampayan, U., Abrams, J. & Darrah, D. et al. (2002). Clin Cancer Res. *Active immunotherapy of metastatic melanoma with allogeneic melanoma lysates and interferon alpha.* (December 2002), Vol. 8, No. 12, pp. 3696–36701.

Varker, K.A., Biber, J.E. & Kefauver, C. et al. (2007). Ann. Surg. Oncol. *A randomized Phase 2 trial of bevacizumab with or without daily low-dose interferon a-2b in metastatic malignant melanoma.* (August 2007), Vol. 14, No. 8, pp. 2367-2376.

Vonderheide, R.H., Flaherty, K. & Khalil, M. et al. (2006). J Clin Oncol. *Clinical activity and immune modulation in cancer patients treated with CP-870,893, a novel CD40 agonist monoclonal antibody.* (March 2006), Vol. 25, No. 7, pp. 876-883.

Von Mos, R., Seifert ,B. & Ochsenbein, A. et al. (2009). Ann Oncol. *Temozolomide combined with bevacizumab in metastatic melanoma. A multicenter phase II trial (SAKK 50/07).* Suppl 20. Abstract 24LBA.

Wallack, M.K., Sivanandham, M. & Balch & C.M. et al. (1998). J Am Coll Surg. *Surgical adjuvant active specific immunotherapy for patients with stage III melanoma: the final analysis of data from phase III, randomized, double-blind, multicenter vaccinia melanoma oncolysate trial.* (July 1998), Vol. 187, No. 1, pp. 69-77.

Walker, P., Saas, P. & Dietrich, P.Y. (1997). J Immunol. *Role of Fas ligand in immune escape.* (May 1997), Vol. 158, No.10: pp. 4521-4524.

Wang, F., Bade, E., Kuniyoshi, C., Spears, L., Jeffery, G., Marty, V., Groshen, S. & Weber, J. (1999). Clin. Cancer Res. *Phase I trial of a MART-1 peptide vaccine with incomplete Freund's adjuvant for resected high-risk melanoma.* (October 1999), Vol. 5, No. 10, pp. 2756-2765.

Ward, P.L., Koeppen, H., Hurteau, T. & Schreiber, H. (1989). J Exp Med. *Tumor antigens defined by cloned immunological probes are hihgly polymorphic and are not detected anautologous normal cells.* (July 1989), Vol. 170, No. 1, pp. 217-32.

Ward, P.L., Koeppen, H., Hurteau, T., Rowley, D.A. & Schreiber, H. (1990). Cancer Res. *Major histocompatibility complex class I and unique antigen expression by murine tumors that escaped from CD8+ T-cell-dependent surveillance.* (July 1990), Vol. 50, No. 13, pp. 3851-8.

Weber, J., Sondak, V.K. & Scotland et al. (2003). Cancer. *Granulocyte-macrophage-colony-stimulating factor added to a multipeptide vaccine for resected Stage II melanoma.* (January 2003), Vol. 97, No. 1, pp. 186-200.

Weber, J., Boswell, W. & Smith, J. et al. (2008). J. Immunother. *Phase 1 trial of intranodal injection of a Melan-A/MART-1 DNA plasmid vaccine in patients with stage IV melanoma.* (February 2008), Vol. 31, No. 2, pp. 215-223.

Wolchok, J.D., Hoos, A. & O'Day, S. (2009). Clin Cancer Res. *Guidelines for evaluation of immune therapy activity in solid tumors: immune-related response criteria.* (December 2009), Vol. 15, No. 23, pp. 7412-7420.

6

Adjuvant Treatment of Melanoma

J. A. Moreno Nogueira[1], M. Valero Arbizu[2] and C. Moreno Rey[3]
[1]*Real Academia de Medicina de Sevilla. Hospital Universitario Virgen del Rocío. Sevilla;*
[2]*Oncologia Médica. Hospital Infanta Luisa. Sevilla;*
[3]*Departamento de Genómica Estructural. Neocodex. Sevilla;*
España

1. Introduction

Melanomas occur in 95% of cases as skin cancer (1.5-7% of all skin cancers) and only 5% in non-skin locations, especially the eye. The incidence has doubled every 10-20 years since the mid 20th century, but the mortality has not increased in the same proportion. Mortality has increased at a slower rate, thus showing that the higher incidence is mainly at the expenses of early lesions leading to early diagnosis and the application of curative surgical treatment. Globocan's data from 2008 shows an incidence of 199.627 cases and a mortality of 46.372 (M: 101.807/25.860 y W: 97.820/20512), when in 2002 the incidente was 160.000 (M:F sex ratio, 0.97) and the mortality 41.000 (M:F sex ratio, 1.2) The majority of melanomas originate in existing nevi, only 30% are new lesions. Radial or spreading growth initially appears (malignant lentingo melanoma, superficial acral lentiginous melanoma) followed by vertical growth that involves lymphatic colonisation. Nodular melanoma only presents vertical growth, without any previous radial growth phase and this is why it has a worse prognosis. The Clark levels of invasion (I, II, III, IV and V) and Breslow's tumour thickness measurements (0.5, 1.0, 1.5, 2.0, 2.5, 3.0, 4.0, 5.0 mm), are based on the growth depth of histopathological studies and enable evaluating the prognosis and estimating the risk after surgery of the primary tumour (Dyson et al.2005). They indicate the risk of metastasis and are the bases and foundations of studies of tumour extension and classification.

One important step is the study of the sentinel lymph node, which enables precise classification of lymph node affectations. This has good prognosis value and influences making later therapeutic decisions such as the use of high dose adjuvant interferon. Furthermore, in cases where these nodes are positive, it indicates the advantages of early lymphadenectomy. Its indication is for stages I-II of the AJCC, which is without evidence of regional or distant lymph node metastases that may include ultrasonography (Saiag et al. 2005). The Breslow degree of millimetric invasion informs about the risk of hidden metastasis at a lymph node and distal level. If this degree of invasion is less than 1 mm, the positivity of the sentinel lymph node is only 0-5% and the cure rates by surgery are 98%. This means that in this group the indication of performing the sentinel lymph node technique is not logical because of its low indicative value. In patients with a degree of invasion between 1 and 4 mm (T2, T3) the positivity ranges from 1 to 14% in T2 and from 11 to 34% in T3. This is why the sentinel lymph node technique would be very important in this group because of its prognostic and therapeutic repercussions.

In patients with a degree of invasion of more than 4 mm (T4), the risk of regional micro-metastasis is very high, between 20-65%, as is that of distant micro-metastasis (>60%). This means that the sentinel lymph node technique would be less informative regarding palliative lymphadenectomy and the indication of treatment with high dose interferon. This procedure would be indicated from the outset, as the patients are high risk. Nevertheless, it would enable to adequate classification and this would be valuable when planning future clinical trials with more homogeneous groups of patients. (Table 1) (Moreno-Nogueira 2008).

1.- Tumour thickness of more than 1 mm.
2.- Clark level higher than III.
3.- Ulceration.
4.- Histological signs of regression.

Table 1. Histological criteria indicating the sentinel lymph node

A histopathological study of the primary lesion and complementary examinations are the basis of the stage classification as a step prior to planning therapy following surgery. The AJCC/UICC classification of 2001 has evident differences compared to that of 1997. It simplifies the Breslow scale to 1, 2 and 4 mm and consider the presence of ulceration. It adequately classifies lymph node affectation and, in the metastatic phase, distinguishes types of metastasis and the prognosis value of high LDH levels. This disease classification finally includes assessment of the sentinel lymph node. All this enables identification of the different stages as well as different risk groups, an important aspect for deciding complementary treatments (Balch et al. 2001).

Patients with stages I and II have no distant lymph node metastases and survival rates of 40% to 95%, as defined by the degree of infiltration and the presence or not of ulceration. This means that sub-stage IIA is only considered of intermediate risk when it is ulcerated (Breslow 1.1-2 mm) or has a thickness of 2.1-4 mm without ulceration. High risk patients include sub-stage IIB (Breslow 2.1-4 mm ulcerated or > 4 mm non-ulcerated) and IIC (Breslow > 4 mm ulcerated). The variability of survival in these stages indicates its heterogeneity, and so other prognostic factors (mitotic rate, serum YKL-40, PTEN and Ki67 expression, etc.) must be included to better discriminate different patient sub-groups (Liu et al. 2006, Schmidt et al. 2006, Mikhain et al. 2005, Gimotty et al. 2005). Stage III patients are also a very heterogeneous group, with high risk and worse prognosis as they always involve lymph node affectation where the number of affected nodes are an indicator of survival, age, location, and the presence of macro or micro metastasis in the lymphatic nodes (67% vs. 43% up to 5 years, p<0.001) etc. also having an influence. (Tables 2 and 3) (Coit et al. 2006, 11. Balch et al. 2010).

In this stage and in the near future, other factors must be considered such as serum a protein S-100B level which is an independent prognostic factor as an initial baseline measurement but also during the follow up, different gene expressions, circulating melanoma cells, etc. They would provide information in addition to standard clinical and histological information, and bring about an improvement in the precision of both, the diagnosis and the prognosis. It will contribute, as already mentioned, to this therapeutic future (Suciu et al. 2007, Mocellin et al. 2006, Fecher et al. 2007, Tarhini et al. 2009).

Factor	Value of "p"
Patient age	<0.0001
Male vs. female	0.12
Primary location	0.002
Ulceration of primary tumour	0.13
Breslow thickness	0.05
No. of positive nodes	<0.0001
Clinical affectation of nodes	0.0003
Micro vs. macro metástasis in the lymphatic nodes	<0.001
Extranodal extension	0.07

Table 2. Prognostic factors in stage III

Low risk melanomas: -Stage I.	
Intermediate risk melanomas: -Stage II A	(Breslow of 1.1- 2 mm Ulcerated) (Breslow of 2.1- 4 mm Non-ulcerated).
High risk melanomas: -Stage IIB.	(Breslow of 2.1- 4 mm Ulcerated) (Breslow >4 mm Non-ulcerated)
-Stage IIC. -Stage III.	(Breslow >4 mm Ulcerated).

Table 3. Melanomas: risk groups

2. Adjuvant treatment

The treatment of choice for localised primary cutaneous melanoma (stages I, II and III) is surgery and if there is regional affectation of the lymph nodes or if the sentinel lymph node is positive, this must be completed with lymphadenectomy. The resection should be deep in accordance to the thickness of the primary lesion. The recommended width of the margins should be 1 cm, for lesions 1 mm thick. In melanomas of 1-4 mm, about 2 cm is recommended and for lesions of more than 4 mm, about 3 cm. Elective regional lymphadenectomy is not recommended unless the study of the sentinel lymph node was positive. Up to 37% of these cases have nodes affected. Therapeutic lymphadenectomy should be performed when lymph nodes metastases have been clinically diagnosed. Surgery should be assessed once again for the metastatic disease, especially for metastases of the skin or those attached to organs, and they would be considering as candidates for adjuvant treatment.

The rationale of adjuvant treatment to surgery is based on the poor prognosis of high-risk melanomas, with a relapse rate of 50-80% and a low five-year survival of 25-70% (Moreno-Nogueira, 2008). Another reason would be that metastatic disease has no efficient treatment capable of significantly prolonging patient survival.

Patients included in the high-risk group should be assessed for adjuvant treatment with high doses of Interferon-α2b, as it is the only treatment shown to significantly improve disease free and possibly global survival.

Different types of adjuvant treatment have been investigated and others are under study and pending results.

2.1 Adjuvant treatment with chemotherapy

In randomised studies, adjuvant chemotherapy has not shown any significant benefits, even at high doses with the support of autologous bone marrow. (Table 4) (Moschos and Kirkwood, 2005).

Authors	No. of cases	Stage	Treatment	Follow-up (years)	Statistical significance
Fisher 1981	181	II-III	CCNU Observation	3 y.	NS
Veronesi 1982	931	II-III	DTIC BCG DTIC+BCG Observation	5 y.	NS
Lejeune 1988	325	I-IIA-IIB	DTIC Levamisole Placebo	4 y.	NS
Meisenberg 1993	39	III	Autologous bone marrow transplant	N.A.	NS

NA: Not announced. NS: Not significant.

Table 4. Melanomas: Adjuvant chemotherapy. Randomised studies

2.2 Adjuvant treatment with biochemotherapy

Various studies, with contradictory results, have been published of combined treatment with chemotherapy and cytokines; nevertheless, this is an interesting line for further investigation. A first study with 138 patients, 71 treated with biochemotherapy (cisplatin + vinblastine + DTIC + IFN + IL2) compared to two treatments with high dose Interferon-α2b, (33 patients.) vs. intermediate doses (33 patients.), did not show any significant differences in the groups regarding GS and RFS (Kin et al. 2006). A second study compared two cycles of DTIC 850 mg/m2 followed by Interferon-α2b 3 mill./3 s.c., during six months, compared to observation in patients with stage IIa, IIb, IIIa and IIIb. There were no significant differences regarding RFS and GS in low risk patients (IIa), but the differences were significant in high risk patients with a RFS at 5 years of 42% vs. 17% (p=0.0018) and a GS at 7 years of 51% vs. 30% (p=0.0077). The benefits were more evident in metastasis free survival and the procedure has an acceptable toxicity (Stadler and Luger, 2005). On the other hand, a wide Phase III study from DeCOG (*Dermatologic Cooperative Oncology Group*) with 441 patients with regional lymphatic clearance after having positive nodes compared: IFN α2a, 3 MU s.c. three times a week (A), (A) plus DTIC 850 mg/m2 every 4-8 weeks for two years (B) and just observation (C). The results showed significant improvement in RFS and OS in group A vs. C, but with no differences between B and C, meaning possibly that DTIC reverts the benefits of adjuvant IFN (Garbe el al. 2008).

There are also some studies of neoadjuvant treatment with biochemotherapy. One in Stage III with 48 patients analysed the association of cisplatin + vinblastine + DTIC + IFL + IL2. At five years the GS was 66% and the RFS was 56%, higher than historic controls (Lewis, 2006).

2.3 Adjuvant treatment with immunostimulants

Seven studies with non-specific immunostimulants did not show any significant benefits (Table 5) (Moschos and Kirkwood. 2005)

Authors	No. of cases	Stage	Treatment.	Follow-up (years).	Statistical significance
Balch 1982	260	III	C. parvum	2 y.	NS
Paterson 1984	199	I-II	BCG	4 y.	NS
Miller 1988	168	II-III	Transfer factor Observation	2 y.	NS
Lipton 1991	262		C. parvum BCG	4 – 9 y.	CS
Quirt 1991	577	I-IIA-IIB-	Levamisole BCG BCG+Levamisole Observation		
Spitler 1991	216	I-IIA-IIB-III-IV	Levamisole Observation	10 y.	NS
Czarnetzki 1993	353	ii	BCG (RIV) BCG (Pasteur) Observation	6 y.	NS

CS: Close to significance. NS: Not significant.

Table 5. Melanomas. Adjuvant treatment with non-specific immune stimulants. Randomised studies

2.4 Adjuvant treatment with vaccines

Various vaccines against melanoma are currently under development, some of them in Phase I, II and III clinical trials, but in general they have not offered any advantages except in one study which only included 38 patients (Table 6) (Moschos and Kirkwood, 2005).

Melacine, a vaccination made from cell lysate was compared to observation by SWOG (*Southwest Oncology Group*) in patients with melanoma of 1.5-4 mm in thickness without lymph node affectation. No benefit was observed but a retrospective analysis showed that the vaccinated patients that had positive HLA-A2 or C3 presented a disease free survival of 77% compared to 64% of patients with the negative marker observed (Sosman et al. 2002). In the ECOG 1694 study, the group that received the vaccination of Ganglioside GM2 activator protein fared worse than the group with high doses of Interferon-α2b after a relatively short

Authors	No. of cases	Stage	Treatment	Follow-up (years.)	Statistical significance
Livingston 1994	123	III	GM2+BCG+CFM BCG+CFM	5 y.	NS
Wallack 1995	250	II	Virus allogeneic polyvalent melanoma cell lysate	2.5 y.	NS
Wallack 1998	250	III	Melanoma cell lysate vaccine	3 y.	NS
Bystryn 2001	38	III	Polyvalent shed antigen Placebo	2.5 y.	S
Sondak 2002	689	IIA	Melacine and DETOX Observation	5.6 y.	NS
Hershey	700	IIB	Cell lysate vaccine Placebo	8 y.	Tendency in RFS/GS

Table 6. Melanomas. Adjuvant treatment with vaccines. Randomised studies

	RFS		DMFS		OS	
	OBS	GM2-KLH/QS-21	OBS	GM2-KLH/QS-21	OBS	GM2-KLH/QS-21
N° events	204	205	143	52	112	124
4-yr %(SE%)	69.4% (1.9%)	68.2%(1.9%)	78.8%(1.7%)	6.1%(1.8%)	83.6%(1.6%)	81.5%(1.6%)
HR (95% CI)*	1.03 (0.84, 1.25)		1.11 (0.88, 1.40)		1.16 (0.90, 1.51)	
P value*	0.81		0.36		0.26	

Abbreviation: HR, hazard ratio. * Cox model, stratified for stratification factors.
OBS: Observation. RFS: Relapse-free survival. DMFS: Distant metastasis-free survival.
OS: Overall survival

Table 7. Final results of study EORTC 18961

median follow-up. However this study did not include a control group without adjuvant treatment, and so it is not possible to determine whether vaccination with ganglioside was equivalent to observation or even prejudicial (Kirkwood et al., 2001). A recently presented randomised trial, where 604 patients in stage III were enrolled between April 1997 and January 2003, studied vaccination of allogeneic melanoma lysates with low doses of Interferon α-2b, compared to high doses of Interferon α-2b. At five years there were no differences in GS (61% vs. 57%) or RFS (50% vs. 48%), between both groups, but these figures were better than those for patients who did not receive any adjuvant treatment. The incidence of important side effects was similar, but the neuropsychiatric toxicity was higher in the second group (Mitchell et al., 2007). The final results of the Phase III Study form EORTC 18961 have been presented in the ASCO 2010 meeting. The study had 1314 patients in stage II (T3-T4N0M0), between March 2002 and December 2005, divided into two groups, the ones with GM2-KLH/QS-21 vaccination after surgery and the ones that were just observed. The study had to be stopped because it did not show good results as supposed and the vaccination could be potentially harmful to patients. (Table 7) (Eggermont et al, 2010).

2.5 Adjuvant treatment with interferon

At present the most common adjuvant treatment in high risk melanomas is Interferon-α2b at high doses according to the Kirkwood scheme (Induction: Interferon-α2b: 20 million/m2, i.v., 5 days a week for four weeks. Maintenance: Interferon-α2b: 10 million/m2, s.c., three times a week for 48 weeks), which should also be assessed after metastasis surgery, without evidence of tumour.

Interferon is a glycoprotein described in 1957 by A. Isaacs and J. Lindemann as a product of virus infected cells that interfered with the replication of live virus in cell cultures. In the eighties, cloning by genetic engineering of a human interferon gene in *Escherichia coli*, enabled the production of large amounts of interferon thus simplifying clinical research into cancer treatments. There are more than 20 varieties, but the three most important are Interferon α, β, and γ, all being used in clinical oncology, especially α.

The genes that code interferon α and β are found in chromosome 9, whereas the gene coding the γ is in chromosome 12. Both α and β are structurally similar, with the same number of amino acids, the homology of the sequence of nucleotides being 45% and 29% for amino acids.

Interferon acts by binding to a specific membrane receptor protein, thus unleashing a cascade of signals whose end result is the expression of a certain number of genes. Interferon α and β share the same receptor, but β has greater affinity. The gene of this receptor has been found in chromosome 21 and for interferon γ in chromosome 6 (Faltynek et al. 1986, Pestka, 1997).

The proteins produced as a result of gene activation and expression, participate in different biological activities such as antiviral and immunomodulating actions, reduction of cell proliferation, suppression of gene expressions, inhibition of angiogenesis, induction of cell differentiation etc.

Oncological pathology essentially uses Interferon α (IFNα-2a and IFNα-2b) as a single agent or in combination with chemotherapy or other cytokines and monoclonal antibodies. Interferon-α2b was the first to be produced using the DNA recombinant technique and approved by the United States FDA. Over the last 15 years numerous studies have been carried out in various neoplasias, including lymphomas, CML, melanomas and kidney cancer.

The antineoplastic activity of interferon has a double mechanism, it inhibits the proliferation and growth of tumour cells, directly affecting all phases of the cell cycle (M, G1 and G2), prolonging the cell cycle and reducing the number of cells that enter phase S and G2. The accumulative effect of prolongation of the cell cycle has cytostatic action and increases apoptosis. In second place it acts indirectly by inducing an increase of the antigen expression of the Class I and II major histocompatibility complex on the surface of tumour cells, exercising an effect on modulation of the immune response to these cells. These antigens play an important role in recognition of neoplastic cells by cytotoxic T-cells together with increasing the effectiveness of all effector immune cells with cytotoxic capacity

(NK cells, macrophages etc.) on these tumour cells. The increased interferon induced expression of TNF-α receptors on the surface of these cells, and increases the cytostatic and cytotoxic action of TNF-α, whose production is also increased. Something similar also occurs with other cytokines (CSF, IL1 etc.) that are involved in immune antitumorigenic cytotoxicity mechanisms (Foss, 2002).

Another effect of interferon is the inhibition of tumour angiogenesis. Systemic treatment with interferon α and β reduces growth endothelial cells, essential for the formation of new vessels, by inhibition of angiogenic factors, thus having an indirect anti-proliferation effect. Interferon α reduces the expression of FGF-2 and the transcription of VEGF. This is further enhanced by another possible mechanism, inhibition of IL-8, which has neo-angiogenic capacity in numerous neoplasias.

Interferon has been widely investigated in melanomas, both as adjuvant to locoregional treatment, as well as in the metastatic phase in the case of a tumour with evident immunogenic activity.

The adjuvant treatment most recognised at present in high-risk melanomas specially in USA is Interferon-α2b at high doses and according to the Kirkwood scheme. This scheme has been used by the *Eastern Cooperative Oncology Group and Intergroup* to perform four randomised studies on 1916 patients whose data was updated in 2004 (Figure 1).

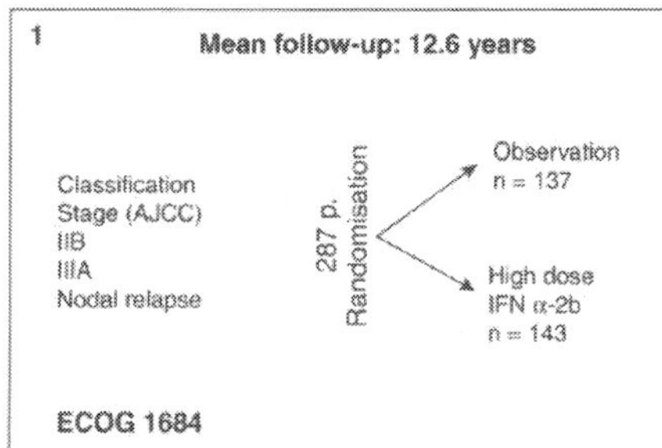

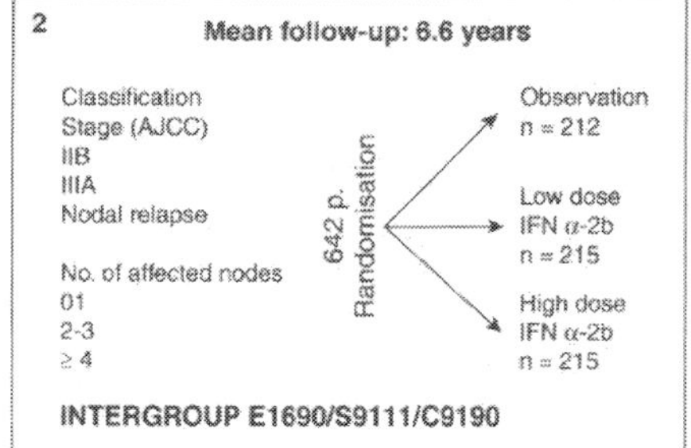

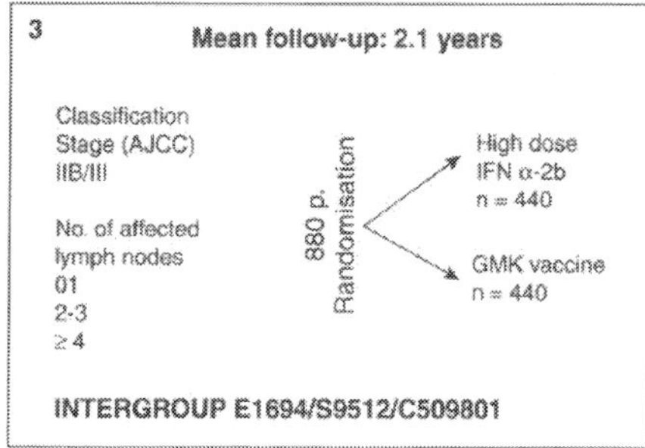

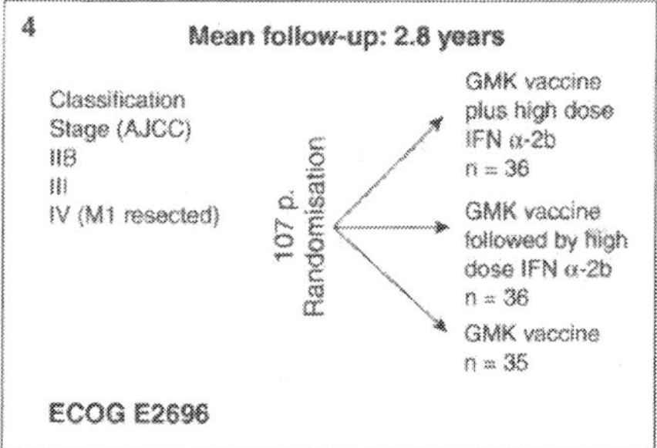

Fig. 1. Eastern Cooperative Oncology Group and Intergroup IFN

The first study, E1684, showed that patients who received adjuvant treatment presented a recurrence free survival (RFS) at five years of 37% compared to 26% (p=0.0023) in the untreated group. The global survival at five years was also significantly better (46% vs. 37%, p=0.0237) and this information enabled approval of IFN-α 2b as adjuvant treatment in high risk melanomas by the United States FDA, as well as the Spanish Ministry of Health.

When this study was updated with a median follow-up of 12.6 years, it maintained the benefits in RFS (HR=1.38, p=0.02). The benefits for GS descended slightly (HR=1.22, p=0.18), but this could be due to deaths by other causes in the elderly population of the study (current mean age of > 60 years).

The second E1690 study also showed benefits in RFS after a follow-up of 6.6 years (HR= 1.24; p2=0.09), but not for GS.

In the combined analysis of these two ECOG studies with 713 patients and a median follow-up of 7.2 years, high doses of Interferon-α2b were better than the observation group in regard to the RFS (HR= 1.30, p < 0.002). However this analysis showed no benefit in global survival (GS) (HR= 1.08, p=0.42). (Figure 2).

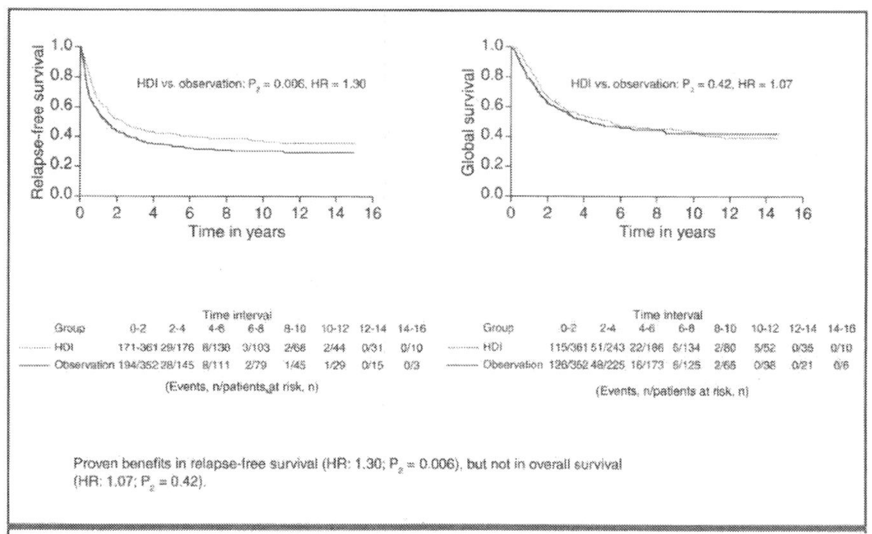

Fig. 2. Joint analysis of the E1683 and E1690 studies recurrence free survival/global survival

Study E1694 showed benefits in RFS and GS compared to GMK vaccine after a median follow-up of 2.1 years. Equally, study E2696 showed that the combination of GMK vaccine and Interferon-α2b at high doses reduced the risk of relapse compared to GMK alone (Figure 3) (Kirkwood et al. 2004).

In view of the above, it is possible to say that in patients with resected high risk melanoma Interferon-α2b at high doses is an adjuvant treatment with clear evidence of increased RFS and moderate, but not significant, improvement of GS. Toxicity should be well assessed and explained to each patient, so that he/she participates in the decision making process. Adequate experience in the use of high dose interferon, with control of its toxicity and recommending good hydration, means that the majority of patients comply with the therapeutic plan and a relatively low number of dropouts. The most outstanding toxicity reactions are asthenia, neuropsychiatric symptoms, myelosuppression, alteration of liver enzymes, etc. The neuropsychiatric effects may appear early or tardive and include signs of depression, anxiety and occasionally suicidal thoughts. (Table 8)

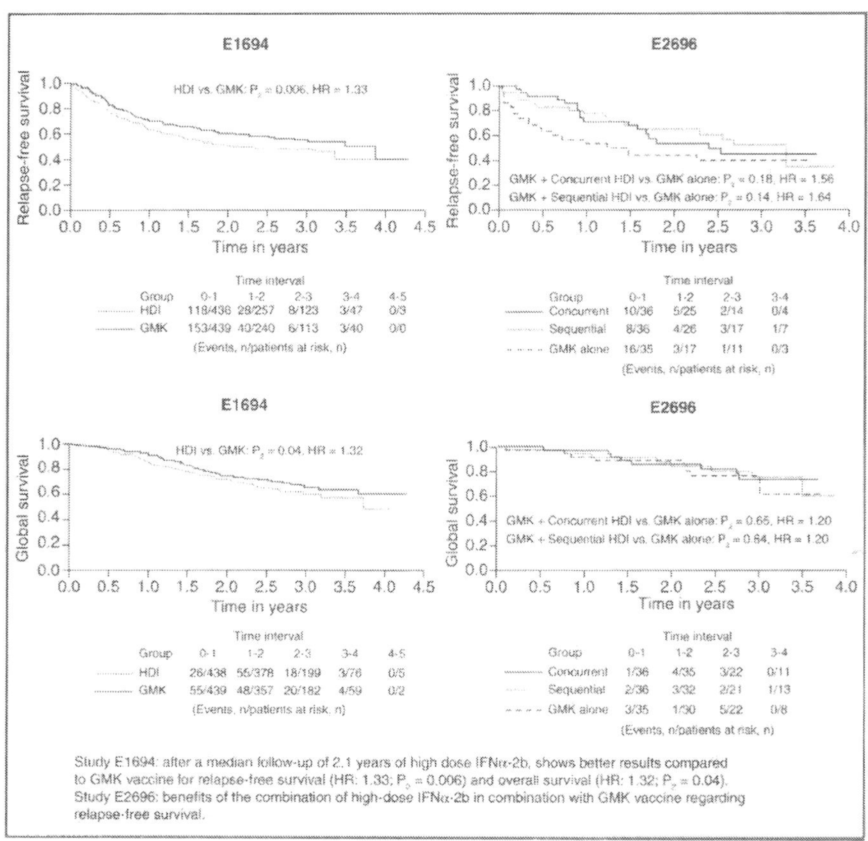

Fig. 3. Studies E1694 and E2696. Recurrence free survival/global survival

In conclusion, there are arguments in favour of the use of high dose Interferon-α2b as this treatment shows improvement of disease free survival in all studies carried out to date, and increased, but not statistically significant, global survival. The toxicity is undoubtedly high, but manageable in services with experience. Furthermore, there is no other therapeutic regimen that has shown benefits in adjuvant treatment of melanoma. However, there are also arguments against high dose Interferon-α2b. In the first place it is not clear which patient population really benefits from adjuvant treatment. The only clear benefit is for disease free survival; no consistent data is available for global survival. In second place the toxicity is considerable and requires a team with experience in its management even though a certain number of patients will abandon or suspend treatment for this reason. Finally the duration and ideal dosage for the treatment is unknown. (Table 9) (Jonasch and Haluska. 2001, Trask et al. 2000).

	Patients (%) *	Patients (%) *
Adverse effects	All degrees	Degree 3-4
Asthenia	96	21-24
Fever	81	18
Myalgia	754	4-17
Nauseas	66	5-9
Vomiting	66	5
Myelosuppression	92	26-60
Elevated AST	63	14-29
Neuropsychiatric symptoms	40	2-10
- Depression. - Anxiety - Suicidal thoughts	0-70%	
* Data taken from the E1684 study of 143 patients. ** Data taken from the E1684, E1690 and E1694 studies.		

Table 8. Most common adverse events (degree III/IV) in patients treated with high dose IFN-α2b

1) ARGUMENTS IN FAVOUR.
• A consistent improvement in disease free survival has been demonstrated • in all studies carried out. • An improvement in global survival has been shown, but without this being statistically significant. • The toxicity is high, but manageable by experienced medical teams. • No other therapeutic regime has shown benefits in the adjuvance of melanoma.
2) ARGUMENTS AGAINST.
• It is not clear which population most benefits from the adjuvant treatment. • The benefit is only clear for disease free survival, there being no consistent information referring to global survival. • The toxicity is considerable. • The ideal duration and dose for the treatment are unknown

Table 9. Arguments for and against high dose interferon as adjuvant treatment

Other favourable arguments are the data from a study that analysed the quality adjusted survival (QAS) using clinical data from the E1684 and E1690 studies which pointed out that the majority of patients showed improvement of the QAS, but the benefit was only significant in 16% of patients in the E1684 study (Kilbridge et al. 2002).

A cost-effectiveness analysis of high dose Interferon-α2b as adjuvant treatment for high-risk melanomas in Spain, shows that it is within established limits for healthcare economy regarding the use of a new treatment (Gonzalez-Larriba et al. 2002). Another recent study of cost effectiveness in node positive melanomas shows, that the treatment was cost effective, even though it varied according to the sub-stage, and also highly effective in terms of quality of life per year in patients under 60 years of age with stage IIIC melanoma (Cormier et al. 2007).

Even more recently a Stage III study was published comparing i.v. induction of Interferon α2b to the classic high dose scheme with induction and maintenance. At 51 months of follow-up, the RFS was 32 months vs. 31 months (p=0.836) and the GS was 61 months vs. 63 months (p=0.444), without being significant differences. There were more dropouts in the classic treatment (p<0.001), mainly because of its duration and signs of recurrence more than for toxicity. This study, which included 355 patients, attempted to show the value of induction (no differences between both groups), but lacked on untreated control group, could not confirm this in a more evident way. However, the existence of this group was not considered after the information published on the benefits of adjuvance (Gogas et al. 2007).

Another similar study presented in ASCO 2010 showed that patients in stage IIB and IIIA have similar RFS and OS in both groups, the ones with induction plus 8 weeks of maintenance dose and the ones with high doses according to Kirkwood regime (Sullivan et al. 2010). In high risk melanomas there is another study in Phase III with 364 patients that compares 4 weeks of induction versus 1 year of treatment with classic high doses of IFN, showing no significant differences in RFS and OS between both regimens (Pectasides et al. 2009). There is also another Phase III randomized study from DeCIG MM-ADJ-5 with 380 patients in stage III that compares 3 treatments with IFN α2b 20 MU/m2 i.v, five days a week for four weeks every four months and the classic regimen of high doses of IFN from Kirkwook, showing no significant differences in DMFS, but with better tolerance and safety with the intermitent treatment (Mohr et al. 2008). Therefore shorter regimens might encourage the use of IFN as an adjuvant treatment in melanoma patients.

As a final summary it can be said that in patients with high risk resected melanoma, high dose interferon is the adjuvant treatment to be proposed, together with background information on its collateral effects, as there is clear and significant evidence of improvement in the RFS and moderate, although not significant improvement of the GS.

New data have recently been published on high dose Interferon-α2b according to the Kirkwood scheme as neoadjuvant treatment prior to lymphadenectomy, in patients with palpable stage IIIB and IIIC adenopathies. After four weeks of intravenous phase among the 20 patients enrolled, 11 (55%) showed response, three of them (15%) pathological complete response. At a median of 18.5 months follow-up, 10 patients continued disease free. In responding patients, cells CD11+ and CD3+ increased on the tumour and CD83+ decreased, indicating a correlation between reactivity of the immune system and the benefit of the treatment. This study also included molecular analysis with activation of STAT3 being observed and related to cell proliferation, high dose Interferon-α2b would reduce this protein and increase STAT1. This enables opening a new approach to adjuvant treatment in high risk patients which should be more widely explored (Moschos et al. 2006).

Low and intermediate doses have not shown any real benefits in the adjuvant treatment of high-risk melanomas (Table 10) (Eggermont et al. 2005).

Trial	No. of cases	SLE	OS
Low dose IFN (3 mU x 3/s x 3 y.):			
-WHO-16 (2001)	426	NS	NS
-UK (2004)	674	NS	NS
-Scottish study (2001)	59	NS	NS
Ultra-low dose IFN (1 mU):			
-EORTC/DKG-80 (2001)	830	NS	NS
Low dose INF + Isotretinoin (IFN: 3 mU x 3/s x 2 y.)			
-ECAMTSG (2005)	407	NS	NS
Intermediate dose IFN.			
-EORTC 18952	1388	NS	NS
(10 mill. 13 m vs 5 mill. 25 m. vs observation)			

Table 10. High risk melanomas: adjuvant treatment with low and intermediate dose interferon

But in the review by A. Verma et al. (2007),patients with high risk melanomas, the results show, that treatment with high doses of IFN constantly improve the SLR and the mortality rate at two years (p<0.03). The authors conclusion is that IFN at high doses is a reasonable option in selected patients. A recent meta-analysis evaluating 6067 patients from 10 trials found significant benefits in RFS and GS (p=0.00006 and p=0.008), even though the absolute benefits on survival are small, just a 3% at five years. This meta-analysis did not clarify the ideal dose of interferon neither the duration of the treatment and found a sub-group where the benefits were greater, the presence of ulceration in the primary tumour, but this needs clarification. (Wheatley et al. 2007).

A recent Phase III randomized study from DeCOG, has compared low doses of IFN α2b (3MU three times a week) for 18 months (group A) versus 60 months (group B), in patients with primary melanoma, a Breslow's thickness ≥ 1.5 mm and negative lymphadenopathies clinically. The 75.6% of them had a sentinel lymph node biopsy, with a positive results in 18% in the group A and 17.5% in the group B. Overall they had 840 patients, with a median follow up of 4.3 years, and it did not show any benefits with prolonged treatments. All this suggest that the optimal length of the treatment with IFN is still nuclear (Hauschild et al. 2010).

It has been published recently some data on adjuvant treatment with pegylated Interferon α2b (PEG-IFN) from the EORTC 18991 study (Induction of 6 µg/Kg/week, s.c. for 8 weeks, followed by maintenance at the dose of 3 µg/Kg/week, s.c., for a total duration of 5 years). The study included 1256 patients in stage III (any T, N1-2, Mo, without metastasis in transit). Patients were randomised into two groups, one for treatment (608 p.) and the other for observation as a control (613 p.). The randomization was divided into positive microscopic lymphadenopathy (N1) versus macroscopic one (N2), number of positive lymph nodes, tumour ulceration and Breslow's thickness, sex of the patients and the referral center, analysing the data according to the intention to treat. The average length of treatment with PEG-IFN was 12 months (IQR: 3.8-33.4). The mean follow up was 3.8 years, and 328 recurrences were observed in the interferon group vs. 368 in the control one (p=0.01), being at four years the RFS value 45.6% in the first group and 38.95 in the second one, showing a risk reduction of 18% (p=0.01). No significant differences were observed between the two groups in OS. Grade 3 adverse event occurred in 246 (40%) patients in the interferon group and 80(10%) in the observation group; grade 4 adverse events occurred in 32 (5%) patients in interferon group and 14 (2%) in the observation group. In the interferon group the most common grade 3 or 4 adverse events were fatigue (97 patients, 16%), hepatotoxicity (66 patients, 11%), and depression (39 patients, 6%). Treatment with PEG-IFN was discontinued because of toxicity in 191(31%) patients. Regarding the quality of life, there was a negative effect in the group treated with IFN with a decrease in social activity and appetite. Knowing that PEG-IFN increases the RFS, the patients should be informed about the negative effects of the treatment and they should be encourage to participate in the planning of it (Table 11). (Eggermont et al., 2008; Bottomley et al., 2009).

	RFS		DMFS		OS	
	Obs.	PEG-IFN	Obs.	PEG-IFN	Obs.	PEG-IFN
No. of events	368	328	325	304	263	262
Rates at 4 years	39%	46%	45%	48%	56%	57%
Mean years	2.1	2.9	3.0	3.8	NR	NR
HR (95% CI)	0.82 (0.71-0.96)		0.88 (0.75-1.03)		0.98 (0.82-1.16)	
Value of "p"	0.01		0.11		0.78	

Table 11. Pegylated interferon. Results of the EORTC 18991 study

The EADO trial is a Phase III study with excised melanomas ≥ 1.5 mm of thickness and no affected lymph nodes clinically. Patients were randomized to received IFNα-2b (3 MU subcutaneously three times a week for 18 months) versus PEG-IFN (100 mcg. Subcutaneously once a week for 36 months). Out of 898 patients included, 896 were evaluated (453 IFN and 443 PEG) with a mean follow up of 4.7 years. Sentinel node biopsy was performed in 68.2% because it was not a standard procedure initially. The recurrence free survival (RFS) was 64.8% vs. 66.2% (p=0.43), the distant metastasis free survival (DMFS) was 72.6% vs. 71.3% (p=0.55), not showing significant differences. Adverse effects of grade 3-4 were seen in 26.6% vs. 44.6% in the first 18 months, which affected the mead length of treatment (17.8 months vs. 19.2 months, completing the full 36 months of treatment 28% of the patients). In summary, low doses of PEG-IFN was no better than low doses of conventional IFNα-2b. Trying to increase the benefits of PG-IFN by increasing the length of the treatment up to three years is not easy, because the high numbers of patients not completing the full treatment due to the side effects is important and therefore would not solve the clinical needs of them (Grob et al. 2010). Advocating the use of IFN in melanomas, a new meta-analysis has recently been published with a large number of patients reviewing the adjuvant treatment with IFN-α in high risk cases, in relation to DFS and OS, and also it has been studied the effect of the doses and the length of the treatment. There were 14 randomized studies included between 1990 and 2008, with a total of 8122 patients, out of which 4362 were treated only with IFN-α, the rest were only observed. The treatment with IFN-α is associated to and improvement of the DFS (p< 0.001/ 18% risk reduction) and also of the SG (p=0.002/ 11% risk reduction) (Figures 4 and 5).
The study has its own limitations according to the authors and therefore it cannot recommend the regime, doses or length of the treatment, neither, which subgroup of patients would respond better the adjuvant therapy. Given the lack of and effective systemic treatment to treat the melanoma, the meta-analysis suggests the use of IFN-α on the daily

clinical bases to offer the patients the best survival opportunities. It is important to remember that other adjuvant therapies well established for other types of cancer like breast, colorectal and ovarian is associated with a risk reduction. These data suggest that it is very important to research the molecular mechanism that could explain the sensibility to the IFN-α to try to identify the group of patients that would benefit most from it (Mocellin et al. 2010).

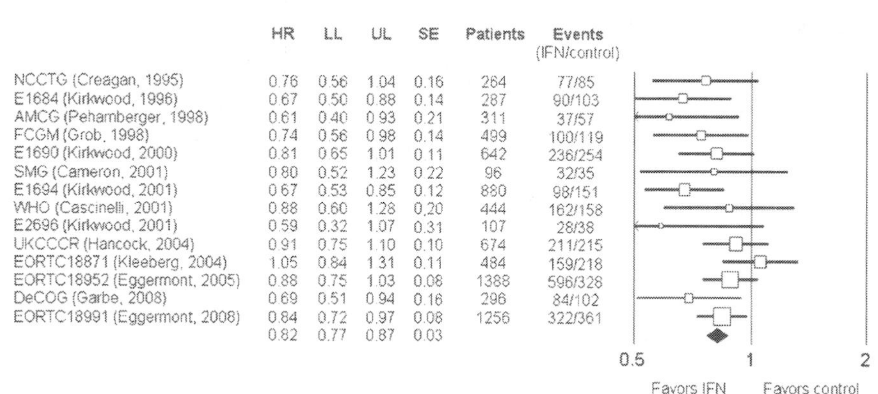

	HR	LL	UL	SE	Patients	Events (IFN/control)
NCCTG (Creagan, 1995)	0.76	0.56	1.04	0.16	264	77/85
E1684 (Kirkwood, 1996)	0.67	0.50	0.88	0.14	287	90/103
AMCG (Pehamberger, 1998)	0.61	0.40	0.93	0.21	311	37/57
FCGM (Grob, 1998)	0.74	0.56	0.98	0.14	499	100/119
E1690 (Kirkwood, 2000)	0.81	0.65	1.01	0.11	642	236/254
SMG (Cameron, 2001)	0.80	0.52	1.23	0.22	96	32/35
E1694 (Kirkwood, 2001)	0.67	0.53	0.85	0.12	880	98/151
WHO (Cascinelli, 2001)	0.88	0.60	1.28	0.20	444	162/158
E2696 (Kirkwood, 2001)	0.59	0.32	1.07	0.31	107	28/38
UKCCCR (Hancock, 2004)	0.91	0.75	1.10	0.10	674	211/215
EORTC18871 (Kleeberg, 2004)	1.05	0.84	1.31	0.11	484	159/218
EORTC18952 (Eggermont, 2005)	0.88	0.75	1.03	0.08	1388	596/328
DeCOG (Garbe, 2008)	0.69	0.51	0.94	0.16	296	84/102
EORTC18991 (Eggermont, 2008)	0.84	0.72	0.97	0.08	1256	322/361
	0.82	0.77	0.87	0.03		

HR: Hazard ratio. LL: Lower limit. UL: Upper limit. SE: Significant estimate.

Fig. 4. Meta-analysis. Disease-free survival

	HR	LL	UL	SE	Patients	Events (IFN/control)
NCCTG (Creagan, 1995)	0.90	0.64	1.25	0.17	264	68/72
E1684 (Kirkwood, 1996)	0.73	0.54	0.99	0.15	287	81/90
FCGM (Grob, 1998)	0.70	0.49	0.98	0.17	499	59/76
E1690 (Kirkwood, 2000)	0.98	0.76	1.24	0.12	642	194/186
SMG (Cameron, 2001)	0.86	0.54	1.35	0.23	96	31/36
E1694 (Kirkwood, 2001)	0.72	0.52	0.99	0.16	880	52/81
WHO (Cascinelli, 2001)	0.95	0.76	1.20	0.12	444	146/138
UKCCCR (Hancock, 2004)	0.94	0.74	1.17	0.12	674	151/156
EORTC18871 (Kleeberg, 2004)	0.98	0.77	1.23	0.12	484	137/202
EORTC18952 (Eggermont, 2005)	0.91	0.76	1.07	0.09	1388	534/292
DeCOG (Garbe, 2008)	0.62	0.44	0.86	0.17	296	65/88
EORTC18991 (Eggermont, 2008)	1.00	0.84	1.18	0.09	1256	256/257
	0.89	0.83	0.96	0.04		

HR: Hazard ratio. LL: Lower limit. UL: Upper limit.

Fig. 5. Meta-analysis. Overall survival

Given the characteristics of adjuvant treatment with Interferon-α2b, it would be extremely important to find factors predicting efficiency and parameters for classification of patients to enable a better choice of therapy. Autoimmunity seems to be a factor predicting efficiency in adjuvant treatment with interferon. A prospective study with high dose interferon analysed the autoimmune response through the appearance of thyroid, anticardiolipins, antinuclear, antiDNA autoantibodies or the presence of depigmentation. A quarter of all patients treated develop autoimmunity phenomena. After a follow-up of 45.6 months, only 13% of those presenting autoimmunity had suffered relapse and 4% had died. In the group that presented no autoimmunity reactions, 73% suffered relapse and 54% died. The mean survival has not been reached among the patients with autoimmunity phenomena and was 37.6 months in the group without these manifestations. Therefore, after multivariate analysis, autoimmunity constitutes a significant predictive factor for global and disease free survival (Gogas et al. 2006).

On the other hand, the trial 18991 from EORTC where adjuvant IFN was compared versus control, the presence or not of autoantibodies (anti-cardiolipin, anti-thyreoglobulin y antinuclear) did not represent an important prognostic factor and did not find a significant relationship with the treatment (Bouwhuis et al. 2010).

The determination of HLA is also a factor predicting recurrence in patients treated with Interferon α2b as adjuvant treatment. The percentage of relapse is significantly lower in patients with HLA genotype A33, HLA B57, HLA-Cw03 and HLA-Cw06. (Gogas et al. 2006).

It therefore seems essential to be able to discriminate those patients who would really benefit from adjuvant treatment with Interferon α2b, thus avoiding all side effects in patients that would not really benefit. In addition, this would also have a considerable economic impact.

2.6 Adjuvant treatment with GM-CSF

The GM-CSF is an important hematopoyetic growth factor, codified by a gene placed in the long arm of chromosome 5 (5q21-q32), present in monocytes, fibroblasts and endothelial cells, with an stimulating action over the developing and maturation of stem cells that will become neutrophils, eosinophils monocytes and macrophages. Is has been use therapeutically to treat QT induced neutopenias. The in-vivo studies have shown that recombinant GM-CSF increases the citotoxic activity of monocytes and lymphocytes, and also increases the activity of macrophages by increasing the production of matrix metaloprotheasas and angiogenesis inhibitors, and therefore an overall anti-tumoral effect, together with the increased inmunogenicicy of the tumoral cell, facilitating the antigen presentation. The reason for its use as an adjuvant therapy in excised high risk melanoma is because it also induces dentritic cell differentiation. In 2000 the first results were published on GM-CSF showing benefits on survival in relation to historic controls in stage III patients with a poor prognosis or stage IV with resected disease. Recent data on 98, high risk patients under treatment for three years, show a mean survival of 58.7 months, longer than the result of 37.5 months obtained in the first study where treatment only lasted one year. The benefits were especially observed in stage IIIc. The conclusion was the superiority of long-term treatment over three years, especially in patients that maintained eosinophilia for a longer period of time.

This study has been reviewed recently and once again they conclude that GM-CSF for three years increases the survival in patients with a high recurrent risk of melanoma (HR = 0,61;

p = 0,047), but those on three years treatment have potentially causing AML, as it did happened in two patients. Immunological studies showed an increase of neopterin related to the macrophages activity that potentially could explain the mechanism of action of the therapy (Spitler et al. 2008). The Phase III study E4697 that compares GM-CSF versus placebo as an adjuvant treatment in staging III-IV melanoma that were excised, did included 815 patients (1999 to 2006), out of which 735 were eligibles. The overall mean survival rate was 72.1 vs. 59.8 months (p = 0.551) and the disease free survival was 11.8 vs. 8.8 months (p-0.034), with a minimum toxicity (Lawson et al. 2010). Undoubtedly the use of GM-CSF as monotherapy or in combination in adjuvance is a line of research that must be confirmed over the next few years.

2.7 Adjuvant radiotherapy

It is an option in melanomas with a high risk of regional recurrence after lymphatic clearance, specially in those cases with extra lymphatic extension, a positive lymph node greater than 3 cm, 4 or more positive nodes, residual disease or a Breslow's thickness equal or greater that 4mm. In a randomized study with 227 patients considered as having high risk of recurrence, 109 were included in the adjuvant radiotherapy group and 108 on the control group. After a mean follow up of 27 months, 20 patients had a recurrence in the radiotherapy group and 34 in the control one (p=0.0410), indicating a better control of the local recurrence with radiotherapy but not affecting the survival rate (Henderson et al. 2009).

3. New treatments

The lack of proven efficient treatments against metastatic melanoma affects the use of the adjuvant treatment. Chemotherapy, cytoquines, vaccines and combination treatments have been studied with little success. Only IFN has shown to be beneficial in DFS and in less degree in OS in high risk patients, therefore it is necessary to continue to research for new therapies. A new line of research has been found in the monoclonal auto-antibodies anti-CTLA-4 that block the interaction between B7 (B7-1 and B7-2 are homologous costimulatory ligands expressed on the surface of antigen presenting cells) and CTLA-4 (Cytotoxic T-Lymphocyte Antigen 4), causing a negative inhibition that increases the citotoxicity of T-lymphocytes with antitumoral activity (Eggermond et al. 2010). At present, there are two monoclonal antibodies on phase II/III trials, use on their own or in combination: Ipilimumab and Tremelimumab.

Early-phase (I/II) clinical studies of tremelimumab demonstrated acceptable toxicity, mostly immune-related adverse events and similar efficacy of 10 mg/kg monthly and 15 mg/kg quarterly doses of the antibody with median survival times of 10.3 and 11 months, respectively. Both phase II regimens generated durable tumor response (Camacho et al. 2009).

Interesting data were presented at the 2010 annual meeting of the ASCO (American Society of Clinical Oncology), regarding the combination of Tremelimumab and HDI (High-dose Interferon alpha-2b) in a phase II trial in patients with metastatic melanoma. With an overall response rate of 30%, a progression-free survival rate at 6 months of 53%, and a median OS of 15.9 months, the results were very encouraging, especially since there seemed to be no added toxicity associated with the combination de Tremelimumab and HDI. Autoimmunity induced by therapy is significantly correlated with therapeutic benefit (Tarhini et al. 2010).

There are several studies in the last few years about metastatic melanoma and Ipilimumab as the only treatment and in combination with DTIC with survival rates of 11.5 and 13 months respectively. The presence of autoimmune reactions (diarrhoea, colitis and dermatitis) that can be controlled with steroids, can be used as a marker to asses the respond and duration of the treatment. A phase III study compares monotherapy with Ipilimumab and placebo (137 p.) versus Ipilimumab and vaccine gp100 (403 P.) versus placebo and vaccine gp100 (136 p.) in patients with stage III melanoma not excised or stage IV previously treated, with the main aim on the overall survival rate (OS). The mean survival was 10.0 months for the group that had Ipilimumab and gp100 and 6.4 months for the group that had gp100 alone (p=0.001). The survival of the patients who only had Ipilimumab was 10.1, also better that the gp100 alone group (p=0.003), not showing any differences between the groups with Ipilimumab. Immune reactions grade 3-4 were seen in about 10-155 of patients treated with Ipilimumab and 7 deaths were related to these side effects. In summary, Ipilimumab is the first drug that increases the survival in patients with advanced melanoma previously treated (Hodi et al. 2010).

The lack of benefit observed in stage IIIB/C with adjuvant IFN therapy was, for the EORTC Melanoma Group, the reason to move to a different drug. Thus, the EORTC 18071 pivotal adjuvant trial in stage IIIB/C, comparing a 3-years treatment with Ipilimumab to placebo in a double-blind randomized setting, was activated in 2009 and is expected to be completed in 2011.

4. Final comments

The reality is that except for data on IFN, no new validated strategies that improve results have come to the fore. The unquestionable increase of our understanding of the cell biology of melanomas leads to the idea of identification of sub-groups where the benefits would be greater. It is therefore absolutely necessary to identify new therapeutic targets, develop new drugs and make an optimal selection of patients. One of the most interesting targets is the analysis of the BRAF gene, mutated in 50-70% of melanomas, and furthermore associated with exposure to ultraviolet light. This mutation gives rise to a protein with a kinase activity about 500 times higher than the un-mutated protein thus enabling greater survival and proliferation of neoplastic cells. Sorafenib, a double target anti-angiogenic which inhibits BRAF on the one hand and VEGFR and PDGFR on the other, in association with CDDP in metastatic melanomas results in 13% PR and 53% SD. PD0325901 is another important inhibitor of the BRAF signal cascade (MEK1 and MEK2) and its efficiency has been tested in preclinical models as well as PLX40323 (Solid and Rosen, 2011). Nevertheless, the use of CTLA-4 inhibitors such as Ipilimumab and Tremelimumab, open new horizons in the treatment of melanomas and the future studies about adjuvant therapies, can change the prognosis, specially in high risk patients.

5. References

Balch, C. M.; Soong, S-J.; Gershenwald, J. E. et al. (2001). Prognostic factor analysis of 17.600 melanoma patients: Validation of the American Joint Committee on Cancer Melanoma Staging System. *J. Clin Oncol*, 2001, 19, 16: 3622-3634.

Balch, C. M.; Gershenwald, J. E.; Soong, S., el al. (2010). Multivariate analysis of prognostic factor among 2.313 patients with stage III melanoma: comparison of nodal micrometastases versus macrometastases. *J Clin Oncol*. 2010, 28, 14: 2452-2459.

Bottomley, A.; Coens, C.; Suciu, S. et al. (2009). Adjuvant therapy with Pregylated Interferon Alfa-2b versus observation in resected stage III melanoma: a phase III randomized controlled trial of Health-Related Quality of Life and symptoms by the European Organisation for Research and Treatment of Cancer Melanoma Group. *J Clin Oncol*, 2009, 27, 18:2916-2923.

Bouwhuis, M.; Suciu, S.; Testori, A. et al. (2010). Phase III trial comparing adjuvant treatment with Pegylated Interferon Alfa-2b versus observation: Prognostic significance of autoantibodies-EORTC 18991. *J Clin Oncol*, 2010, 28, 14: 2460-2466.

Camacho, L. H.; Antonia, S.; Jeffrey, S. et al. (2009). Phase I/II trial of Tremelimumab in patients with metastatic melanoma. *J Clin Oncol*, 2009, 27, 7:1075-1081.

Coit, D. G.; Zhou, Q.; Patel, A. et al. (2006) « Estimating survival probability in stage III melanoma: A multivariable individualized patient risk assessment nomogram ». *J Clin Oncol*. ASCO. 2006, 24, 18S, Abst. 8020

Cormier, J. N. ; Xing, Y. ; Ding, M. et al.(2007). Cost effectiveness of adjuvant Interferon in node-positive melanomas. *J Clin Oncol*. 2007, 25, 17: 2442-2448.

Dyson, S. W.; Bass, J.; Pomeranz, J. et al. (2005) "Impact of thorough block sampling in the histological evaluation of melanoma". *Arch Dermatol*. 2005, 141: 734-736.

Eggermont, A. M.; Suciu, S.; Mackie,R. et al. (2005). Post-surgery adjuvant therapy with intermediate doses of Interferon alpha-2b versus Observation in patients with IIB/III melanoma (EORTC18952): randomised controlled trial. *The Lancet*, 2005, 366, 9492: 1189-1196.

Eggermont, A. M.; Suciu, S.; Santimani, M. et al. (2008). Adjuvant therapy with pegylated interferon alfa-2b versus observation alone in resected stage III melanoma: final results of EORTC 18991, a randomised phase III trial". *The Lancet*. 2008, 372, 9633: 117-126.

Eggermont, A.M.; Suciu, S.; Rutkowski, P. et al. (2010). Randomized phase III trial comparing postoperative adjuvant ganglioside GM2-KLH/QS-21 vaccination versus observation in stage II (T3-T4N0M0) melanoma: Final results of study EORTC 18961. *J Clin Oncol*. ASCO, 2010, 28, 15s, Abst. 8505.

Eggermont, A. M.; Testori, A.; Maio, M. et al. (2010). Anti-CTLA-4 antibody adjuvant therapy in melanoma. *Semin Oncol*, 2010, 27, 5: 455-459

Faltynek, C. R.; Princler, G. L.; Rossio, J. L. et al.(1986). Relationship of the clinical response and binding of recombinant interferon-alpha in patients with lymphoproliferative diseases. *Blood*, 1986, 67:1077-1082.

Fecher, L. A.; Cummings, S. D.; Keefe, M. J. et al. (2007). Towards a molecular classification of melanoma. *J. Clin Oncol*. 2007, 25, 12: 1606-1620.

Foss, F. M. (2002). Immunologic mechanisms of antitumor activity. *Semin. Oncol*. 2002, 29, 3, 7, 5-11.

Garbe, C.; Radny, P.; Linse, R. et al. (2008). Adjuvant low-dose interferon α2a with or without dacarbazine compared with surgery alone: a prospective-randomized phase III DeCOG trial in melanoma patients with regional lymph node metastasis. *Ann Oncol*, 2008, 19, 6: 1195-1201.

Gimotty, Ph. A.; Van Belle, P.; Elder, D. E. et al. (2005). Biologic and prognostic significance of dermal Ki67 expression, mitoses, and tumorigenicity in thin invasive cutaneous melanoma. *J Clin Oncol*. 2005, 23, 31: 8084-8056.

Gogas, H.; Dafni, U.; Bafaloukos, D. et al. (2007). A randomized phase III trial of 1 month versus 1 year adjuvant high-dose Interferon alfa-2b in patients with resected high risk melanoma. *J Clin Oncol*, ASCO, 2007, 25, 18S, Abst. 8505.

Gogas, H.; Ioannovich, J.; DafnI, U. et al. (2006). Prognostic significance of autoimmunity during treatment of melanoma with interferon. *N. Engl. J. Med*. 2006, 354: 709-718.

Gogas, H.; Spyropoulou-Vlachou, U.; Dafni, D. et al. (2006). Correlation of molecular HLA typing and outcome in high-risk melanoma patients receiving adjuvant interferon. *J Clin Oncol*. ASCO. 2006, 24, 18S, Abst. 8029.

Gonzalez-Larriba, J. L.; Serrano, S.; Alvarez-Mon, M y col. (2001). Análisis coste-efectividad de interferón como tratamiento adjuvante en pacientes con melanoma de alto riesgo en España. *Eur. J. Cáncer* (Ed. Esp.) 2001, 1: 191-199.

Grob, J. J.; Jouary, T.; Dreno, B. et al. (2010). Adjuvant therapy with pegylated interferon alfa-2b (36 months) versus low-dose interferon alfa-2b (18 months) in melanoma patients without macro-metastatic nodes: EADO trial. *J Clin Oncol*, ASCO, 2010. 28, 15S, Abst. LBA8506

Hauschild, A.; Weichenthal, M.; Rass, K. et al. (2010). Efficazy of low-dose interferon α2b 18 versus 60 months of treatment in patients with primary melanoma of ≥ 1.5 mm tumor thicknes: Results of a randomized phase III DeCOG trial. *J Clin Oncol*, 2010, 28, 5:841-846.

Henderson, M. A.; Burmeister, B.; Thompson, J. F. et al. (2009). Adjuvant radiotherapy and regional lymph node field control in melanoma patients after lymphadenectomy: Results of an intergroup randomized trial (ANZMTG 01.02/TROG 02.01). *J Clin Oncol*. ASCO 2009, 27, 18S, Abst. LBA9084.

Hodi, F. S.; O'Day, S. J.; McDermott, D. F. et al. (2010). Improved survival with Ipilimumab in patients with metastatic melanoma. *N Engl J Med* 2010, 363, 8: 711-723.

Jonasch, E. & Haluska, F. G.(2001). El interferón en la practica clínica oncológica: revisión de la biología, las aplicaciones practicas y los efectos tóxicos del interferón. *The Oncologist*. (Ed. Esp.) 2001, 6, 1, 37-59.

Kin, K. B.; Legha, S. S.; Gonzalez, R. et al. (2006). A phase III randomized trial of adjuvant biochemotherapy versus interferon-α2b in patients with high risk for melanoma recurrence. *J Clin Oncol*, ASCO, 2006, 24, 18S, Abst.8003

Kirkwood, J. M.; Ibrahim, J. G.; Sosman, J. A. et al. (2001). High-dose interferon alpha-2b significantly prolongs relapse-free and overall survival compared with the GM2-KLH/QS-21 vaccine in patients with resected stage IIB-III melanoma: Results of Intergroup Trial E1694/S9512/C509801. *J Clin Oncol* 2001, 19, 9: 2370-2380.

Kirkwood, J. M.; Manola, J.; Ibrahim, J. et al. (2004). Análisis conjunto de los estudios del Eastern Cooperative Oncology Group e Intergroup sobre altas dosis de IFN como adjuvante para el melanoma. *Clinical Cancer Research*. 2004, 10, 1670-1677.

Kilbridge, K. L.; Cole, B.F.; Kirkwood, J. W. et al. (2002). "Quality-of-Life-Adjusted Survival Analysis of High-dose Adjuvant Interferon Alfa-2b for High-Risk Melanoma Patients Using Intergroup Clinical Trial Data. *J Clin Oncol* 2002, 20, 6: 1311-1318.

Lawson, D. H.; Lee, S. J.; Tarhini, A. A. et al. (2010). E4697: Phase III cooperative group study of yeast-derived granulocyte macrophage colony-stimulating factor (GM-

CSF) versus placebo as adjuvant treatment of patients with completely resected stage III-IV melanoma. *J Clin Oncol*, ASCO. 2010, 28, 15S, Abst. 8504.

Lewis, K. D.; Robinson, W. A.; McCarter, M. et al. (2006). Phase II study neoadjuvant biochemotherapy for stage III malignant melanoma: Results of long-term fallow-up. *J Clin Oncol*, ASCO 2006, 24, 18S, Abst.8035.

Liu, W.; Dowling, J. P.; Murray, W. K. et al. (2006). Rate of growth in melanoma. *Arch Dermatol*. 2006, 142: 1551-1558.

Mikhain, M.; Velazquez, E.; Shapiro, R. et al. (2005). PTEN expression in melanoma: Relationship with patient survival, bcl-2 expression, and proliferation. *Clin Cancer Research*. 2005, 11: 5153-5157.

Mitchell, M. S.; Abrams, J.; Thompson, J. A. et al. (2007). Randomized trial of an allogeneic melanoma lysate vaccine with low-dose interferon alpha-2b compared with high-dose interferon alfa-2b for resected stage III cutaneous melanoma. *J Clin Oncol* 2007, 25, 15: 2078-2085.

Mocellin, S.; Hoon, D.; Ambrosi, A. et al. (2006). The prognostic value of circulating tumor cells in patients with melanoma: A systematic review and meta-analysis. *Clin Cancer Research*. 2006, 12: 4605-4613.

Mocellin, S.; Paquali, S.; Rossi, C. R. et al. (2010). Interferon alfa adjuvant therapy with high-risk melanoma: A systematic review and meta-analysis. *J. Natl Cancer Inst*. 2010. 102, 493-501.

Mohr, P.; Hauschild, a.; Enk, A. et al. (2008). Intermittent high-dose intranenous interferon alpha 2b for adjuvant treatment of stage III malignant melanoma: An interim analysis of a randomized phase III study (NCT226408). *J Clin Oncol*, ASCO 2008, 26, Abst. 9040.

Moreno-Nogueira, J. A.; Valero Arbizu, M & Moreno Rey, C. (2008). Adjuvant treatment melanoma. *Cancer & Chemotherapy Rev*. 2008, 3: 10-22.

Moreno-Nogueira, J. A.; Sancho Márquez, P.; Corral Jaime, J. y col. (2008). Tratamiento. Melanomas. Ed. J. A. Moreno-Nogueira, P. Sancho Márquez, J. Corral Jaime y P. Ramírez Daffos. Ed. ARAN ediciones S.L. ISNB 978-84-96881-35-8. Madrid. 2008, 50-74.

Moschos, S.J; Edington, H. D.; Land, S. R. et al. (2006). Neoadjuvant treatment of regional stage IIIB melanoma with High-Dose Interferon-alpha 2b induce objective tumor regression in association with modulation of tumor infiltrating host cellular immune responses. *J. Clin. Oncol*. 2006, 24, 19 : 3164-3171.

Moschos, S. J. & Kirkwood, J. M. (2005). Adjuvant therapy for cutaneous melanoma. Chapter 52. Cancer of the skin. Ed. D. S. Rigel, R. J. Friedman, L. M. Dzubow, D. S. Reinterg, J-C. Bystryn and R. Marks. Ed. Elsevier Saunders. ISBN 0 7216 0544 3. Philadelphia. 2005, 641-654.

Pectasides, D.; Dafni, U.; Bafaloukos, D. et al. (2009). Randomized phase III study of 1 month versus 1 year of adjuvant high-dose interferon añfa-2b in patients with resected high-risk melanoma .*J Clin Oncol*, 2009, 27, 6: 939-944.

Pestka, S. (1997). The interferon receptors. Semin. Oncol. 1997, 24, 3, 9: 18-40.

Saiag, PH.; Bernard, M.; Beauchet, A. et al. (2005). Ultrasonography using simple diagnostic criteria vs. palpation for the detection of regional lymph node metastases of melanoma". *Arch Dermatol*, 2005, 141: 183-189.

Schmidt, H.; Johansen, J. S.; Sjoegren, P. et al. (2006). Serum YKL-40 predicts relapse-free and overall survival inpatients with American Joint Committee on Cancer stage I and II melanoma. *J Clin Oncol.* 2006, 24, 5: 798-804.

Solid, D. B. & Rosen, N. (2011). Resistance to BRAF inhibition in melanoma. *N Engl J Med* 2011, 364, 8:772-774

Sosman, J. A.; Unger, J. M.; Liu, P. Y. et al. (2002). Adjuvant immunotherapy of resected, intermediate-thickness, node-negative melanoma with an allogeneic tumor vaccine: Impact of HLA class I antigen expression on outcome. *J Clin Oncol.* 2002, 20, 8: 2067-2075.

Spitier, L.E.; Weber.; R.W.; Cruickshank, S. et al. (2008). Granulocyte-macrophage colony stimulating factor as adjuvant therapy of melanoma. *J Clin Oncol* .ASCO. 2008, 26, Abst.20006.

Stadler, R and Luger, T. (2005). Long term survival benefit adjuvant treatment of high risk cutaneous with dacarbazine and low dose natural interferon alpha: a controlled, randomised, multicentre trial. *J Clin Oncol,* ASCO, 2005, 23, 16S, Abst. 7516.

Suciu, S.; Ghanem, G.; Kruit, W. et al. (2007). Serum S-100B protein is a strong independent prognostic marker for distant-metastasis free survival in stage III melanoma patients: An evaluation of the EORTC randomized trial 18952 comparing IFNα versus observation. *J Clin Oncol,* ASCO 2007, 25, 18S, Abst. 8518.

Sullivan, R. J.; Frankenthaler, A.; Wang, W. et al. (2010). A retrospective comparison of 12 weeks versus 52 weeks of adjuvant interferon for patients with stage IIB, IIC and IIIA melanoma. *J Clin Oncol* ASCO, 2010, 28, 15S, Abst. 19013.

Tarhini, A.A.; Stuckert, J.; Lee, S. et al. (2009). Prognostic significance of serum S100B protein in high-risk resected melanoma patients participating in Intergroup Trial ECOG 1694. *J Clin Oncol,* 2009, 27, 1: 38-43.

Tarhini, A.A.; Moschos, S. J.; Tawbi, H. et al. (2010). Phase II evaluation of tremelimumab combined with high-dose interferon alpha-2b for metastatic melanoma. *J Clin Oncol,* ASCO 2010, 28, 15S. Abstr. 8524.

Trask, P. C.; Esper, P.; Riba, M. et al. (2000). Psychiatric side effects of Interferon therapy: Prevalence, proposed mechanisms, and future directions. *J Clin Oncol* 2000, 18, 11:2316-2326.

Verma, S.; Quirt, I.; McCready, D. et al. (2007). Systematic review of systemic adjuvant therapy for patients at high risk for recurrent melanoma. *Arch Dermatol.* 2007, 143, 6: 779-782.

Wheatley, K.; Ives, N.; Eggermont, A. M. et al. (2007). Interferon-α as adjuvant therapy for melanoma: An individual patient data meta-analysis of randomized trial. *J Clin Oncol,* ASCO, 2007, 25, 18S, Abst.8526.

7

Photodiagnosis and Photodynamic Therapy of Cutaneous Melanoma

Ekaterina Borisova[1], Vanya Mantareva[2], Irina Bliznakova[1],
Ivan Angelov[2], Latchezar Avramov[1] and Elmira Pavlova[3]
[1]Institute of Electronics, Bulgarian Academy of Sciences
[2]Institute of Organic Chemistry with Center on Phytochemistry,
Bulgarian Academy of Sciences
[3]Medical Center of University Hospital "Tsaritza Yoanna-ISUL"
Bulgaria

1. Introduction

Skin cancer is one of the most widespread tumours. However, despite the progress achieved in all clinical diagnostic techniques, the most severe of those tumours - cutaneous melanoma, continues to be an important problem of social health. A large number of optical techniques have been recently applied in the clinical practice in view of obtaining qualitatively and quantitatively new data from cutaneous neoplasia. Due to their high sensitivity in detecting small changes, spectroscopic techniques are now widely used for detection of early changes in biological tissues. Fluorescence detection of normal and abnormal tissues is among the most promising such approaches as it makes use of naturally existing fluorescent molecules (in the case of autofluorescence) or added fluorescent markers (in the case of exogenous fluorescence) of high importance. Fluorescent markers are introduced wherever native fluorescence is not informative enough to be used for diagnostic goals due to the absence or non-specificity of the changes in the tumour vs. the normal tissues.

The fluorescent diagnostic techniques are particularly suitable in diagnosing melanin-pigmented cutaneous pathologies. Melanin is a pigment which absorbs strongly within practically entire visible spectral range. Its high content in these lesions leads to low penetration depth of the excitation light and a small amount of re-emitted fluorescent light that can be collected and used for fluorescent analysis of the pathology under investigation. Therefore, fluorescent diagnosis of melanin-pigmented neoplasia, such as cutaneous malignant melanoma and its differentiation vs. dysplastic precursors and similar benign skin pathologies, such as nevi, is an elaborate and challenging task for all researchers working in the field of biomedical photonics. Photodiagnosis (PD) and photodynamic therapy (PDT) have been established as emerging modalities for a variety of pathogenic conditions including pigmented melanoma (Awan et al., 2006; Davids and Kleemann, 2010). The number of cases of pigmented malignancies has been steadily increasing during the last decades in general, and, in particular, malignant melanoma (MM) incidence has also increased. Melanomas are the most aggressively developing form of dermatological cancers due to the difficulty of diagnosis at an early stage combined with the low rate of success of the treatment at the late stage. The key factor of success with melanoma disease is an early detection followed by effective treatment procedures. PD and PDT could be the proper answer in achieving this goal.

1.1 Autofluorescence of cutaneous melanoma

Autofluorescence has been proven to be a very sensitive and accurate method for detection of early changes in many cancer types; however, due to the specific optical properties of melanin, fluorescence spectroscopy application to malignant melanoma detection is still a matter of debate. A few attempts have been made to detect fluorescence of melanin itself based on natural and synthetic melanin solutions. The authors reported that a major part of the excitation energy (>99,9%) in melanin molecules dissipates through non-radiative pathways (Lohmann and Paul, 1988; Meredith and Riesz, 2004). The natural fluorescence of melanin related to its oligomeric units is of extremely low intensity, with emission spectrum in the range 450 – 550 nm (Nighswander-Rempel et al., 2005; Perna et al., 2009). The first reports on using fluorescence spectroscopy for diagnostics of melanin-pigmented neoplasia were published in the late 80's and early 90's (Leffel et al., 1988; Lohmann et al., 1991).

There is still no universal procedure for photodiagnosis and differentiation between malignant melanoma and other melanin-pigmented pathologies. Melanin is known to have unique light absorption behaviour, completely different from that of the other organic fluorophores, namely, an exponential decrease of the absorption from the UV to the near infrared region (Nighswander-Rempel et al., 2005). A great number of studies have been carried out in this field obtaining promising results based on autofluorescence and on exogenous fluorescence detection of these cutaneous malignancies. Interesting approaches for diagnosis have been employed based on the autofluorescence properties of melanoma and its subtypes using additional analysis of the spectra detected, or specific algorithms, some of which allow relatively high sensitivity and specificity of tumour detection and evaluation (Chiwot et al. 2001; Borisova, 2006). The authors reported values for sensitivity of 82.5% and specificity of 78.6% after ultraviolet irradiation of the tumours (Chwirot et al., 1998).

In our investigations with excitation light with wavelength 337 nm used in autofluorescence measurements, the sensitivity obtained was about 77,8% and the specificity of 93,3% (Borisova et al., 2008b). Whether melanoma autofluorescence is an appropriate diagnostic tool is still debatable. Our investigations did not reveal any significant spectral shape changes (Borisova, 2006), only a significant fluorescent signal intensity decrease in the case of melanoma. While Lohmann and co-authors (Lohmann et al. 1991) concluded that autofluorescence spectroscopy is capable of differentiating melanoma from normal tissue using ultraviolet excitation (365 nm), Sterenborg and co-authors (Sterenborg et al., 1995) reported that they did not observe a significant correlation between the fluorescence emission and the histopathological examination of the lesions studied. Thus, melanoma remains a work in progress for non-invasive diagnosis.

Low-level fluorescent signals distorted by the melanin absorption can be detected in spite of the pigment influence on the spectra registered by the means of high-sensitivity detectors, which appeared recently in the market (Borisova et al., 2005).The signals detected from melanoma lesions originate mainly from co-enzymes and structural proteins (Borisova et al., 2008a).

A promising approach based on femtosecond two-photon excitation of melanin was also proposed (Teuchner et al. 1999). Despite its potential, this method is very expensive and inconvenient to be introduced into the standard clinical practice.

1.2 Exogenous fluorescence (photodiagnosis) of cutaneous melanoma

Another possible way of detection is based on introducing exogenous fluorescent markers in the lesions, as melanoma lesions exhibit very low autofluorescence signals. The conventional application of a fluorescent contrast agent as a positional marker for detection of malignancies appears to be commonly used for diagnosis of pigmented melanoma tumours.

The exogenous fluorophores called photosensitizers (PS) have found the widest application; they are used to improve the fluorescent detection of melanin-pigmented neoplasia. These compounds could be used for photodiagnosis, as well for initiation of a photodynamic effect in the tumour cell, so that one could combine photodiagnosis with a subsequent photodynamic therapy of the lesion.

Bearing in mind the specific optical properties of melanin, especially its strong absorption in the shorter wavelengths' spectral range, scientists have focused their efforts on the synthesis and study of long-wavelengths photosensitizers, such as phthalocyanines and naphthalocyanines, which absorb in the 670-760 nm range and fluoresce in the 680 – 800 nm range (Woehrle et al., 1999; Peeva et al., 1999; Shopova et al., 1999; Mantareva et al., 2005).

The incident light must be of appropriate wavelength to ensure deep penetration in order to excite the native tissue chromophores of the malignant tissue. The diagnostic light usually covers the part of visible spectra (488-635 nm) where the so called endogenous sensitizers absorb strongly. The fact that the absorption spectra for normal vs. pathogenic tissues are different is a useful tool allowing fast diagnosis (Borisova et al., 2005). The application of exogenous chromophores can enhance the images and can further assist the therapy. It is important that the applied light's wavelength to be shifted away from the absorption peak of the tumour localizing photosensitizers, so that detection at both wavelengths should be possible. Recently, PSs that possess the properties of good tumour tissues uptake and retention for fluorescent detection and relatively high photochemical parameters of singlet oxygen generation and other ROSs were defined as theranostic drugs (Rai et al., 2005). The appropriate use of the competitive approaches after light excitation is limited by the absorption coefficients of the native chromophores of tumour cells and by the light scattering properties of the constituents of the tumour tissue. External to the tissue natural or synthetic photosensitizers that would allow large intensity fluorescence demarcation and powerful photosensitizing processes are still under development.

1.3 Photodynamic therapy of cutaneous melanoma

Besides the initial diagnosis of the pathology, an important clinical aspect is related to the following treatment and therapeutic modalities, which could be applied on sensitive and severe skin lesion, such as malignant melanoma. The photodynamic therapy modality is a curvative tool developed and applied in the clinical practice in the last few decades, whereby photosensitizers absorbing in the near-infrared spectral region and selectively accumulated in tumour tissue transfer their energy after light irradiation to the surrounding oxygen and produce singlet oxygen, which then reacts with and destroys adjacent proteins and lipids in the cell membrane structures, or switches on the processes of apoptosis in the tumour cells. These compounds can also fluoresce; this combination of a possibility for photodetection and the following photodynamic effect of the drugs developed for photodynamic therapy applications is very promising and useful for the clinical practice.

The photodynamic approach appears as a complementary methodology which is not developed for pigmented melanomas (Mac Donald et al., 2001). The PDT is based on a photoactive compound (photosensitizer, PS) and a proper light excitation, together with the presence of molecular oxygen (Dougherty, 1992). As soon as selective localization of PS into the tumour tissue occurs, visible light must be applied locally to provoke the photophysical mechanisms of excitation of the singlet and triplet states of PS, the latter being metastable and can be involved in chemical reactions. The transfer of the light energy absorbed by the tissue or only by the PS can take place through radiative decay of the singlet state (fluorescence), which is used in non-invasive diagnosis. The same PS can undergo non-radiative relaxation to the lower energy triplet exited state of PS, which can participate in chemical reactions with the surrounding molecules. Basically, two mechanisms of photosensitization have been established (Foote, 1991). The more important one takes place via an energy transfer from the triplet PS to the ground state of molecular oxygen from atmospheric air, which results in the formation of highly cytotoxic singlet oxygen. The process is known as mechanism type II of photooxidation. Concurrently, the mechanism takes place of an electron or proton transfer from the excited triplet PS to the surrounding tissue molecules. As a result, reactive oxygen species (ROSs) are generated. This is known as mechanism type I of photosensitization.

Diverse results have been reported on the application of exogenous photosensitizers.

PDT appears to be a promising new approach for an early detection and sufficient therapy of the most aggressive forms of cancer, such as pigmented melanoma tumours. The clinically approved photosensitizers are the porphyrin derivatives (Photofrin® and Haematoporphyrin derivative) and aminolevulinic acid (ALA) which is a precursor of the porphyrin-like compound protoporphyrin IX. However, the so-called first generation sensitizers exhibit the disadvantage of optical limitation which precludes the application of the existing drugs to the diagnosis and treatment of pigmented melanomas. The difference in the ALA-induced protoporphyrin IX autofluorescence (excitation at 365 and 405 nm, emission at 635 nm) from malignant melanoma as compared with healthy skin in humans appears to be related to the different oxygenation rather than to the specificity of the fluorophores of malignancies. The fluorescence-based detection of abnormal tissues during the therapy is based on temporary differences in the kinetics of drug uptake between normal and malignant cells. At present, 5-aminolevulinic acid (ALA, with commercial name Levulan®) is used for the formation of protoporphyrin IX. The product of the haem biosynthesis is being considered as a drug for fluorescent diagnosis. The further development and evaluation of advanced fluorescent contrast agents is an important research topic which could lead to a successful solution of many fundamental scientific problems. Unlike other primary cutaneous malignancies, melanoma has a strong tendency for proliferation; some authors (Allison et al., 2006) even consider that local treatment by photodynamic therapy or any other local treatment modality prior to sentinel node procedure for evaluation of lymphatic metastasis is contraindicated. As the survival is based generally on the successful immunomodulation on a system level, local photodynamic therapy would only be a part of the treatment procedures. The photodynamic therapeutic immunomodulatory effect achieved seems to be very important in the evaluation of the PDT effect in the local control of the lesion and on the survival rate in general (Saczko et al., 2005; Allison et al., 2006; Kaplan et al., 2008). This effect is still under investigations and a large amount of work remains to be done.

The further development of PDT agents leading to the development of a second generation of far-red absorbing photosensitive dyes with improved spectral properties was the aim of our research in recent years (Borisova et al., 2005; Wohrle et al., 1999, Mantareva et al., 2005). The new photodynamic drugs were designed to become more efficient contrast agents for fluorescence diagnosis of early-stage malignancies, and especially of pigmented melanomas. Other researchers have also reported very promising results from PDT treatment of pigmented melanoma with a new generation of photosensitizers making melanoma cells highly sensitivity to the PDT (Davids and Kleemann, 2010; Kolarova et al., 2007a; Kolarova et al., 2007b). PDT treatment with a new generation of photosensitizers was also proposed to be used as an additional palliative procedure for patients with malignant melanoma (Kubler, 2005).

A part of our own research interests were the highly conjugated macrocyclic complexes from the group of tetra-isoindoles, such as phthalocyanines and naphthalocyanines. Phthalocyanines are characterized by a red-shifted and strong absorption maximum (> 670 nm) as compared to porphyrins (~ 630 nm). The zinc(II) coordinated complexes were studied as efficient fluorescent contrast agents of an experimental B16 pigmented melanoma on mice. Several cationic Zn(II)-phthalocyanines (ZnPcRs) with different hydrophilic/ lipophilic balance were synthesized and studied as promising diagnostic agents for pigmented melanoma. It was shown that the long wavelength absorption together with a high fluorescence intensity at the wavelength over 680 nm as well as the selective tumour cells uptake as compared to the surrounding normal tissue result in two advantages over the porphyrins and derivatives. The additional benzene rings lead to extended Pc analogues such as naphthalocyanines. They have the advantage of a stronger and deeper far-red absorption (760-790 nm) than phthalocyanines. A number of in vivo studies on B16 pigmented melanoma treated with Si(IV)- and Zn(II)-naphthalocyanines at different therapeutic protocols showed the potential value of the PDT approach when combined with some other methodology.

The clinical acceptance of the method was achieved in 1998 for treatment of non-pigmented tumour localizations with porphyrin derivatives (Haematoporphyrin derivative, Photofrin) and aminolevulinic acid (ALA) by application of visible light at 635 nm (Brown et al., 2004). The porphyrin derivatives and ALA, which is a precursor in the biosynthesis of protoporphyrin IX, have shown low efficiency for pigmented melanomas (Ibbotson, 2010). This was explained by the overlapping of the absorption spectra of the melanin pigment and porphyrins. The low transparency of the pigmented tissue at the excitation wavelength typical for porphyrins (around 630 nm) minimized the photosensitizing process efficiency. The pigmented melanomas are known as being weakly affected by the so called first generation photodynamic sensitizers, which are porphyrin based molecules (Kalka et al., 2000). An ideal PS for tumours needs to absorb at longer wavelengths to be suitable for treating melanomas with pigments. The so-called second-generation PSs were developed to have improved physical, chemical and spectral properties. The representative groups of PSs are the pheophorbide derivative, chlorine-type molecules like benzoporphyrin monoacid derivative (Verteporfin), and more extended macrocycles such as phthalo- and naphthalo-cyanines (sulfonated MPcs, Photosense). These PSs have energy absorption band in the far red spectral region (> 660 nm) with high absorption coefficients which allows a deeper tissue penetration of the excitation light, enabling it to penetrate blood, melanin and fibrotic tissue.

The studies in our laboratory on highly pigmented variety of malignant melanoma B16 demonstrated an effective diagnosis and PDT response by using phthalocyanine and naphthalocyanines metal complexes (MPcs and MNcs) with intensive far red absorption band (Michailov et al., 1997; Peeva et al, 1999; Mantareva et al., 1997; Woehrle et al., 1999). The competition for the absorption of melanin with the applied light decreases as a single-exponent when the wavelength is increased (Mantareva et al., 2005). These photosensitive compounds are characterized by a large molar extinction coefficient ($1\text{-}5 \times 10^{5}$ M^{-1} cm^{-1}) in the spectral range around 675 nm (MPcs) and 770 nm (MNcs) where the pigmented melanomas have minimal absorption (Sounik et al., 1990).

1.4 PD and PDT of melanoma – applications

In view of improving the early diagnosis and the differentiation of risk lesions, we proposed a method of evaluating the autofluorescent characteristics of several common cutaneous benign and malignant lesions. Pigmented melanoma may simulate benign lesions, including seborreic keratoses, heamangioma, compound and dysplastic nevi. Amelanotic malignant melanoma may clinically mimic a basal cell carcinoma. All these pathologies were investigated and their fluorescent spectra and specific features were evaluated vs. malignant melanoma pathologies for development of a broad clinically valuable algorithm for melanoma detection based on the autofluorescent properties of skin lesions. The origins of diagnostically significant spectral features were discussed. The differentiation algorithm of benign/dysplastic/ malignant pigmented skin melanin-pigmented lesions proposed allowed us to differentiate MM with sensitivity about 78% and specificity more than 90 %. These numbers give a diagnostic accuracy of about 70% using the autofluorescence signals received.

To improve the diagnostic accuracy, exogenous photosensitizers need to be applied. A large number of experiments have been already carried out using photosensitizers from the phthalocyanines group (Mantareva et al., 2005). These compounds have very promising optical properties in terms of fluorescence quantum yield and photodynamic properties and high selectivity to the tumour cells. Cationic phthalocyanines differing in their lipophylicity were studied as long-wavelength absorbing fluorescent markers for pigmented melanoma tumour on a model animal (mice) (Fig. 1). In order to study the transport through the cellular membranes, lipophilic and hydrophilic Pcs were prepared. Their fluorescence behaviour was studied in solutions (dimethylsulfoxide) (Fig. 2) and in turbid media (incorporated into the cells). In vivo fluorescence detection studies showed a higher in situ discrimination of the tumour from the healthy surrounding tissue compared with the commonly used drugs. The limitations of pigmented melanomas detection when using ALA can be avoided by using cationic phthalocyanine complexes with a proper hydrophilic/ lipophilic balance. The proposed experimental fluorescence spectroscopy technique (Fig. 3) is suitable for clinical application in fluorescence detection of pigmented malignancies. In vivo fluorescent diagnostic potential of the studied compounds concerning pigmented melanoma was demonstrated, so that clinical studies on humans are foreseen in our long-term plans with the purpose of introducing photodiagnostics and photodynamic therapy of malignant melanoma.

Both autofluorescence and exogenous fluorescent detection have their place in the clinical practice. The former method could be used as a screening tool for initial detection and evaluation of cutaneous pathologies, while the latter must be applied on suspicious cases, where it could be used as an affirmative test of the initial diagnosis, as well as a tool for photodynamic therapy of the neoplasia, if such is diagnosed as cutaneous pigmented melanoma.

2. Chemistry of phthalocyanines as photosensitizers for pigmented melanoma

During the last decades of intensive research on PDT with phthalocyanines, several of them were proposed as potential candidates for second generation photosensitizers. In concerns of their chemistry, the strong lipophilic and aggregation properties of the macrocycle facilitate the proper tailoring of the Pcs structure.

Most of the well-known Pcs under physiological conditions are insoluble, unstable to light and tend to form dimers and higher aggregates which leads to a dramatic decrease of photochemical properties of the generation of ROSs and, in turn, the PDT effectiveness. Overcoming these limitations is the crucial factor for potential clinical applications. A number of suitable substitutions on the peripheral position of the ring, as well as axially to the coordinated metal ion have been devised and tested by in vitro/ in vivo experiments.

Several Zn(II) naphthalocyanines with differing substituents (amino-, amide-, sulfuric acid - groups) and Si(IV) with methoxyethylenglycol axial substitution were studied in our group (Mantareva and co-authors, 1997, 1999, 2005). The results showed that after incorporation of liposome vesicles ZnNcA, which has four benzamido-substituents, had a high photodynamic response for B16 pigmented melanomas.

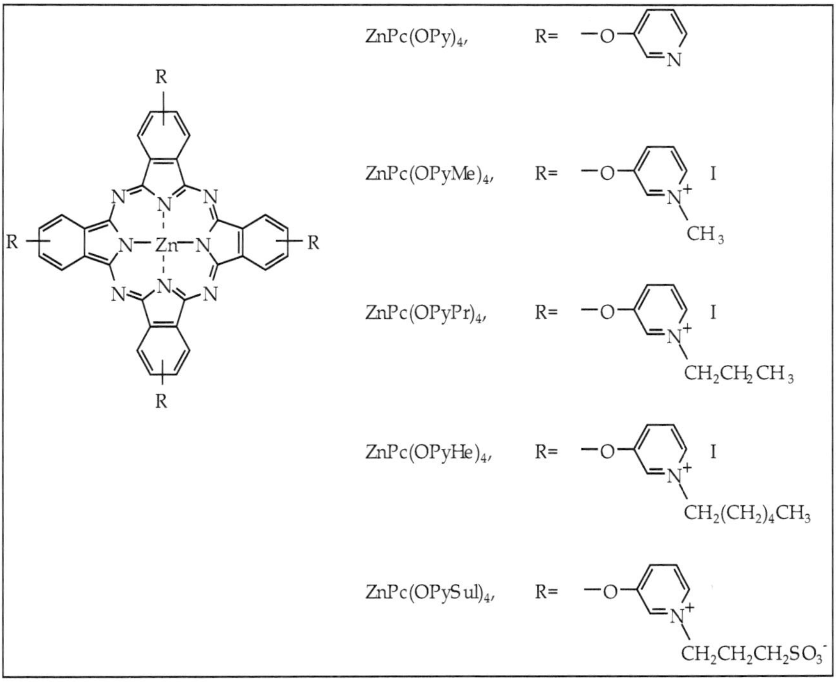

$ZnPc(OPy)_4$,   R=   (pyridyloxy)

$ZnPc(OPyMe)_4$,   R= CH_3

$ZnPc(OPyPr)_4$,   R= $CH_2CH_2CH_3$

$ZnPc(OPyHe)_4$,   R= $CH_2(CH_2)_4CH_3$

$ZnPc(OPySul)_4$,   R= $CH_2CH_2CH_2SO_3^-$

Fig. 1. Chemical structure of Zn(II)-phthalocyanine with pyridyloxy substituents with increasing hydrocarbon chain to N-atom

The coordinated with silicon (IV) naphthalocyanine axially substituted with polyethyleneglycol (SiNc) was synthesized and studied as promising for PDT of B16 pigmented melanoma (Mantareva et al., 1997; Woehrle et al., 1999). Other authors have studied Si(IV) naphthalocyanine (isoBO-SiNc) for PDT of B16 pigmented melanoma with pretreatment by high-peak-power (HPP) laser 1064 nm irradiation, which enhanced the tumour susceptibility to conventional PDT (Sounik et al., 1990; Busetti et al., 1998).

3. Absorbance of melanin and other tissues' chromohores vs. phthalocyanines

The strong absorption in the red and far-red region of the visible spectrum ensures deeper light penetration that does not depend on the melanin pigment. The typical absorption spectrum of Pcs is characterized by a strong Q-band around 675 nm and with a half as intensive Soret band, which lies around 350 and 360 nm (Fig. 1). By adding substituents, the position of the maxima can vary by 5-8 nm, to the red with increase of the molar absorption coefficients. We studied the absorption spectra of endogenous chromophores which are good absorbers of visible light (Mantareva et al., 2005). Figure 2 presents the spectra of natural chromophores such as riboflavin, hemoglobin, cytochrome C and melanin extracted from B16 pigmented melanoma.

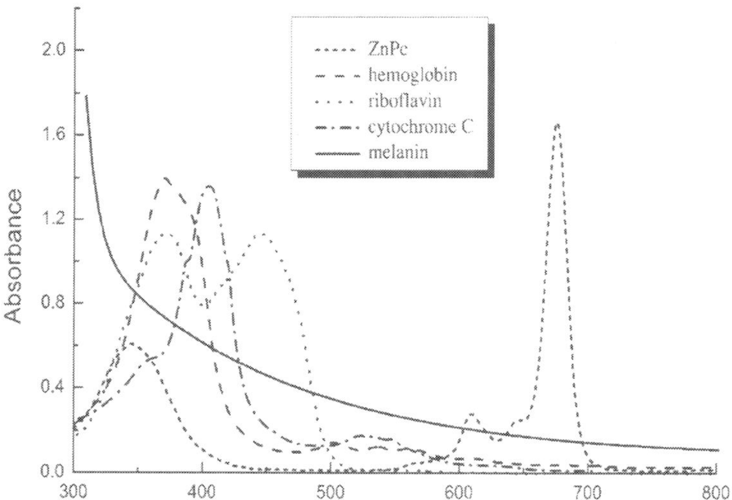

Fig. 2. Absorption spectra of Zn(II)-phthalocyanine (DMSO) and native tissues chromophores (hemoglobin, riboflavin, cytochrome C, all in saline) vs. melanin (1N NaOH) (Mantareva et al., 2005)

Melanin showed a mono-exponential decrease of the absorption from the UV to the near IR region (300-800nm). The absorbance of unsubstituted ZnPc is typical for phthalocyanines. There is only a limited overlapping of the spectra of native chromophores and ZnPc as a photosensitizer. When the excitation light is not in the region of the absorbance of the tissue, light is not interacting with the tissue pigments, all light energy can be absorbed by the photosensitizer localized in a pigmented melanoma tumour. Two optical processes that influence these effects must be taken into account, namely, malignant tissue's absorption and light scattering. Both are known to decrease while the wavelength is increased (635-850nm). In the case of a deeply pigmented tumour tissue, such as B16 pigmented melanoma, the absorption by melanin even in the far-red region (>700nm) is not negligible. The melanin absorption reduces the depth of light penetration and further limits the effect of photodiagnosis and therapy. The depth of light penetration and the light scattering are recognized as crucial for to controlling the response of tumours to PDT. In our previous work with naphthalocyanines, we showed the strong absorbance (776 nm, 5 x 10^5 M^{-1} cm^{-1}) of these compounds and a successful treatment of B16 pigmented melanoma implanted in mice (Mantareva et. al., 1997; Peeva et. al., 2001). However, the PDT effect was still incomplete, probably as a result of the low drug selectivity and the insufficient light penetration to the deeper pigmented melanoma layers.

4. Photobiology of B16 pigmented melanoma

4.1 Uptake study

The uptake study of the group of phthalocyanines with increased hydrophobicity depending on the attached hydrocarbon chain to the methypyridyloxy group (ZnPcMe, ZnPcPr, ZnPcHe and ZnPcDo) was carried out by the experimental set-up, which is presented on Fig. 3.

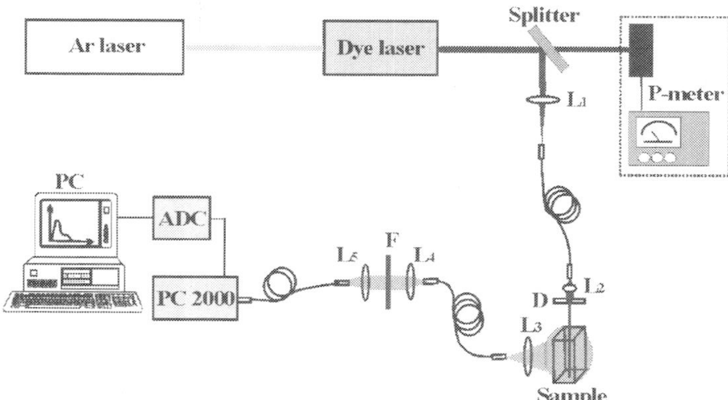

Fig. 3. The experimental set-up for fluorescence determination of photosensitizer uptake (Mantareva et. al., 2005)

The samples of B16 melanoma cells were incubated with respect to ZnPcs (1.6 µM and 2.3 µM) and the fluorescence was measured after tissue chemical extraction. The data showed the amount of dye per mg tumour mass (Fig 4). The time-dependence curves were obtained within a 6-hour follow-up period. The results showed that the maximal amounts of ZnPcs in the pigmented melanomas tissue (between 2.3-7.1 nmol mg^{-1}) as compared to the surrounding skin/ epithelial cells were reached 90 min after injection.

Considering the hydrophilic vs. hydrophobic nature of the studied ZnPcs, which were evaluated by their partitition coefficients, the uptake results showed a highest uptake in the case of an amphiphilic compound (ZnPcHe with 7.1 nmol at 90 min)). The most hydrophobic ZnPcDo and the hydrophilic ZnPcMe showed similar accumulation behaviour (2.3 nmol and 3.1 nmol). The water-soluble photosensitizer ZnPcMe showed the lowest tumour accumulation and the longest retention period (6h).

The lipophilic ZnPcDo was evaluated with low accumulation during the studied period (1-6h). The phenomenon of precipitation of a lipophilic drug under physiological condition (pH~7) can provoke an insufficient accumulation into the cells. We found that cationic ZnPcs differing in lipophilicity have specific uptake into B16 pigmented melanoma in dependence on their hydrophilic/lipophilic nature.

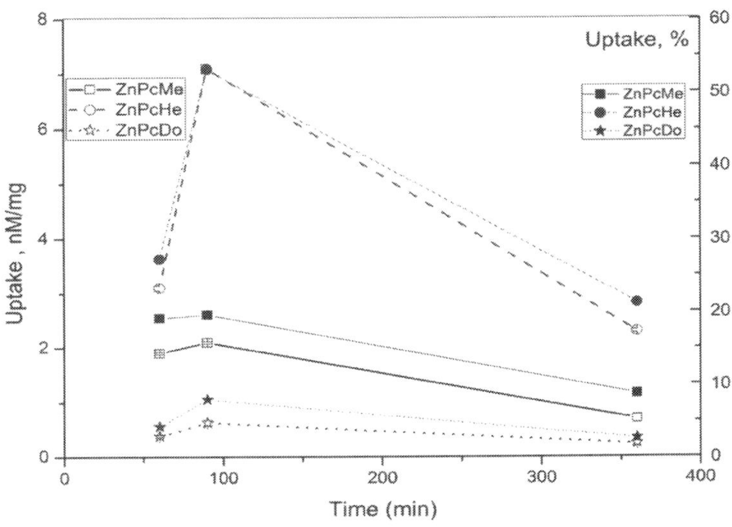

Fig. 4. Tumour uptake of cationic ZnPcs into B16 pigmented melanoma cells presented by ZnPcs concentration

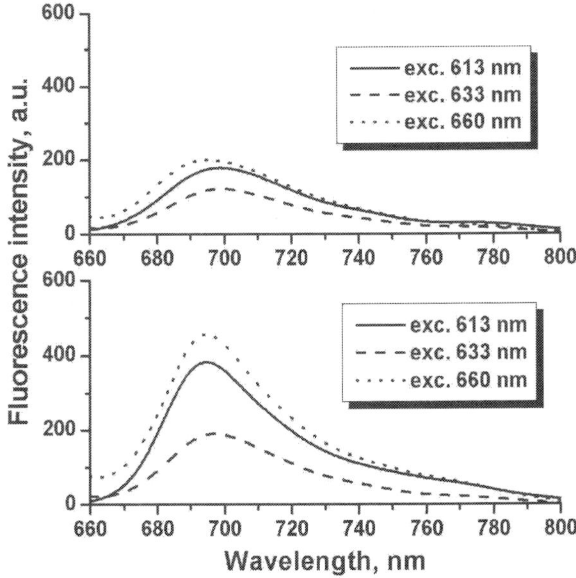

Fig. 5. In vivo fluorescence spectra of healthy (up) and tumour (down) tissues recorded 24 h after i.p. injection of ZnPcHe-DPPC liposomes. The fluorescence spectra are taken at different excitation wavelengths using an Ar-dye laser source (insets)

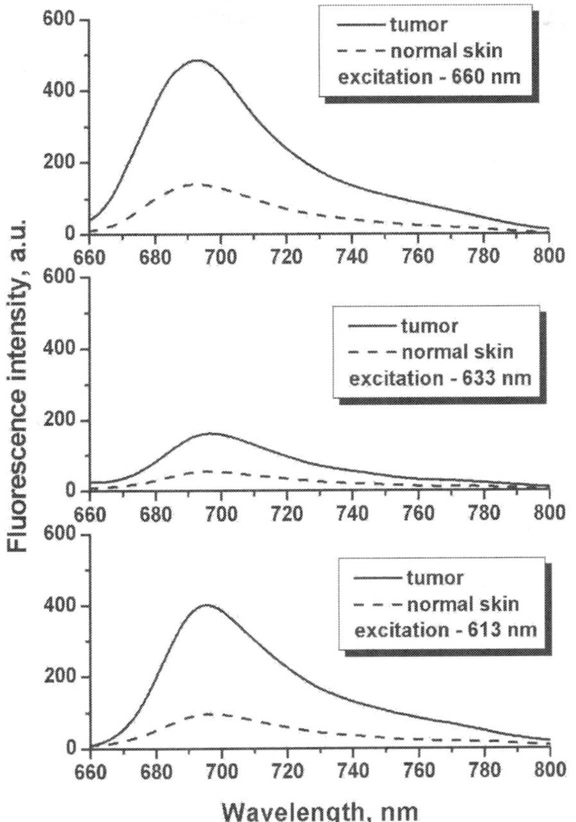

Fig. 6. Comparison of the spectral signals obtained by in vivo fluorescence detection of tumour and healthy tissues recorded 24 h after i.p. injection of ZnPcHe-DPPC liposomes, using different excitation wavelengths (Mantareva et al., 2005)

4.2 Photodiagnosis and photodynamic therapy studies on B16 pigmented melanoma

In the recent photodynamic studies, we prepared differently substituted Zn(II)-phthalocyanines (ZnPcs) to be studied as selective B16 pigmented melanoma cells agents. The hydrophobicity of ZnPcs was evaluated with respect to their selective localizing properties on a B16 tumour model. We were able to demonstrate the effective diagnosis at the early stage of development of pigmented melanoma in an in vivo experiment (Fig. 5 and Fig. 6).

The PDT response of B16 pigmented melanoma implanted on mice was compared for different generations of photosensitizers by varying the treatment parameters. The treatment of pigmented melanomas with naphthalocyanines was successful. The phototoxicity studies performed with liposome-incorporated Zn(II)-phthalocyanine (Ciba-Geigy, Switzerland) and tetrabenzamido-substituted Zn(II)-naphthalocyanine, ZnPcA synthesized for PDT studies revealed a high PDT response (Peeva et al., 1999; Soncin et al., 1998).

4.3 Light dose effects

The effectiveness for treatment of B16 pigmented melanoma of the long-wavelength absorbing benzamido-substituted naphthalocyanine (ZnNcA) was examined due to its strong absorption around 774 nm, which allowed light penetration into the pigmented tissue. It was demonstrated that the phototoxicity of ZnNcA increased as the irradiance was increased up to 380 mW cm^{-2}, which caused extensive tumour necrosis and substantial delay in the rate of tumour growth with 40 % cure rate (Michailov et al., 1997). A moderate increase of the tumour temperature above the basal value during the treatment can contribute to a better phototherapeutic effect (Fig. 7). The temperature increased above 41 °C at 440 mW.cm-2 and above the higher irradiance of 440 and 500 mW.cm^{-2} led to a lower PDT response and the possibility of hyperthermia.

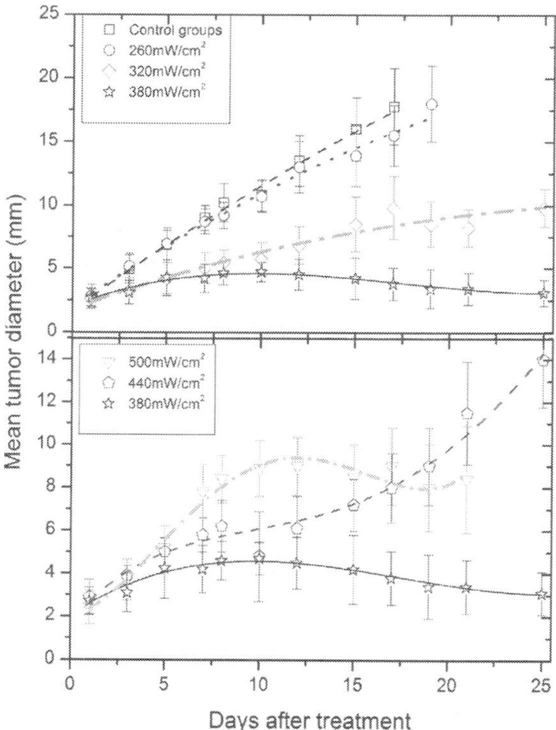

Fig. 7. PDT with ZnNcA (0.5 mg.kg^{-1} b.w.) on mice with implanted B16 pigmented melanoma as a function of the fluence (exc: 774 nm 24 h after sensitizer administration). Tumour response in mice after PDT treatment at a fluence of 360 J cm^{-2} performed 24 h after sensitizer administration (0.5 mg kg^{-1} b.w.) and 30 min after anesthesia (490 µg/g chloral hydrate). (a) Tumours exposed to 774 nm at fluences of 260, 320 and 380 mW cm^{-2}. Control groups without sensitizer and irradiation. (b) Tumors exposed to 774 nm at fluencs of 440 and 500 mW cm^{-2}. To facilitate the comparison, the PDT curve for 380 mW cm^{-2} irradiation is also given (Michailov et al., Copyright 1997, Elsevier)

5. Conclusions

Photodiagnosis and photodynamic therapy are based on the native tissue chromophores and on the exogenous photosensitizers, which are deposed preferentially into malignant tissues. Excitation with light with appropriate wavelength catalyzes the production of ROSs which induces cytotoxic effects causing irreversible photodamage to tumour tissues (Awan and Tarin, 2006; Davids and Kleemann, 2010; MacDonald, 2011; Foote, 1991). The data collected from preclinical and some clinical observations suggest that the PDT approach appears to be useful in numerous oncological malignances (Dougherty, 1992; Allison, 2006). Pigmented melanoma is one of the malignancies that are highly aggressive, while the known treatment procedures have poor prognosis. In our in vitro/ in vivo studies on B16 pigmented melanomas, we focused on the improvement of the photosensitizing agents from the group of phthalocyanines and naphthalocyanines and on the applied treatment protocols (Borisova et al., 2005; Rai et al., 2010; Brown et al., 2004). The principal factor which influences the susceptibility of pigmented melanoma to the PDT is the competition between the absorbance of melanin from B16 melanoma and the absorbance of the photosensitizing agent at the excitation wavelength. The porphyrin derivatives Photofrin and HpD have low absorbance at 630 nm where the pigmented tissue absorbs sufficiently; as a result, the PDT response of B16 pigmented melanoma was insignificant (Rai et al., 2010). The studies with photosensitizers absorbing in the far-red region, namely, phthalocyanines and especially naphthalocyanines suggested that the significant level of pigmentation is not an obstacle to applying PDT for diagnosis and therapy of highly pigmented tumours, such as B16 pigmented melanoma. The combined action of the photosensitizing process and the photoinduced hyperthermia can boost the anti-tumour effect. The optimization of the treatment modality concerning pigmented melanoma involves the photodegradation of the pigment as a first step of treatment and further application of PDT with naphthalocyanines or other far-red absorbing sensitizers.

6. Acknowledgements

The studies were supported by EC grants (G5RD-CT-2000-00372, IMPECABLE) and by the National Science Fund, Bulgaria (L 403, DO-02-112/08, DO-02-177/08).

7. References

Allison R.; Sibata C.; Downie G.; Cuenca R. (2006). A clinical review of PDT for cutaneous malignancies. *Photodiagnosis and Photodynamic Therapy* vol. 3, pp. 214-226, ISSN: 1572-1000.

Awan, M. A.; Tarin, S. A.; (2006). Review of Photodynamic therapy, *Surgeon*, Vol.4 (4), pp. 231-236. ISSN 1479-666X.

Borisova E. (2006). Fluorescence detection makes malignant melanoma diagnosis more precise and easier. *SPIE Newsroom*, DOI: 10.1117/2.1200610.0470].

Borisova E.; Nikolova E.; Troyanova P.; Avramov L. (2008a). Autofluorescence and diffuse reflectance spectroscopy of pigment disorders in human skin, *Journal on optoelectronics and advanced materials* Vol.10 No.3, pp. 717-722, ISSN 1454-4164.

Borisova E.; Troyanova P.; Pavlova P.; Avramov L. (2008b). Diagnostics of pigmented skin tumours based on laser-induced autofluorescence and diffuse reflectance spectroscopy, *Quantum Electronics* Vol. 38, No.6, pp. 597-605, ISSN 1063-7818.

Borisova, E.; Angelov, I.; Mantareva, V.; Petrova, D.; Townsend, P.; Valberg, L.; Avramov, L.; (2005). Tumor detection by exogenous fluorescent dyes using new generation photo-multiplier tubes. *Proceedings of SPIE, The International Society of Optics and Photonics*, Vol.5830, pp. 399-403. ISBN: 9780819458223.

Brown, S. B.; Brown, E. A.; Walker, I.; (2004). The present and the future role of photodynamic therapy in cancer treatment. *Lancet Oncology*, Vol.5, pp. 497-508, ISSN 1470-2045.

Busetti, A.; Soncin, M.; Jori, G.; Kenney, M. E.; Rodgers, M.A.J.; (1998). Treatment of malignant melanoma by high-peak-power 1064 nm irradiation followed by photodynamic therapy, *Photochemistry and Photobiology*, Vol.68. No.3, pp. 377-381. ISSN 1751-1097.

Chwirot B.; Chwirot S.; Redzinaski J.; Michniewicz Z. (1998). Detection of Melanomas by Digital Imaging of Spectrally Resolved Ultraviolet Light-induced Autofluorescence of Human Skin. *European Journal of Cancer*, Vol. 34, No. 11, pp. 1730-1734, ISSN 0959-8049.

Chwirot B.; Chwirot S.; Sypniewska N.; Michniewicz Z; Redzinski J.; Kurzawski G.; Ruka W. (2001). Fluorescence In Situ Detection of Human Cutaneous Melanoma: Study of Diagnostic Parameters of the Method. *Journal of Investigative Dermatology* Vol. 11, pp.1449-1451, ISSN: 0022-202X.

Davids, L. M.; Kleemann, B.; (2010). Combating melanoma: The use of photodynamic therapy as a novel, adjuvant therapeutic tool, *Cancer Treatment reviews*, ISSN 0305-7372.

Dougherty, T. J.; (1992). Photochemistry in the treatment of cancer. *Advances in Photochemistry*. Vol.17, pp. 275-311. ISSN 1934-4570.

Foote, C. S.; (1991). Definition of type I and type II photosensitized oxidation. *Journal of Photochemistry and Photobiology*, Vol.54, pp. 659-668. ISSN 1010-6030.

Ibbotson, S. H.; (2010). An overview of topical photodynamic therapy in dermatology. *Photodiagnosis and Photodynamic Therapy*, Vol.7, No.1, pp. 16-23. ISSN 1572-1000.

Kalka, K.; Merk, H.; Mukhtar, H.; (2000). Photodynamic therapy in dermatology. *Journal of the American Academy of Dermatology*, Vol.42, pp. 389-413. ISSN 0190-9622.

Kaplan M.; Borgul O.; Zakurdyaeva I.; Spichenkova I. (2008). Photodynamic therapy in combined treatment modalities of disseminated melanoma. *Photodiagnosis and Photodynamic Therapy*, Vol. 5, Suppl. 1 - Abstracts of 13th EMLA Congress ed. A. Makela, L. Gasparyan, pp. S9, ISSN: 1572-1000.

Kolarova H.; Nevrelova P.; Bajgar R.; Jirova D.; Kejlova K.; Strnad M. (2007a) In vitro photodynamic therapy on melanoma cell lines with phthalocyanines. *Toxicology in Vitro* vol. 21, pp. 249–253, ISSN 0887-2333.

Kolarova H.; Lenobel R.; Kolar P.; Strnad M. (2007b) Sensitivity of different cell lines to phototoxic effect of disulfonated chloroaluminium phthalocyanines. *Toxicology in Vitro*, vol. 21, pp.1304–1306, ISSN 0887-2333.

Kubler A. (2005) Photodynamic therapy. *Medical Laser Applications* Vol.20, pp.37-45, ISSN 1615-1615.

Leffel D.; Stetz M.; Milstone L.; Deckelbaum L. (1988). In vivo fluorescence of human skin. *Archives in Dermatology* Vol. 124, pp.1514-1518, ISSN 0003-987X.

Lohmann W.; Nilles M.; Boedeker R. (1991). In situ differentiation between nevi and malignant melanomas by fluorescence measurements. *Naturwissenschaften* Vol. 78, pp. 456-457, ISSN 0028-1042.

Lohmann W.; Paul E. (1988). In situ detection of melanomas by fluorescence measurements. *Naturwissenschaften*, Vol. 75, Issue 4, pp. 201-202, ISSN 0028-1042.

MacDonald, I. J.; Dougherty, T. J.; (2001). Basic principles of photodynamic therapy, *Journal of Porphyrines and Phthalocyanines*, Vol.5, pp.105-129. ISSN 1099-1409.

Mantareva, V.; Petrova, D.; Avramov, L.; Angelov, I.; Borisova, E.; Peeva, M.; Wöhrle, D.; (2005). Long wavelength absorbing cationic Zn(II)-phthalocyanines as fluorescent contrast agents for B16 pigmented melanoma, *Journal of Porphyrins and Phthalocyanines*, Vol.9, No.1, pp.47-53. ISSN 1088-4246.

Mantareva, V.; Shopova, M.; Spassova, G.; Wöhrle, D.; Muller, S.; Jori, G.; Ricchelli, F.; (1997). Si(IV)-methoxyethylene-glycol-naphthalocyanine: synthesis and pharmacokinetic and photosensitizing properties in different tumour models, *Journal of Photochemistry and Photobiology B: Biology*, Vol.40, pp. 258-262. ISSN 1011-1344.

Meredith P.; Riesz J. (2004). Radiative relaxation quantum yields for synthetic eumelanin. *Photochemistry and Photobiology*, Vol. 79, issue 2, pp. 211-216, ISSN 1751-1097

Michailov, N. ; Peeva, M. ; Angelov, I. ; Woehrle, D. ; Mueller, S. ; Jori, G.; Riccelli F. & Shopova, M.; (1997). Fluence rate effects on B16 pigmented melanoma. *Journal of Photochemistry and Photobiology B: Biology*, Vol.37, pp. 154-157, ISSN 1011-1344.

Nighswander-Rempel S.P.; Riesz J., Gilmore J., Meredith P. (2005). A Quantum Yield Map for Synthetic Eumelanin. *The Journal of Chemical Physics*, Vol. 123, pp. 194901-6, ISSN 1089-7690.

Peeva, M.; Shopova, M.; Stoichkova, N.; Michailov, N.; Woehrle, D.; Mueller, S.; (1999). Comparative photodynamic therapy of B16 pigmented melanoma with different generations of sensitizers, *Journal of Porphyrines and Phthalocyanines*, Vol.3, pp. 380-387. ISSN 1088-4246.

Perna G.; Frassanito M.C.; Palazzo G.; Gallone A.; Mallardi A.; Biagi P.F.; V.Capozzi (2009). Fluorescence spectroscopy of synthetic melanin in solution. *Journal of Luminescence* Vol. 129, pp. 44–49, ISSN 0022-2313.

Rai, P.; Mallidi, S.; Zheng, X.; Rahmanzadeh, R.; Mir, Y.; Elrmington, S.; Khurshid, A.; Hasan, T.; (2010). Development and applications of photo-triggered theranostic agents. *Advanced Drug Delivery Reviews*, Vol.62, pp. 1094-1124. ISSN 0169-409X.

Saczko J.; Kulbacka J.; Chwilkowska A.; Drag-Zalesinska M.; Wysocka T.; Lugovski M.; Banas T. (2005). The influence of photodynamic therapy in apoptosis in human melanoma cell line. *Folia Histochemica Cytobiologica* Vol. 43 issue 3, pp. 129–132, ISSN 1897-5631.

Shopova, M.; Woehrle, D.; Mantareva V.; & Mueller, S. (1999). Naphthalocyanine-complexes as potential photosensitizers for PDT of tumours, *Journal Biomedical Optics*, Vol.4, No.3, pp. 276-285. ISSN: 1083-3668.

Soncin, M.; Busetti, A.; Biolo, R.; Jori, G.; Kwag, G.; Li, Y.S.; Kenney, M. E.; Rodgers, M.; (1998). Photoinactivation of amelanotic and melanotic melanoma cells sensitized by axially substituted Si-naphthalocyanines, *Journal of Photochemistry and Photobiology B: Biology*, Vol.42, pp.202-210. ISSN 1011-1344.

Sounik, J.R.; Schechtman, L.A.; Rihter, B.D.; Ford, W.E.; Rodgers, M.A.J.; Kenney, M.E.; (1990) Synthesis and characterization of naphthalocyanines and phthalocyanines of use in sensitizers studies in: Photodynamic therapy: Mechanisms II, *Proceedings of SPIE, The International Society of Optics and Photonics*, Vol.1203, T.J. Dougherty and A. Katzir (eds.), 224-232. DOI: 10.1117/12.17668.

Sterenborg H.; Thomsen S.; Jacques S.; Motamedi M. (1995). In vivo autofluorescence of an unpigmented melanoma in mice. Correlation of spectroscopic properties to microscopic structure. *Melanoma Research* Vol.5 No.4, pp. 211-216, ISSN 0960-8931.

Teuchner K.; FreyerW.; Leupold D.; VolkmerA.; Birch D.; Altmeyer P.; Stucker M.; Hoffmann K. (1999). Femtosecond Two-photon Excited Fluorescence of Melanin. *Photochemistry and photobiology* Vol. 70, pp.146–151, ISSN 1751-1097.

Woehrle, D.; Mueller, S.; Shopova, M.; Mantareva, V.; Spassova, G.; Vietric, F.; Ricchellid, F.; Jori, G.; (1999). Pharmacokinetic and PDT efficacy of Bis(methyloxyethyleneoxy)silicon-phthalocyanine as function of delivery system *Journal of Photochemistry & Photobiology Biology*, Vol.50, pp. 124-128, ISSN 1011-1344.

8

Update on Current Phase III Clinical Trials in Melanoma

Amy Q. Cao[1] and Ming Yu Cao[2]
[1]Queen's University School of Medicine
[2]200 Tunney's Pasture
Canada

1. Introduction

Melanoma is the deadliest form of skin cancer and responsible for 4% of all cancer deaths and 86% of skin cancer-related deaths in the United States (Losina et al., 2007). Melanoma is caused by malignant growth of the melanocytes, which are melanin-producing cells found in the skin's epidermis, hair, and eyes. In melanoma, these cells undergo an uncontrollable cell growth that manifests in the skin, the nail bed, and sometimes although rarely in the eyes and mucous membrane (Garbe et al., 2010).

Melanomas can be classified clinically into four major classes (Table 1). Most melanomas are superficially spreading malignant melanoma. Rare melanomas include amelanotic melanoma, splitzoid melanoma, desmoplastic melanoma, malignant blue nevus, ocular melanoma, and mucosa melanoma. Melanomas usually have an initial radial growth phase followed by a vertical growth phase. The radial growth is mostly intraepidermal, and is considered preinvasive or minimally invasive. In contrast, the vertical growth is invasion

TYPE	CHARACTERISTICS	RADIAL GROWTH	VERTICAL GROWTH	PROGNOSIS
Superficially spreading malignant melanoma	Occurs at any site, frequently at the torso in males and the legs in females	Months – 2 years	Delayed	Variable
Nodular melanoma	Occurs at any site, frequently at trunk, head, neck Most rapidly growing and aggressive melanoma	Not clinically observable	Rapid	Poor (due to advance stage at diagnosis)
Lentigo maligna melanoma	Tends to occur on sun-damaged skin in the elderly, particularly at the head and neck Mostly slow growth	Years	Much delayed	Favourable
Acral lentiginous melanoma	Occurs at the palms, soles, and subungual	Months – years	Early	Poor (due to advance stage at diagnosis)

Table 1. The four major clinical classifications of melanoma (Wolff & Johnson, 2009; Duncan, 2009)

into the dermis, and allows for a higher risk of metastasis due to its proximity to blood vessels (Wolff & Johnson, 2009).

1.1 Diagnosis

Typically, melanomas are detected as changes in the skin, often in or near an already existing mole. Normal moles are round to oval in shape with a homogeneous colour, and have a distinctive border. In contrast, melanoma can present as a change in the colour, shape, or diameter of a mole, which might also be painful, bleeding, or itchy. When suspecting melanoma, lesions can be characterized by the 'ABCDE rule' (Wolff & Johnson, 2009). This is accomplished by first, determining whether there is asymmetry in the shape of the lesion by comparing one-half to the other, then by inspecting whether the border of the lesion is irregular or poorly defined, as well as if the colour is heterogeneous and varying from one area to another. Also, there is reason for suspicion if the diameter is greater than 6 mm, and if the lesion is elevated or has a history of enlargement. However, it should be noted that these rules are more sensitive than specific (Marsden et al., 2010; Wolff & Johnson, 2009). The gold standard for diagnosing melanoma continues to be histopathology from an excision biopsy. Features on the histopathology that are useful for determining the prognosis include the thickness measured by the Breslow depth, whether there is ulceration, vascular invasion, microscopic satellites, and the mitotic count (Dummer et al., 2010). Breslow method of determining the tumour thickness is the greatest single prognostic variable, and is therefore of importance when choosing treatment options (see other chapters). Ulceration also usually indicates a worst prognosis. Once the diagnosis is confirmed, melanoma staging is useful when determining the treatment options. Staging usually follows the tumour-node-metastasis (TNM) classification endorsed by the American Joint Committee on Cancer (AJCC), which evaluates the primary tumour, regional nodes, and metastases (Table 2). Recently, dermoscopy by experienced and trained physicians have shown to enhance diagnostic accuracy (Garbe et al., 2010). Additionally, a sentinel lymph node biopsy (SLNB) is often used to stage melanoma because cancer cells frequently travel to the closest lymph nodes when they first spread.

1.2 Treatment

Melanoma *in situ* is the earliest stage and is 99% curable with just surgical removal of the tumour. With increasing melanoma stages, other treatments in addition to surgery need to be considered. They include radiation therapy, chemotherapy, immunotherapy, and other interventions. Patients will often receive a combination of these treatments in more advanced melanomas (Garbe et al., 2010). Table 3 summarizes current treatment options in the United States (American Cancer Society, 2011; Kingham et al. 2010). Surgery usually is the first choice for the treatment of malignant melanoma if it is resectable. A safety margin around the border of the primary tumour is an important factors for consideration. The safety margin during excision is made in effort to avoid spread of the primary tumour to the surrounding skin. The size of the margins for optimal care is still debatable. Five trials were recently reviewed, and examined to determine whether a narrow margin, defined as 1 cm to 2 cm, had better outcome survival than a wide margin of 3 cm to 5 cm. The reviewed trials only involved those with invasive melanoma, and not melanoma *in situ*. No significant difference was found in the overall survival between the narrow or wide excision margins, although there is an estimated small increase in survival in the wide

STAGE	PRIMARY TUMOUR	REGIONAL NODES	METASTASES
0; *in situ*	Confined to the epidermis	None	None
IA	Confined to skin Tumour thickness of ≤1.0mm Without ulceration	None	None
IB	Confined to skin AND Tumour thickness of ≤1.0mm, with ulceration OR Tumour thickness of 1.01 – 2.0mm, without ulceration	None	None
IIA	Tumour thickness of 1.01 – 2.0mm, with ulceration Tumour thickness of 2.01 – 4.0mm, without ulceration	None	None
IIB	Tumour thickness of 2.01 – 4.0mm, with ulceration Tumour thickness of > 4.0mm, without ulceration	None	None
IIC	Tumour thickness of > 4.0mm, with ulceration	None	None
IIIA	Any tumour thickness, without ulceration	Micrometastases	None
IIIB	Any tumour thickness, with ulceration OR Any tumour thickness, without ulceration OR Any tumour thickness, with or without ulceration	Micrometastases Up to 3 macrometastases None, but satellite metastases and/or in-transit metastases	None
IIIC	Any tumour thickness, with ulceration OR Any tumour thickness, with or without ulceration	Up to 3 macrometastases 4 or more macrometastases or capsule transgressing lymph node metastases, or satellite and/or in-transit metastases affecting the lymph nodes	None
IV	Has spread to internal organs, beyond the nearest lymph node to other lymph nodes, or areas of skin far from original tumour	Any nodal involvement	Including distant metastases

Table 2. The TMN classification of melanoma (Balch et al., 2009)

excision group. Therefore, these trials provide insufficient evidence for defining the most favourable surgical excision margin in primary cutaneous melanoma (Sladden et al., 2010).

Unfortunately, metastatic forms of melanoma still have a high mortality rate due to its lack of response to systemic treatments. Numerous novel methods and approaches have been studied for the management of melanoma and although they were associated with increased toxicity and cost of treatment, some of the results showed potential for treatment of melanoma. Chemoimmunotherapy (or biochemotherapy), which is a combination of chemotherapy and immunotherapy, is one such approach that resulted in improvements although it still remains unclear whether it is clinically beneficial as compared to the standard chemotherapy alone. A Cochrane review found that there is currently inconclusive evidence to support the use of chemoimmunotherapy in treating metastatic malignant melanoma as trials have not shown a difference in survival rates. In addition, there is also an increase risk of toxic effects (Sasse et al., 2007).

STAGE	TREATMENT
0; *in situ*	- Surgical excision with safety margin of 0.5 cm - Use of imiquimod cream is controversial
I	- Surgical excision with safety margin of 1 cm if tumour thickness is less than 1 mm, 1 – 2 cm if tumour thickness is 1 – 2 mm - Consider a SLNB
II	- Surgical excision with safety margin of 1 – 2 cm if tumour thickness is 1 – 2 mm, 2 cm if tumour thickness is greater than 2 mm - SLNB - If tumour is greater than 4 mm thick, or lymph nodes is cancerous, adjuvant therapy with interferon is considered
III	- Surgical excision of all melanoma (safety margin as in stage II) with lymph node dissection - Adjuvant therapy with interferon - If not all melanomas are excised, consider injections of bacilli Calmette-Guerin (BCG) vaccine or interleukin-2 (IL2) - If melanoma of the limbs, consider chemotherapy with a heated solution of melphalan - Radiation therapy for the area of excised lymph nodes may be offered after surgery, especially if nodes contained cancerous cells - Consider chemotherapy, immunotherapy with cytokines, and chemoimmunotherapy
IV	- Surgical excision of tumours and metastases - Surgical excision of internal organ metastases may be possible - If surgery is not possible, may be treated with chemotherapy, immunotherapy, or radiation

Table 3. Melanoma treatments according to stage

1.3 Prevention

Melanoma is a serious disease. Although prognosis is excellent for melanoma *in situ*, it decreases with increasing stages. Thus, methods of prevention and early detection should be considered in efforts to decrease the risk of melanoma. Early detection in melanoma is a key since melanomas have a tendency to metastasize early relative to the tumour mass (Garbe et al., 2010). As incidences increases, early prevention and treatment is becoming more crucial. Ultraviolet radiation has been implicated as a major environmental factor in the pathogenesis of melanoma. Protection from skin damage by ultraviolet radiation may play an important role in the prevention of melanoma.

2. Recently published phase III clinical studies

Numerous clinical trials have attempted to find novel ways of targeting malignant melanoma, and to extend overall survival of patients. Although many clinical trials investigating melanoma have been completed, there has been a lack of real conclusive evidence to change current treatment options. A search of the recent literature was performed for the recent trials conducted on melanoma. The search was limited to only phase III clinical trials, published in English in the last five years. Due to limited space for this chapter, some of results from recent clinical studies in the field are summarized in the following section.

2.1 Monoclonal antibodies

Recently, the United States Food and Drug Administration (FDA) has approved ipilimumab (Yervoy), a fully human monoclonal antibody, as adjuvant immunotherapy for the treatment of metastatic melanoma. It is the first new drug approved for melanoma in over 13 years. Dacarbazine was approved in 1975, and interleukin-2 was approved in 1998 (U. S. Food and Drug Administration, 2011). Ipilimumab was approved by the FDA mainly based on an increase in overall survival in patients with late-stage melanoma in phase III clinical trials (Hodi et al., 2010). This is considered to be a significant improvement since there are limited options for patients with metastatic melanoma. Ipilimumab acts by inhibiting the cytotoxic T-lymphocyte associated-antigen 4 (CTLA-4). The antigen is thought to slow down or inactivate the body's immune system, and thus limiting its effect on cancerous cells. Therefore, ipilimumab may enhance the antitumour T-lymphocyte response to attack the tumours of melanoma patients (Hodi et al., 2010).

During the trial, ipilimumab was administered intravenously at 3 mg/kg of body weight, with or without a glycoprotein 100 (gp100) peptide vaccine, every 3 weeks for up to four treatments in the induction phase of the treatment. Additionally, a maintenance dose at every 12-week intervals was given in some studies (Hodi et al., 2010). It is interesting to note that the trial compared ipilimumab against an experimental vaccine, and not a placebo or standard treatment. The drug's safety and effectiveness was determined from a single international study of 676 patients, all of whom had metastatic melanoma that may have not been surgically removed, and that were refractive to other treatment methods. Since ipilumumab is a monoclonal antibody and immunogenic, side effects commonly associated with the novel compound include fatigue, diarrhea, pruritis, endocrine deficiencies, and colitis. In 12.9% of patients studied, there was severe to fatal autoimmune reactions (Hodi et al., 2010). Thus adjuvant immunotherapy with ipilimumab is approved with a Risk Evaluation and Mitigation Strategy (U. S. Food and Drug Administration, 2011). Physicians must be vigilant in detecting patients with these serious side effects.

Due to ipilimumab's effect on the immune system, it may take some time to have an effect in a melanoma patient. Thus patients with rapidly progressive metastatic melanoma may not benefit from the treatment (Hodi et al., 2010). Currently, research efforts to identify biomarkers that predict the outcome due to ipilimumab is being conducted in hopes of determining a selectively way to conduct the adjuvant therapy.

Ipilimumab was hypothesized to act through a human leukocyte antigen (HLA) independent mechanism, and thus most trials enrolled subjects into their study without regards to HLA subtype. It should be noted that the phase III trial restricted enrolment of subjects to class-I-HLA-A*0201-positive because of the use of HLA-A*0201-restricted gp100 vaccine in two of the three arms. Thus a retrospective analysis was conducted to determined whether ipilimumab could treat patients regardless of their HLA-A*0201status. The pooled efficacy and safety data were analyzed according to HLA-A*0201 status and found no difference in the overall survival using ipilimumab in advanced melanoma (Wolchok et al., 2010). However, the interpretation of the results should be made with caution because of the nature of the analysis.

2.2 Cytokines
2.2.1 Interferon alpha-2b
It is postulated that the benefits of interferon alpha-2b is dependent on the dose and duration of the treatment. A high-dose interferon alpha (IFN-α) regimen with an induction phase of maximally tolerated dosages (20 MU/m^2 per day) by intravenous (IV) therapy for the initial 4 weeks has shown prolongation of overall survival (OS) and relapse-free survival (RFS) in comparison with observation in study E1684 (Kirkwood et al., 2009). Following this study, a prospective randomized study was conducted to compare intravenous induction therapy versus a full year of high-dose interferon, with primary endpoints of RFS and OS for patients with stage IIB, IIC, and III melanoma. Treatment was initiated within 56 days of curative surgery. Patients were randomly assigned to receive IFN-α-2b 15 MU/m^2 IV for five times a week for 4 weeks (arm A) versus the same regimen followed by IFN-α-2b 10 MU (flat dose) administered subcutaneously three times a week for 48 weeks (arm B). Between 1998 and 2004, 364 patients were enrolled (353 eligible: arm A, n = 177; arm B, n = 176). At a median follow-up of 63 months (95% CI, 58.1 to 67.7), the median RFS was 24.1 months versus 27.9 months ($P = 0 .9$) and the median OS was 64.4 months versus 65.3 months ($P = 0.49$). Patients in arm B had more grade 1 to grade 2 hepatotoxicity, nausea, vomiting, alopecia, and neurologic toxicity. Thus the study concluded that there is no difference between a one month and a one year treatment in terms of relapsed-free or overall survival (Pectasides et al., 2009).

High dose interferon alpha-2b is however associated with toxic effects. To investigate whether the use of an intermediate-dose of the interferon alpha-2b improves the overall benefit-risk ratio, a study was conducted in 855 patients in Nordic countries, who had either stage IIB, IIC, or III resected cutaneous melanoma. The data did not find intermediate adjuvant therapy to be significant in improving the overall survival of patients (Hansson et al., 2011).

Low dose interferon alpha has been shown to provide patients with disease-free survival benefits in clinical trials in which patients had clinically lymph-node negative melanoma. Since there is a lack of knowledge on the proper duration of adjuvant treatment, a Dermatology Cooperative Oncology Group (DeCOG) trial investigated whether extending low dose interferon treatment from 18 months to 60 months would be beneficial. The trial found no significant clinical benefit in patients suffering from intermediate and high-risk primary melanoma (Hauschild et al., 2010).

The DeCOG trial also evaluated the patients' psychiatric symptoms before and during the adjuvant therapy. A higher pretreatment depression score, as determined by the Beck Depression Inventory and the Symptom Check List 90-Revised, was determined to be a risk factor for early drop-out during treatment. Therefore, it is recommended that pretreatment screening be completed and an interdisciplinary care be considered when treating patients (Heinze et al., 2010).

2.2.2 Pegylated interferon alpha-2b

The European Organisation for Research and Treatment of Cancer (EORTC) 18991 trial was conducted in order to compare adjuvant pegylated interferon alpha-2b therapy to observation alone in resected stage III melanoma (Eggermont et al., 2008). The purpose was to establish whether pegylated interferon alpha-2b could be tolerated over long exposures. The randomised phase III trial enrolled 1256 patients, and had stratified random assignment to either the treatment or observation group. The treatment group (n = 627) received 6 mug/kg of pegylated interferon alpha-2b per week for 8 weeks in the induction phase, then 3 mug/kg per week for 5 years in the maintenance phase of the trial. The primary endpoint was recurrence-free survival. The data were analyzed for intention-to-treat population. Results showed a statistically significant and sustained effect on recurrence-free survival with patients assigned to the adjuvant therapy. However, there was no difference found between the groups in overall survival. Additionally, patients receiving the pegylated interferon alpha-2b were at a higher risk of therapy related adverse events, such as hepatotoxicity and depression, and thus the treatment was discontinued (Eggermont et al., 2008, 2010).

In a clinical trial by the EORTC Melanoma Group, the health-related quality of life (HRQOL) effects of adjuvant therapy with pegylated interferon alpha-2b versus observation in resected stage III melanoma patients was assessed by the EORTC Quality of Life Questionnaire C30 (Bottomley et al., 2009). It found that although pegylated interferon alpha-2b lead to a sustained and significant improvement in relapse-free survival, there was no significant difference in the overall survival. Additionally, there was a negative effect on global HRQOL and selected symptoms in melanoma patients undergoing the treatment. Patients on adjuvant therapy suffered from fatigue and loss of appetite statistically more so than the observation group. The effect was also clinically significant. Additionally, they also had statistically higher rates of dyspnea, as found at 3 months and 3 years after baseline. Patients also reported statistically greater frequency of fevers, headaches, and sore muscle or stiffness as compared with the observation group. A limitation in this trial was the drop-out rate in which few patients remained in the trial at 4 and 5 years after baseline. The high drop-out rate seriously undermines the long-term HRQOL analysis (Bottomley et al., 2009).

The prognostic significance of autoantibodies in the EORTC 18991 trial was analyzed by comparing the long-term administration of pegylated interferon with observation. The study analyzed 220 patients (out of 296 that were initially tested) for anticardiolipin, antithyroglobulin, and antinuclear antibodies by an enzyme-linked immunosorbent assay at 6 months intervals throughout the trial. Results found that there was no significance in the appearance of autoantibodies as a prognostic or predictive factor for outcomes in melanoma patients treated with pegylated interferon (Bouwhuis et al., 2010).

2.2.3 Biochemotherapy with interferon alpha-2b

A randomized trial was conducted to compare the clinical benefits of biochemotherapy to adjuvant interferon-alpha-2b in high risk recurrent melanoma patients (Kim et al., 2009). This study enrolled 138 patients, and divided them into three groups: biochemotherapy (n = 71), high-dose interferon (n = 34), and intermediate-dose interferon (n = 33). The biochemotherapy group received cisplatin at 20 mg/m^2 IV on days 1–4, vinblastine at 1.5 mg/m^2 IV on days 1–4, dacarbazine at 800 mg/m^2 IV on day 1, interferon-alpha-2b at 5MU/m^2 s.c. on days 1–5 and interleukin-2 at 9MU/m^2 for a daily continuous IV infusion over days 1 - 4. The high-dose interferon-alpha-2b group received 20 MU/m^2 IV for 5 days a week for 4 weeks, followed by 10 MU/m² s.c. injection three times a week for 48 weeks. The intermediate-dose interferon-alpha-2b group received 10 MU/m² s.c. injection three times a week for 52 weeks. The study found that biochemotherapy is not more effective than adjuvant therapy with interferon. Also, there was no significant difference between the high-dose and intermediate-dose interferon in terms of RFS or OS. Thus, the findings precipitated the early termination of the trial (Kim et al., 2009).

Another study on patients with metastatic malignant melanoma was conducted in order to compare cisplatin, vinblastine, and dacarbazine (CVD) either alone or concurrently with interleukin-2 and interferon alfa-2b (biochemotherapy). The treatments were given at every 21-day intervals, for a maximum of 4 cycles, and the tumour response was measured after the second and fourth cycles, and every 3 months thereafter. The study assessed 395 patients, who were initially randomized and balanced for stratification factors and other prognostic factors. The patients receiving biochemotherapy had a slightly better response rate and longer median progression-free survival than with chemotherapy, but it did not translate to overall survival. Therefore, the study concluded that biochemotherapy should not be considered as a standard of care for metastatic melanoma due to its high toxicity and complexity in comparison to standard chemotherapy (Atkins et al., 2008).

A multicenter trial was conducted to compare the effect of polychemotherapy through a CVD regimen against CVD with interleukin-2 and interferon-alpha-2b in patients with metastatic melanoma. A total of 151 patients were randomized in the study to two arms: 75 participants on arm A which received cisplatin 30 mg/m² on days 1-3, vindesine 2.5 mg/m² on day 1 and dacarbazine 250 mg/m² on days 1-3, while 76 participants on arm B which received the same CVD scheme plus s.c. interleukin-2 on days 1-5 and 8-15 and interferon-alpha-2b on days 1-5. Both arms ran on a 21-day cycle. The study was conducted in patients with untreated metastatic melanoma, and response was assessed every two cycles. Measures included the response rate, median time to progression, and median OS. Although biochemotherapy showed a better response rate, it is not better than chemotherapy alone since it did not improve median time to progression or OS. Therefore, this study also concluded that biochemotherapy should not be a standard of care for metastatic melanoma (Bajetta et al., 2006).

In a German phase III trial, adjuvant low-dose interferon alpha-2a with or without dacarbazine, was compared to surgery alone in an observation group. A total of 444 patients who had received a complete lymph node dissection for pathologically proven regional node involvement were recruited in 42 centers (Garbe et al., 2008). Patients were either given 3 MU of interferon alpha-2a subcutaneously 3 times a week for 2 years or the same doses of interferon alpha-2a plus dacarbazine 850 mg/m² every 4-8 weeks for 2 years or observation alone. A total of 441 patients results were used in intention-to-treat analysis, and disease-free survival (DFS) and OS were assessed. Results found that patients on the low-dose interferon had significantly better DFS and OS. Additionally, results showed that dacarbazine reversed the advantageous effect of the low-dose interferon alpha-2a therapy (Garbe et al., 2008).

In a retrospective study of the EORTC 18951 biochemotherapy trial, results were used to determine whether pretreatment levels of neutrophils and leukocytes in a blood count could be independent predictors for short overall survival for stage IV melanoma patients undergoing interleukin-2 based immunotherapy. Patients in the trial were treated with dacarbazine, cisplatin, and interferon alpha, with or without interleukin-2. Results showed that elevated pretreatment neutrophils in the blood were an independent prognostic factor for short OS, while elevated leukocytes counts were prognostic for short OS and progression-free survival. Therefore, both neutrophils and leukocytes counts may be used as stratification factors in future clinical trials (Schmidt et al., 2007).

2.3 Vaccines

Vitespen is an autologous tumour-derived heat shock protein gp96 peptide complex vaccine. An open-label phase III trial was conducted in which vitespen was compared with the physician's choice for treatment for stage IV melanoma patients (Testori et al., 2008). Patients (n = 322) were randomly assigned in a 2:1 ratio to receive vitespen or physician's choice of a treatment containing one or more of the following: dacarbazine, temozolomide, interleukin-2, or complete tumor resection. Temozolomide was found to have comparable activity as dacarbazine in a systematic review. It also has the additional advantage of being an oral therapy that can cross the blood-brain barrier (Quirt et al., 2007). Patients were monitored for safety and overall survival. Patients in the vitespen vaccine group received a variable number of injections (ranging from 0 to 87, with a median of 6). Intention-to-treat analysis showed that OS in the vitespen group is not statistically different from that of the physician's choice group. Exploratory landmark analyses show that patients in the M1a and M1b substages receiving a larger number of vitespen immunizations survived longer than those receiving fewer such treatments. Such difference was not detected for substage M1c patients (Testori et al., 2008).

Another randomized phase III trial was conducted for demonstrating the superiority of autologous peptide-loaded dendritic cell (DC) vaccination over standard dacarbazine chemotherapy in stage IV melanoma patients. Dacarbazine was given at 850 mg/m^2 intravenously at a 4-week interval. DC vaccines loaded with MHC class I and II-restricted peptides were applied subcutaneously at a 2-week interval for the first five vaccinations and every 4 weeks thereafter. The primary endpoint was objective response, while secondary measures included toxicity, OS, and progression-free survival. At the time of the first interim analysis for the intention-to-treat population, 55 patients had been enrolled into the dacarbazine-arm and 53 into the DC-arm. The objective response was low (dacarbazine: 5.5%, DC: 3.8%), but not significantly different in the two arms. The Data Safety & Monitoring Board recommended closure of the study. Thus, DC vaccination could not be demonstrated to be more effective than dacarbazine in stage IV melanoma patients (Schadendorf, et al, 2006).

In the last decade, most published clinical trials on vaccines for melanoma were conducted at an early stage of development (e.g. phase I and phase II). Chi and Dudek (2011) conducted a systematic review and meta-analysis on the clinical trials pertaining to melanoma vaccine published between January 1, 1990 and May 1, 2010. The authors concluded that a melanoma-specific immune response predicted longer overall survival, although no evidence was found that vaccine therapy provides better overall disease control or overall survival compared with other treatments (Chi & Dudek, 2011).

2.4 Small molecules

Lenalidomide is a new compound under investigation for the treatment of metastatic malignant melanoma. Lenalidomide has shown effective antitumour activity against metastatic melanoma in an animal model (Payvandi et al., 2009). It was studied in a phase II/III trial that compared the efficacy and safety at two different doses (5 mg or 25 mg) for patients with relapsed metastatic melanoma refractory to previous treatments including dacarbazine, interleukin-2, interferon alpha, and temozolomide. The results did not find a difference in the overall survival, response rate, or time to progression between the different dosing regimes. In addition, treatment with lenalidomide caused an observable myelosuppression (Glaspy et al., 2009).

An international multicenter, randomized, double-blind phase II/III trial was also undertaken to assess the efficacy and safety of lenalidomide, given at 25 mg per day for 21 days in a 28-day cycle, as compared to placebo in 306 patients with refractory stage IV metastatic malignant melanoma. The treatment was continued until there was progression of disease or an unacceptable toxicity. Results found that there was no significant difference between the use of lenalidomide and placebo in overall survival of the patient. Statistically, there was also no benefit in tumour response and time to progression (Eisen et al., 2010).

Sorafenib is a multikinase inhibitor that prevents tumor cell proliferation and angiogenesis through receptor tyrosine kinases, vascular endothelial growth factor receptor (VEGFR)-1, -2, -3, and platelet derived growth factor receptor-α and -β, and the Raf/MEK/ERK pathway at the level of Raf kinase (Wilhelm, et al, 2004). A phase III trial was conducted in 270 patients to evaluate the efficacy and safety of sorafenib with carboplastin and paclitaxel in comparison with placebo and paclitaxel in advanced melanoma patients who had previously received dacarbazine or temozolomide therapy. The primary efficacy endpoint was progression-free survival, with secondary and tertiary endpoints included overall survival and incidence of best response, respectively. As the results did not find any improvements with sorafenib plus paclitaxel over placebo plus paclitaxel, the regimen cannot be recommended for second-line treatment in advanced melanoma (Hauschild et al., 2009).

2.5 Adoptive therapy using tumor infiltrating lymphocytes

Benlalam et al. (2007) reported a study on the adoptive therapy of cancer using tumour infiltrating lymphocytes (TIL) in stage III melanoma patients. The patients received autologous interleukin-2 or TIL with interleukin-2 after complete tumour resection. They discovered that infusion of Melan-A/MART-1 reactive TIL is correlated with a longer relapse-free survival for patients with HLA-A2. The authors indicate that Melan-A/MART-1 antigen may serve as a target for melanoma immunotherapy (Benlalam et al., 2007).

3. Recently completed or ongoing phase III clinical trials

In the last five years, there were over 700 registered trials using 'melanoma' as a search term in the United States clinical trial registry. When the search was refined to phase III trials that started from 2006 – 2010, inclusive, it narrowed down the field to 40 studies. Out of the 40 trials: 7 were completed, 24 were active or recruiting, 3 have an unknown status, 1 was no longer available, 2 were suspended, and 3 were terminated. The following briefly summarize some of the phase III clinical trials registered on clinicaltrials.gov in the last five years (U. S. National Institute of Health, 2011). All the following information was obtained from the registry unless otherwise noted.

3.1 Interferon-alpha

A Nordic adjuvant interferon trial was completed by giving patients an intermediate dose of interferon-alpha-2b after surgery for high risk melanoma. High risk melanoma patients were defined as T4N0M0 or TxN1-2M0. The study had three arms: control, adjuvant interferon

TRIAL	THERAPIES COMPARED (REGIMEN)		TARGET POPULATION	SAMPLE SIZE	STATUS
NCT01259934	Interferon alpha2b (1 year: s.c. 10 MU for 5 days a week for 4 weeks, with a maintenance dose of 10 MU 3 days a week for 1 year Or, 2 year: s.c. 10 MU for 5 days a week for 4 weeks, with a maintenance dose of 10 MU 3 days a week for 1 year)	Observation	High risk melanoma	855	Completed
NCT00447356	High dose interferon alpha (dosing not available)	Observation	Resected stage II and III	1420	Unknown

Table 4. Studies on interferon-alpha for the treatment of melanoma

for one year, and adjuvant interferon for two years. It aimed to study overall survival as a primary end point, as well as relapse-free survival, side effects and quality of life for secondary endpoints. The results of the study were summarized in section 2.

Another study was designed to determine the use of high dose interferon-alpha in patients with stage II or stage III melanoma that have been completely removed by surgery. The status is currently unknown since the information has not been verified recently.

3.2 Ipilimumab

TRIAL	THERAPIES COMPARED (REGIMEN)		TARGET POPULATION	SAMPLE SIZE	STATUS
NCT00324155	Ipilimumab and dacarbazine (10 mg/kg once every 3 weeks for 10 weeks, then once every 12 weeks at week 24; 850 mg/m^2 once every 3 weeks for 22 weeks, respectively)	Placebo and dacarbazine (0 mg once every 3 weeks for 10 weeks, then once every 12 weeks at week 24; 850 mg/m^2 once every 3 weeks for 22 weeks, respectively)	Unresectable stage III or IV	500	Active, but not recruiting
NCT00636168	Ipilimumab (IV 10 mg/kg four times every 21 days, then once every 12 week starting at week 24 for 3 years)	Placebo (IV 0 mg/kg four times every 21 days, then once every 12 week starting at week 24 for 3 years)	High risk stage III	950	Recruiting

Table 5. Studies on ipilimumab for the treatment of melanoma

Ipilimumab is an anti-CTLA-4 monoclonal antibody that was recently approved by the U.S. FDA for use in melanoma. Currently, a phase III trial (NCT00324155) is designed to assess the efficacy of ipilimumab at 10 mg/kg with dacarbazine against a control group of placebo and dacarbazine in patients with unresectable stage III or IV melanoma. Another ipilimumab trial (NCT00636168) is attempting to investigate whether the therapy is effective as compared to placebo for stage III melanoma patients as adjuvant immunotherapy. The primary outcome measure is recurrence free survival, and secondary outcomes include OS, distant metastases-free survival, quality of life, and adverse events of ipilimumab as compared to placebo.

3.3 Small molecules - tyrosine kinase inhibitors
3.3.1 Targeting melanoma with a BRAF V600E mutation

TRIAL	THERAPIES COMPARED (REGIMEN)		TARGET POPULATION	SAMPLE SIZE	STATUS
NCT01006980; BRIM3	RO5185426 (oral 960 mg, twice daily)	Dacarbazine (IV 1000 mg/m² every 3 weeks)	Stage IIIc or IV with BRAF V600E positive mutation	680	Recruiting
NCT01227889	GSK2118436 (oral 150 mg, twice daily)	Dacarbazine (IV 1000 mg/m² every 3 weeks)	Stage III and IV with BRAF mutation-positive tumour	200	Recruiting
NCT01245062	GSK1120212 (dosing not available)	Chemotherapy (dacarbazine or paclitaxel; dosing not available)	Stage IIIc and IV with BRAF mutation-positive tumour	297	Recruiting

Table 6. Studies on compounds targeting melanoma with BRAF mutations

BRAF belongs to the RAF family of protein kinases. The BRAF V600 mutation is seen in as high as 60% of melanoma patients. Small molecules RO5185426, GSK2118436 and GSK1120212 are developed to inhibit the RAS/RAF/MEK/ERK signalling system, and thus inhibit cellular growth of melanoma. These molecules are currently in clinical trials to assess their efficacy.
RO5185426 is being studied for efficacy, safety, and tolerability as compared to dacarbazine in previously untreated patients with unresectable stage IIIC or stage IV melanoma with BRAF V600E mutation. This is a randomized, open-label study using overall survival and progression-free survival as a primary outcome. The participants will be followed for approximately three years.
An randomized trial is comparing the efficacy, safety, and tolerability of the oral agent GSK2118436, a BRAF inhibitor, against standard chemotherapy. It is conducted in patients with BRAF mutant-positive tumours in stage IIIc or stage IV malignant cutaneous melanoma. Subjects will be followed for two years to determine the progression-free survival. Secondary endpoints include OS, rate of treatment, overall response rate, duration of response, and validation of the BRAF mutation assay. This is another study trying to determine whether an agent could stop or slow melanoma progression in BRAF V600 mutant patients by altering the MAP kinase pathway.
Study NCT00796445 is an open-label randomized trial comparing the single agent GSK1120212 (a MEK inhibitor) against standard chemotherapy, in patients with BRAF mutant-positive tumours in stage IIIc or stage IV malignant cutaneous melanoma. The study intends to measure progression free survival of patients.

3.3.2 Targeting melanoma with a c-Kit mutation
Nilotinib (AMNN107) is a selective *BCR-ABL* inhibitor. Currently, a phase III trial also known as the TEAM (Tasigna Efficacy in Advanced Melanoma) trial is recruiting

TRIAL	THERAPIES COMPARED (REGIMEN)		TARGET POPULATION	SAMPLE SIZE	STATUS
NCT01028222; TEAM	Nilotinib (dosing not available)	Dacarbazine (dosing not available)	Ureseactable Stage III, and IV with c-Kit mutation	120	Recruiting
NCT01280565	Masitinib (7.5 mg/kg perday)	Dacarbazine (IV 1000 mg/m² once every three days)	Unresectable stage IIIb or IIIc, or IV with mutation at juxta membrane domain of c-Kit	200	Recruiting

Table 7. Studies on compounds targeting melanoma with c-Kit mutations

metastastic and/or inoperative melanoma patients that also have a c-Kit mutation for the study. This interventional study will be compared against dacarbazine, and is intended to have crossover assignment. The primary outcome measures will be progression free survival.

Mastinib is another novel tyrosine kinase inhibitor that has been implicated in pre-clinical trial results for the treatment of advanced melanoma patients with a c-Kit juxtamembrane mutation. It is currently undergoing a prospective randomized trial for safety and efficacy in stage III and stage IV melanoma patients with a mutation in the juxtamembrane domain of c-Kit.

3.4 Treatment for choroidal melanoma

TRIAL	THERAPIES COMPARED		TARGET POPULATION	SAMPLE SIZE	STATUS
NCT00680225	Ranibizumab with Transpupillary Thermotherapy (TTT) - Indocyanine Green (ICG) based photodynamic therapy (PDT) (0.5 mg ranibizumab once a month for 6 months, TTT-ICG once or twice a month starting at month 2)	Not applicable	Choroidal melanoma	10	Active, but not recruiting
NCT00811200; TORR	Ranibizumab (intravitreal injections of 0.5 mg, three times for a month) or triamcinolone acetonide (intravitreal injection of 4.0 mg)	Placebo	Choroidal melanoma	220	Not yet recruiting

Table 8. Studies on choroidal melanoma treatments

A currently active study is undertaken to study the safety and tolerability of intravitreal injection of ranibizumab combined with Transpupillary Thermotherapy (TTT) - Indocyanine Green (ICG) based photodynamic therapy (PDT) for use as adjuvant treatment in choroidal melanoma. The primary outcome is reduction in tumour size.

Another study plans to research the change in visual acuity after treatment with ranibizumab or triamcinolone acetonide in patients with radiation retinopathy after irradiation of choroidal melanoma. This is important as many patients lose visual acuity after treatment of uveal melanoma using radiation therapy and TTT because of the radiation retinopathy. This study postulated a decrease in such complication with administration of ranibizumab or triamcinolone acetonide.

3.5 Vaccines

TRIAL	THERAPIES COMPARED (REGIMEN)		TARGET POPULATION	SAMPLE SIZE	STATUS
NCT00477906	M-Vax with BCG, cyclophosphamide, and IL2 (M-Vax vaccine: intradermal injection of 4 to 20 million cells, weekly for 7 weeks, with a booster at month 6; cyclophosphamide at 300 mg/m²; IL2 at 3 MU/m² for 5 days with a 16-day rest period)	Placebo vaccine with BCG, cyclophosphamide, and IL2 (placebo vaccine: intradermal injection of 4 to 20 million cells, weekly for 7 weeks, with a booster at month 6; cyclophosphamide at 300 mg/m²; IL2 at 3 MU/m² for 5 days with a 16-day rest)	Stage IV	387	Suspended
NCT00395070	Allovectin-7 (intralesional injection at 2 mg, weekly for 6 consecutive weeks in a 8-week cycle)	Dacarbazine (IV 1000 mg/m² for one hour every 28 days) or temozolomide (oral 150 – 200 mg/m2 daily for five consecutive days in 28-day cycle)	Recurrent stage III or IV	375	Active, but not recruiting
NCT00769704	OncoVex GM-CSF (4 ml of 10⁸ pfu/ml per injection)	GM-CSF (s.c. 125 µg/m² for 14 days in 28-day cycle)	Unresectable Stage IIIb, IIIc, and IV	430	Recruiting

Table 9. Studies on vaccines for the treatment of melanoma

The M-Vax vaccine is an autologous hapten (dinitrophenyl) modified melanoma vaccine derived from a patients' own cancer cells. In previous studies, the vaccine was shown to be able to stimulate the immune system of the patient to react against the melanoma. This study was designed to see whether the vaccine, with administration of low dose interleukin-2 to increase effectiveness, could shrink stage IV melanomas. The vaccine is being studied for best overall anti-tumour response and percent of patients' survival at two years as the primary endpoint, and for safety as a secondary endpoint. Eligible participants must have at least one melanoma tumour that can be resected to be made into a vaccine, and have stage IV metastatic melanoma of the lung and/or soft tissues.

OncoVex GM-CSF is an oncolytic vaccine that contains oncolytic herpes simplex type 1 virus encoding granulocyte macrophage colony-stimulating factor (GM-CSF) and has shown durable complete remission in melanoma patients in phase II clinical trial. The product has commenced phase III clinical trials for metastatic melanoma. The Onco Vex (GM-CSF)

Pivotal Trial in Melanoma (OPTIM) trial is a phase III study on the effects of the vaccine for the treatment of unresectable stage III or stage IV melanoma. (Kaufman & Bines, 2010).

Allovectin-7® is a plasmid-based vaccine expressing two genes (HLA-B7 and β2 microglobulin) that together form an MHC class-1 complex. The product is claimed to train the immune system (both innate and adaptive) to destroy tumour cells. The minimum treatment time for patients is 16 weeks, and involves weekly injections. The progression free survival, as well as the safety and tolerability of the product will be compared to that of dacarbazine.

3.6 Antisense oligonucleotides

TRIAL	THERAPIES COMPARED (REGIMEN)		TARGET POPULATION	SAMPLE SIZE	STATUS
NCT00518895; AGENDA	Genasense and dacarbazine (IV: Genasense at 7 mg/kg per day for 5 days in a 21-day cycle, with dacarbazine at 1000 mg/m² for 1 hour after Genasense, for up to 8 cycles)	Placebo and dacarbazine (IV: 0.9% sodium chloride at 7 mg/kg per day for 5 days in a 21-day cycle, with dacarbazine at 1000 mg/m² for 1 hour after placebo, for up to 8 cycles)	Unresectable or stage IV and low LDH	300	Unknown

Table 10. Studies on antisense oligonucleotides for the treatment of melanoma

Genasense is oblimersen sodium, which is a Bcl-2 antisense oligonucleotide that is currently being studied for use in advanced melanoma. Genasense with dacarbazine as compared to placebo and dacarbazine is being compared in patients that have never received chemotherapy treatment and have a low baseline LDH. The primary endpoints are progression-free survival and overall survival. The secondary endpoints are response rate, durable response rate, duration of response, and safety. The estimated enrollment was 300 patients with unresectable or stage IV and low LDH. Its current status is unknown as the information has not been updated recently.

3.7 Other small molecules

The study on ABI-007, which is a new preparation of paclitaxel (a mitotic inhibitor), is being conducted to determine its activity, safety, and tolerability in comparison to dacarbazine. This study is limited to patients that have metastatic melanoma, and were not previously treated with chemotherapy. ABI-007 contains the same medication as Abrazane, a chemotherapeutic agent approved by the FDA for metastatic breast cancer.

An uncontrolled prospective study is currently studying the effects of imiquimod in patients who received surgical excision for lentigo maligna or lentigo maligna melanoma. Imiquimod cream contains an imidazoquinoline (a class of compounds first synthesized in 1980) as the active ingredient. The imiquimod cream treatment starts 6 weeks post-surgery and will last up to 12 weeks. The cream is to be applied once daily for three times per week and after 2 weeks of treatment, may be increased to five times per week if there is no or minor inflammation. If no or little inflammation is detected at 4 weeks, the treatment will become a daily application. Patients will be followed up to five years for any recurrence of disease.

TRIAL	THERAPIES COMPARED (REGIMEN)		TARGET POPULATION	SAMPLE SIZE	STATUS
NCT00864253	ABI-007 (IV at 150 mg/m^2 at day 1, 8, and 15 of 4 week cycle)	Dacarbazine (IV at 1000 mg/m^2 every 21 days)	Stage IV	514	Recruiting
NCT01088737 (non-randomized)	Imiquimod (5% cream applied once daily, three times per week)		Lantigo maligna or lantigo maligna melanoma	60	Recruiting
NCT01264874; MelaViD	Vitamin D3 (100000 IU every 50 days for 3 years)	Placebo (matched placebo)	Resected stage II	878	Not yet recruiting
NCT00522834; SYMMETRY	Elesclomol and paclitaxel (IV at213 mg/m^2; 80 mg/m^2 for once a week for 3 weeks in a 4-week cycle, respectively)	Paclitaxel (IV at 80 mg/m^2 once a week for 3 weeks in a 4-week cycle)	Stage IV	630	Terminated
NCT01006252; SUMMIT-1	Tasisulam (IV individualized dose at day 1 of 28-day cycle)	Paclitaxel (IV at 80 mg/m^2 at day 1, 8,15 of 28-day cycle)	Stage IV	323	Terminated
NCT00779714; ChemoSensMM	Paclitaxel and cisplatin (200 mg/m^2; 50 mg/ m^2 on day 1 of a 21 day cycle, respectively) Or treosulfan and cytarabine (2500 mg/m^2 on day 2; 100 mg/ m^2 on day 1to 3 of a 21 day cycle, respectively)	Dacarbazine (1000 mg/m^2 on day 1 of a 21 day cycle)	Stage IV	360	Recruiting

Table 11. Studies on other small molecules for treatment of melanoma

The European Institute of Oncology is currently investigating vitamin D3 (cholecalciferol) supplementation as compared to placebo in a double blind trial for its effects in the recurrence of resected stage II melanoma patients. This study will determine whether vitamin D can be used as a preventative and therapeutic cancer agent.

Eclesclomol is a synthesized chemical entity that induced the oxidative stress response of cells. The double blind trial was designed to assess the efficacy of Elesclomol with paclitaxel in progression free survival in stage IV melanoma patients who have never received chemotherapy. The study was terminated. The reason for the termination is unknown.

Trials on Tasisulam as compared to paclitaxel have also been terminated for fear of greater mortality risks with the experimental drug. The study was designed to study the effect of Tasisulam on overall survival in metastatic melanoma patients.

Dacarbazine is the standard chemotherapy offered to melanoma patients for stage IV melanoma as other therapies have yet been proven more effective in a randomized clinical trial. A currently recruiting trial is attempting to establish the efficacy of an individualized combination chemotherapy that is sensitivity-directed. The combination chemotherapy being studied in stage IV melanoma patients are either paclitaxel with cisplatin, or treosulfan with cytarabine. The study also aims at determining whether an individual chemosensitivity index can be used as a prognostic biomarker for chemotherapy. The primary outcome measure is overall survival.

3.8 Surgery and radiotherapy

Table 12 lists some clinical trials on surgery and radiotherapy for melanoma described below.

A currently active study is trying to investigate the effect sentinel lymph node dissection following a wide surgical excision on patients with cutaneous invasive melanoma. The trial has three arms: surgical excision only, surgical excision with SLNB, and surgical excision with SLNB and complete lymph node biopsy. The last of which will be given offered to subjects that have a positive sentinel lymph node detected. The research will determine if surgical resection with intraoperative lymphatic mapping and SLNB prolongs overall survival of subjects as compared to receiving only surgical resection. Patients will be followed for 10 years to determine the OS, as well as the disease-free survival as a secondary outcome measure.

A currently active study by the Trans-Tasman Radiation Oncology Group (TROG) is trying to determine the effect of adjuvant radiotherapy for patients that have resected melanoma involving the lymph nodes, and that are at a high risk of having a recurrence of the disease. The trial intends to determine whether radiotherapy will result in adequate locoregional control of the disease, with secondary outcomes including disease-free survival, overall survival, toxicity, and quality of life. The stage III melanoma patients will be divided into two arms: one who will receive immediate radiotherapy after surgical resection, and one who will be observed with a delay offer of radiotherapy.

In another TROG study, patients that have received a surgical intervention for melanoma and show histological features of neurotropism will be assessed for efficacy of radiation therapy as compared to observation. Neurotropism have been shown in uncontrolled studies to result in a higher risk of local reoccurrence of the disease. The radiation received will encompass the surgical bed with a margin, and starts three month after the surgery. The patient population studied is limited to neurotropic melanoma of the head and neck. The primary outcome will measure time to local relapse for five years, with secondary outcomes including relapse free survival, overall survival, time to relapse, cancer specific survival, patterns of relapse, and toxicity. Patients in the observational group will be offered radiotherapy if there is recurrence of the disease.

Stage IV melanoma is difficult to treat, despite all the research on the subject. A surgical intervention is effective in certain population with solitary metastases, but not in patients with multiple metastases. Currently, a trial is attempting to establish a standardized initial approach for stage IV melanoma patients in hopes of prolonging survival and augment their quality of life. Medical therapy is currently the favoured approach as to prevent numerous patients from undergoing unnecessary surgery for what may turn into a rapidly invasive melanoma with occult metastases at multiple sites. Patients in the trial will be divided into three arms: one that receives a surgical intervention alone, one that receives a surgical intervention and the bacillus Calmette-Guerin (BCG) vaccine as adjuvant immunotherapy, and one that receives best medical therapy. Patients receiving the BCG will receive a dose based on their pre-study tuberculin-reactivity with those that have a greater or equal to 10 mm reactivity receiving half the standard dose of BCG, and those with greater or equal to 20 mm receiving a quarter of the standard BCG dose. The last group will be treated at the discretion of their medical oncologist and surgeons, and will not initially receive a surgical intervention. The treatment they receive can range from standard treatment to experimental

TRIAL	THERAPIES COMPARED		TARGET POPULATION	SAMPLE SIZE	STATUS
NCT00275496	Wide excision, sentinel lymph node dissection, and potential complete lymph node dissection	Wide excision of primary melanoma	Melanoma	2001	Active, but not recruiting
NCT00287196	Radiotherapy (48 Gy at five fractions per week for twenty fractions, for a maximum of 30 days of treatment time)	Observation, with delayed radiotherapy (48 Gy at five fractions per week for twenty fractions, for a maximum of 30 days of treatment time)	Melanoma involving lymph nodes	236	Active, but not recruiting
NCT00975520	Surgery and radiation therapy (48 Gy in twenty fractions over 4 weeks)	Observation after surgery	Completely resected primary melanoma with neurotropism	100	Recruiting
NCT01013623	Surgery, or surgery with 2 adjuvant doses of bacillus Calmette-Guerin (BCG given four weeks after surgery: eight separate intradermal injections, dosing determined by pre-study tuberculin-reactivity, with two doses given two weeks apart)	Best medical therapy	Resectable stage IV	399	Recruiting
NCT00297895	Completion lymphadenectomy	Observation with nodal ultrasound	Molecular or histopathologic al evidence of metastases in sentinel node	1925	Recruiting

Table 12. Studies on surgery and radiotherapy for the treatment of melanoma

therapy in clinical trial. The subjects will be followed for their lifespan to determine overall survival. The study will also measure time to progression of metastatic sites, melanoma-specific survival, and time to development of new metastatic disease sites.

In another study on sentinel lymph node biopsy, melanoma patients that are sentinel node positive will be studied for melanoma-specific survival after receiving a complete lymphadenectomy in comparison with monitoring by nodal ultrasound. Subjects enrolled need to demonstrate either molecular or histopathological evidence of metastases in the sentinel lymph node, and will be followed for ten years. The observation group that receives monitoring by ultrasound will receive delayed complete lymphadanectomy if there is recurrence of disease. The completion lymphadenectomy involved complete dissection of the lymph nodes of the positive lymph node basin.

4. Conclusion

Melanoma is the deadliest form of skin cancer. Melanoma *in situ* is the earliest stage and is 99% curable with just surgical removal of the tumour. With increasing melanoma stages, the prognosis of melanoma becomes worse and the mortality rate increases. Although many trials have been conducted, there has been a lack of real conclusive evidence for any major change to current treatment options based on published results. Many current clinical trials at the late stage of development are now ongoing in order to find novel ways of targeting malignant melanoma, and to extend overall survival of patients. These trials will provide additional information on the treatment of melanoma and may potentially lead to the development of newer, more effective therapies.

5. Acknowledgment

This work received no specific grant from any funding agency in the public, commercial, or not-for-profit sectors. All information is based on published literature and information in the public domain. Due to the limited space in the chapter, the authors regret that not all the interesting papers and information on melanoma clinical trials are cited.

6. References

American Cancer Society. (April 2011). Treatment of melanoma by stage, In: *American Cancer Society*, 28.4.2011, Available from http://www.cancer.org/Cancer/SkinCancer-Melanoma/DetailedGuide/melanoma-skin-cancer-treating-by-stage

Atkins, M., Hsu, J., Lee, S., Cohen, G., Flaherty, L., Sosman, J., Sondak, V., Kirkwood, J., & Eastern Cooperative Oncology Group. (2008). Phase III trial comparing concurrent biochemotherapy with cisplatin, vinblastine, dacarbazine, interleukin-2, and interferon alfa-2b with cisplatin, vinblastine, and dacarbazine alone in patients with metastatic malignant melanoma (E3695): a trial coordinated by the Eastern Cooperative Oncology Group. *Journal of Clinical Oncology*, Vol.26, No.35, (December 2008), pp. 5748-5754, ISSN 0732-183X

Balch, C., Gershenwald, J., Soong, S., Thompson, J., Atkins, M., Byrd, D., Buzaid, A., Cochran, A., Coit, D., Ding, S., Eggermont, A., Flaherty, K., Gimotty, P., Kirkwood, J., McMasters, K., Mihm, M., Morton, D., Ross, M., Sober, A., & Sondak, V. (2009).

Final version of 2009 AJCC melanoma staging and classification. *Journal of Clinical Oncology*, Vol.27, No.36, (December 2009), pp. 6199-6206, ISSN 0732-183X

Bajetta, E., Del Vecchio, M., Nova, P., Fusi, A., Daponte, A., Sertoli, M., Queirolo, P., Taveggia, P., Bernengo, M., Legha, S., Formisano, B., & Cascinelli, N. (2006). Multicenter phase III randomized trial of polychemotherapy (CVD regimen) versus the same chemotherapy (CT) plus subcutaneous interleukin-2 and interferon-alpha2b in metastatic melanoma. *Annals of Oncology*, Vol.17, No.4, (April 2006), pp. 571-577, ISSN 0923-7534

Benlalam, H., Vignard V., Khammari, A., Bonnin, A., Godet, Y., Pandolfino, M., Jotereau, F., Dreno, B., & Labarrière N. (2007). Infusion of Melan-A/Mart-1 specific tumor-infiltrating lymphocytes enhanced relapse-free survival of melanoma patients. *Cancer Immunology and Immunotherapy*, Vol.56, No.4, (April 2007), pp. 515-526, ISSN 0340-7004

Bottomley, A., Coens, C., Suciu, S., Santinami, M., Kruit, W., Testori, A., Marsden, J., Punt, C., Salès, F., Gore, M., Mackie, R., Kusic, Z., Dummer, R., Patel, P., Schadendorf, D., Spatz, A., Keilholz, U., & Eggermont, A. (2009). Adjuvant therapy with pegylated interferon alfa-2b versus observation in resected stage III melanoma: a phase III randomized controlled trial of health-related quality of life and symptoms by the European Organisation for Research and Treatment of Cancer Melanoma Group. *Journal of Clinical Oncology*, Vol.27, No.18, (June 2009), pp. 2916-2923, ISSN 0732-183X

Bouwhuis, M., Suciu, S., Testori, A., Kruit, W., Salès, F., Patel, P., Punt, C., Santinami, M., Spatz, A., Ten Hagen, T., & Eggermont, A. (2010). Phase III trial comparing adjuvant treatment with pegylated interferon alfa-2b versus observation: prognostic significance of autoantibodies – EORTC 18991. *Journal of Clinical Oncology*, Vol. 28, No.14, (May 2010), pp. 2460 – 2466, ISSN 0732-183X

Chi, M., & Dudek, A. (2011). Vaccine therapy for metastatic melanoma: systematic review and meta-analysis of clinical trials. *Melanoma Research*, Vol.21, No. 3 (June 2011), pp. 165-74, ISSN: 0960-8931

Dummer, R., Hauschild, A., Guggenheim, M., Jost, L., & Pentheroudakis, G. (2010). Melanoma: ESMO clinical practice guidelines for diagnosis, treatment and follow-up. *Annals of Oncology*, Vol.21, Supp.5, (May 2010), pp.v194-197, ISSN 0923-7534

Duncan, L. (2009). The classification of cutaneous melanoma. *Hematology/Oncology Clinics of North Americal*, Vol.23, No.3, (June 2009), pp. 501 – 513, ISSN 0889-8588

Eggermont, A., Bouwhuis, M., Kruit, W., Testori, A., ten Hagen, T., Yver, A., & Xu, C. (2010). Serum concentrations of pegylated interferon alpha-2b in patients with resected stage III melanoma receiving adjuvant pegylated interferon alpha-2b in a randomized phase III trial (EORTC 18991). *Cancer Chemotherapy and Pharmacology*, Vol.65, No.4, (March 2010), pp. 671-677, ISSN 0344-5704

Eggermont, A., Suciu, S, Santinami, M., Testori, A., Kruit, W., Marsden, J., Punt, C., Salès, F., Gore, M., Mackie, R., Kusic, Z., Dummer, R., Hauschild, A., Musat, E., Spatz, A., Keilholz, U, & EORTC Melanoma Group. (2008). Adjuvant therapy with pegylated interferon alfa-2b versus observation alone in resected stage III melanoma: final results of EORTC 18991, a randomised phase III trial. *The Lancet*, Vol. 372, No.9633, pp. 117-126, ISSN 0140-6736

Eisen, T., Trefzer, U., Hamilton, A., Hersey, P., Millward, M., Knight, R., Jungnelius, J., & Glaspy, J. (2010). Results of a multicenter, randomized, double-blind phase 2/3 study of lenalidomide in the treatment of pretreated relapsed or refractory metastatic malignant melanoma. *Cancer*, Vol.116, No.1, (January 2010), pp. 146-54, ISSN 1097-0142

Garbe, C., Peris, K., Hauschild, A., Saiag, P., Middleton, M., Spatz, A., Grob, J., Malvehy, J., Newton-Bishop, J., Stratigos, A., Pehamberger, H., & Eggermont, A. (2010). Diagnosis and treatment of melanoma: European consensus-based interdisciplinary guideline. *European Journal of Cancer*, Vol.46, No.2, (January 2010), pp.270-283, ISSN 0959-8049

Garbe, C., Radny, P., Linse, R., Dummer, R., Gutzmer, R., Ulrich, J., Stadler, R., Weichenthal, M., Eigentler, T., Ellwanger, U., & Hauschild, A. (2008). Adjuvant low-dose interferon {alpha}2a with or without dacarbazine compared with surgery alone: a prospective-randomized phase III DeCOG trial in melanoma patients with regional lymph node metastasis. *Annals of Oncology*, Vol.19, No.6, (June 2008), pp. 1195-1201, ISSN 0923-753

Garbe, C., Terheyden, P., Keilholz, U., Kölbl, O., & Hauschild, A. (2008b). Treatment of mmelanoma. *Deutsches Ärzteblatt International*, Vol.105, No.49, (December 2008), pp.845-851, ISSN 1866-0452

Glaspy, J., Atkins, M., Richards, J., Agarwala, S., O'Day, S., Knight, R., Jungnelius, J., & Bedikian, A. (2009). Results of a multicenter, randomized, double-blind, dose-evaluating phase 2/3 study of lenalidomide in the treatment of metastatic malignant melanoma. *Cancer*, Vol.115, No.22, (November 2009), pp. 5228-5236, ISSN 1097-0142

Green, A., Williams, G., Logan, V., & Strutton, G. (2011). Reduced melanoma after regular sunscreen use: randomized trial follow-up. *Journal of Clinical Oncology*, Vol.29, No.3, (January 2011), pp. 257-263, ISSN 0732-183X

Hansson, J., Aamdal, S., Bastholt, L., Brandberg, Y., Hernberg, M., Nilsson, B., Stierner, U., von der Maase, H., & Nordic Melanoma Cooperative Group. (2011). Two different durations of adjuvant therapy with intermediate-dose interferon alfa-2b in patients with high-risk melanoma (Nordic IFN trial): a randomised phase 3 trial. *The Lancet Oncology*, Vol.12, No.2, (February 2011), pp. 144-152, ISSN 1470-2045

Hauschild, A., Agarwala, S., Trefzer, U., Hogg, D., Robert, C., Hersey, P., Eggermont, A., Grabbe, S. Gonzalez, R., Gille, J., Peschel, C., Schadendorf, D., Garbe, C., O'Day, S., Daud, A., White, J., Xia, C., Patel, K., Kirkwood, J., & Keilholz, U. (2009). Results of a phase III, randomized, placebo-controlled study of sorafenib in combination with carboplatin paclitaxel as a second-line treatment in patients with unresectable stage III or stage IV melanoma. *Journal of Clinical Oncology*, Vol.27, No.17, (June 2009), pp. 2823-2830, ISSN 0732-183X

Hauschild, A., Weichenthal, M., Rass, K., Linse, R., Berking, C., Böttjer, J., Vogt, T., Spieth, K., Eigentler, T., Brockmeyer, N., Stein, A., Näher, H., Scadendorf, D., Morh, P., Kaatz, M., Tronnier, M., Hein, R., Schuler, G., Egberts, F., & Garbe, C. (2010). Efficacy of low-dose interferon {alpha}2a 18 versus 60 months of treatment in patients with primary melanoma of >= 1.5 mm tumour thickness: results of a randomized phase III DeCOG trial. *Journal of Clinical Oncology*, Vol.28, No.5, (February 2010), pp. 841-846, ISSN ISSN 0732-183X

Heinze, S., Egberts, F., Rötzer, S., Volkenandt, M., Tilgen, W., Linse, R., Boettjer, J., Vogt, T., Spieth, K., Eigentler, T., Brockmeyer, N., Hinzpeter, A., Hauschild, A., & Schaefer, M. (2010) Depressive mood changes and psychiatric symptoms during 12-month low-dose interferon-alpha treatment in patients with malignant melanoma: results from the multicenter DeCOG trial. *Journal of Immunotherapy*, Vol.33, No.1, pp. 106-114, ISSN 1524-9557

Hodi, F., O'Day, S., McDermott, D., Weber, R., Sosman, J., Haanen, J., Gonzalez, R., Robert, C., Schadendorf, D., Hassel, J., Akerley, W., van den Eertwegh, A., Lutzky, J., Lorigan, P., Vaubel, J., Linette, G., Hogg, D., Ottensmeier, C., Lebbé, C., Peschel, C., Quirt, I., Clark, J., Wolchok, J., Weber, J., Tian, J., Yellin, M., Nichol, G., Hoos, A., & Urba, W. (2010). Improved survival with ipilimumab in patients with metastatic melanoma. *The New England Journal of Medicine*, Vol.363, No.8, (August 2010), pp. 711-723, ISSN 0028-4793

Kaufman, H., & Bines, S. (2010). OPTIM trial: a phase III trial of an oncolytic herpes virus encoding GM-CSF for unresectable stage III or IV melanoma. *Future of Oncology*, Vol.6, No.6, (June 2010), pp. 941-949, ISSN 1479-6694

Kim, K., Legha, S., Gonzalez, R., Anderson, C., Johnson, M., Liu, P., Papadopoulos, N., Eton, O., Plager, C., Buzaid, A., Prieto, V., Hwu, W., Frost, A., Alvarado, G., Hwu, P., Ross, M., Gershenwald, J., Lee, J., Mansfield, P., Benjamin, R., & Bedikian, A. (2009). A randomized phase III trial of biochemotherapy versus interferon-alpha-2b for adjuvant therapy in patients at high risk for melanoma recurrence. *Melanoma Research*, Vol. 19, No.1, (February 2009), pp. 42-49, ISSN: 0960-8931

Kirkwood, J., Strawderman, M., Ernstoff, M., Smith, T., Borden, E., & Blum, R. (1996). Interferon alfa-2b adjuvant therapy of high-risk resected cutaneous melanoma: the Eastern Cooperative Oncology Group Trial EST 1684. *Journal of Clinical Oncology*, Vol.14, No.1, (January 1996), pp. 7-17, ISSN 0732-183X

Kingham, T., Karakousis, G., & Ariyan, C. (2010). Randomized clinical trials in melanoma. *Surgical Oncology Clinics of North America*, Vol.19, No.1, (January 2010), pp. 13-31, ISSN 1055-3207

Losina, E., Walensky, R.., Geller, A., Beddingfield, F., Wolf, L., Gilchrest, B., & Freedberg, K. (2007). Visual screening for malignant melanoma: a cost-effectiveness analysis. *Archives of Dermatology*, Vol.143, No.1, (January 2007), pp. 21-28, ISSN 0003-987X

Marsden, J., Newton-Bishop, J., Burrows, L., Cook, L., Cook, M., Corrie, P., Cox, N., Gore, M., Lorigan, P., MacKie, R., Nathan, P., Peach, H., Powell, B., & Walker C. (2010). Revised U.K. guidelines for the management of cutaneous melanoma 2010. *British Journal of Dermatology*, Vol.163, No.2, (July 2010), pp. 238 – 256, ISSN 0007-0963

Mocellin, S., Pasquali, S., Rossi, C., & Nitti, D. (2010). Interferon alpha adjuvant therapy in patients with high-risk melanoma: a systematic review and meta-analysis. *Journal of the National Cancer Institute*, Vol.102, No. 7, (February 2010), pp. 493 – 501, ISSN 1460-2105

Payvandi, F., Wu, L., Zhang, L., Muller, G., Cohen, L., Chen, R., Harriri, R., & Stirling, D. (2003). CC-1503 inhibits the expression of adhesion molecules ICAM-1 and CD44 and prevents metastasis of B16 F10 mouse melanoma cells in an animal model [abstract]. *Proc Am Soc Clin Oncol*, Vol.22, abstract 992, (2003)

Pectasides, D., Dafni, U., Bafaloukos, D., Skarlos, D., Polyzos, A., Tsoutsos, D., Kalofonos, H., Fountzilas, G., Panagiotou, P., Kokkalis, G., Papadopoulos, O., Castana, O.,

Papadopoulos, S., Stavrinidis, E., Vourli, G., Ioannovich, J., & Gogas, H. (2009). Randomized phase III study of 1 month versus 1 year of adjuvant high-dose interferon alfa-2b in patients with resected high-risk melanoma. *Journal of Clinical Oncology*, Vol.27, No.6, (February 2009), pp.939-944, ISSN 0732-183X

Quirt, I., Verma, S., Petrella, T., Bak, K., & Charette, M. (2007). Temozolomide for the treatment of metastatic melanoma: a systematic review. *The Oncologist*, Vol.12, No. 9, (September 2007), pp. 1114 – 1123, ISSN 1083-7159

Sasse, A., Sasse, E., Clark, L., Ulloa, L., & Clark, O. (2007). Chemoimmunotherapy versus chemotherapy for metastatic malignant melanoma. *Cochrane Database of Systematic Reviews*, Vol.1, (2007), ISSN 1469-493X

Schadendorf, D., Ugurel, S., Schuler-Thurner, B., Nestle, F., Enk, A., Bröcker, E., Grabbe, S., Rittgen, W., Edler, L., Sucker, A., Zimpfer-Rechner, C., Berger, T., Kamarashev, J., Burg, G., Jonuleit, H., Tüttenberg, A., Becker, J., Keikavoussi, P., Kämpgen, E., Schuler, G. & DC study group of the DeCOG (2006). Dacarbazine (DTIC) versus vaccination with autologous peptide-pulsed dendritic cells (DC) in first-line treatment of patients with metastatic melanoma: a randomized phase III trial of the DC study group of the DeCOG. *Annals of Oncology*, Vol. 17, No. 4 (April 2006), pp. 563-70, ISSN 0923-7534

Schmidt, H., Suciu, S., Punt, C., Gore, M., Kruit, W., Patel, P., Lienard, D., von der Maase, H., Eggermont, A., Keilholz, U., & American Joint Committee on Cancer Stage IV Melanoma:EORTC 18951. (2007). Pretreatment levels of peripheral neutrophils and leukocytes as independent predictors of overall survival in patients with American Joint Committee on Cancer Stage IV Melanoma: results of the EORTC 18951 Biochemotherapy Trial. *Journal of Clinical Oncology*, Vol.25, No.12, (April 2007), pp. 1562-1569, ISSN 0732-183X

Sladden, M., Balch, C., Barzilai, D. Berg, D., Freiman, A., Handiside, T., Hollis, S., Lens, M., & Thompson, J. (2010). Surgical excision margins for primary cutaneous melanoma. *Cochrane Database of Systematic Reviews*, Vol.1, (2009), ISSN:1469-493X

Testori, A., Richards, J, Whitman, E., Mann, G., Lutzky, J., Camacho, L., Parmiani, G., Tosti,G., Kirkwood, J., Hoos, A., Yuh, L., Gupta, R., Srivastava, P., & C-100-21 Study Group. (2008). Phase III comparison of vitespen, an autologous tumor-derived heat shock protein gp96 peptide complex vaccine, with physician's choice of treatment for stage IV melanoma: the C-100-21 study group. *Journal of Clinical Oncology*, Vol.26, No.6, (February 2008), pp. 955-962, ISSN 0732-183X

U. S. Food and Drug Administration. (March 2011). FDA approves new treatment for a type of late-stage skin cancer, In: U. S. Food and Drug Administration, 25.3.2011, Available from www.fda.gov/NewsEvents/Newsroom/PressAnnouncements/ucm1193237.htm

U. S. National Institute of Health. (2011). In: *Clinical Trials Registry*, 20.4.2011, Available from http://clinicaltrials.gov

Wilhelm, S., Carter, C., Tang, L., Wilkie, D., McNabola, A., Rong, H., Chen, C., Zhang, X., Vincent, P., McHugh, M., Cao, Y., Shujath, J., Gawlak, S., Eveleigh, D., Rowley, B., Liu, L., Adnane, L., Lynch, M., Auclair, D., Taylor, I., Gedrich, R., Voznesensky, A., Riedl, B., Post L, Bollag, G., & Trail, P. (2004). BAY 43-9006 exhibits broad spectrum oral antitumor activity and targets the RAF/MEK/ERK pathway and receptor tyrosine kinases involved in tumor progression and angiogenesis. *Cancer Research*, Vol.64, pp. 7099–7109, ISSN 0008-5472

Wolchok, J., Weber, J., Hamid, O., Lebbé, C., Maio, M., Schadendorf, D., de Pril, V., Chen, T., Ibrahim, R., Hoos, A., & O'Day, S. (2010). Ipilimumab efficacy and safety in patients with advanced melanoma: a retrospective analysis of HLA subtype from four trials. *Cancer Immunity: a journal of the Academy of Cancer Immunology*, Vol. 10, (October 2010), pp. 9, ISSN 1424-9634

Wolff, K., & Johnson, R. (2009). *Fitzpatrick's Color Atlas and Synopsis of Clinical Dermatology* (6th edition), McGraw Hill, New York, ISBN 978-0-07-163342-0

9

Uvel Melanoma

Ozlem Yenice and Eren Cerman
Marmara University School of Medicine Department of Ophthalmology, Istanbul,
Turkey

1. Introduction

The eye's uveal tract consists of the iris, ciliary body, and choroid. It contains a population of melanocytes. Uveal melanomas develop from melanocytes that reside within the stroma of the choroid, ciliary body or iris.

The choroid is the vascular part of the human eye between retina and sclera. Though accurate measurements of the choroidal blood flow is difficult, it is known that choroid is one of the most vascular tissues in the body and its blood flow is one of highest (1). It is a feared condition because it is potentially lethal and the treatment of metastatic melanoma is ineffective.

2. Epidemiology

Uveal melanomas are found in 3% of cases in the iris, in 5–10% of cases in the ciliary body and in 90% of cases in the choroid in about 40% of cases within 3 mm of optic disc and/or fovea.

Metastatic tumors of the choroid are the most common intraocular malignancy but they are only slightly more common than choroidal melanoma. Choroidal melanoma is the most common primary intraocular malignancy in adults. It has an estimated annual incidence in the United states of 6 cases permillion people (2). Before the age 50 it has an incidence of 3 per million people and after the age 50 it reaches to 21 per million people (3). Sixty five percent of patients are above the age 50 (4). There is no sex predominance. Choroidal melanoma is typically unilateral and unifocal (1). Whites are eight times more likely to have melanoma than African-Americans and three times more likely than Asians. Most melanomas arise from pre-existing, benign choroidal nevi. The prevalence of nevi is 1-2% and the incidence of malignant degeneration into melanoma is less than 1% (5). Exposure to sunlight has been implicated in the development of iris melanomas but there is no convincing evidence to show that sunlight causes choroidal melanomas. Pregnancy accelerates the growth of existing melanoma perhaps through endocrine factors such as excess melanocyte-stimulating hormone (6). Exposure to UV light or other agents is not a risk factor for choroidal melanoma (7).

The most common predisposing factor for choroidal melanoma is ocular melanositosis. Still in congenital ocular melanocytosis the incidence of choroidal melanoma does not exceed %5 (8). In the white population a lifetime risk of developing uveal melanoma increases from 1 in 13000 to 1 in 400 when there is an underlying congenital melanocytosis (9).

3. Diagnosis

Mostly the patients are asymptomatic and the tumor is discovered on ophthalmic examination. On ophthalmoscopy choroidal melanoma usually present as dome shaped tumor with variable pigmentation and sometimes with serous detachment. Tumors are generally pigmented but one fourth are relatively non-pigmented or amelanotic (Figure 1). Symptomatic patients have may have distorted and/or reduced vision when the tumor develops next to or in the macula. Vision field defects may occur   due to exudative detachment or corresponding to the tumor. Exudative retinal detachments are usually seen with tumors more that 4 mm thick. Flashes floaters or photosias may occur due to retinal pathology. Pain is rare but occur when there is angle closure or neovascular glaucoma.

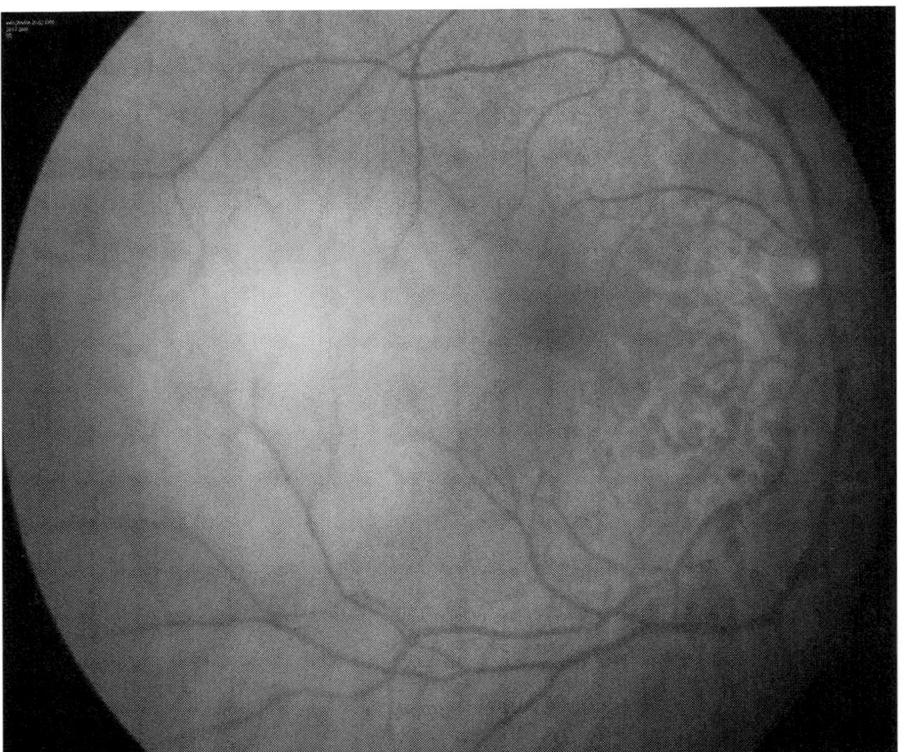

Fig. 1. An amelonocytic choroidal melanoma of the posterior pole

An examination consisting of indirect ophthalmoscopy, fluorescein angiography, scleral transillumination, b-scan ultrasonography has a diagnostic accuracy rate of 99.7% as reported by the Collaborative Ocular Melanoma Study (COMS) (10). In the same study an examination with indirect ophthalmoscopy, revealing a choroidal tumor with orange pigment on its surface and subretinal fluid is correctly diagnosed as choroidal melanoma in 99.6% of cases (10).

Flourescein angiography is reported to have a diagnostic accuracy rate of %36.6 (11). Early hypofluorescence is seen in pigmented melanomas and late hyperfluorescent areas can be seen depending on the interaction of the tumor with the retina pigment epithelium. With changes in RPE early dot-like areas of hyperfluorescence become prominent and they increase in intensity in late phases. Fluorescein angiography may also reveal a typical double circulation seen in choroidal melanomas, a characteristic image caused by simultaneusly retinal and tumor circulation.

For tumors greater than 3 mm thick a combined A-mode and B-mode ultrasonography is more than 95% accurate in diagnosing choroidal melanoma. B-mode ultrasonography might reveal a typical acoustically silent zone within the melanoma, choroidal excavation and acoustic shadowing of the orbit. With A-mode medium to low internal reflectivity might be seen.

Fine needle biopsy is usually not suggested for seeding of the needle tract is reported (12, 13).

4. Prognosis

Long-term follow-up reveals that eventually more than 50% of patients die of disseminated disease (14). About 30-50% of patients with choroidal melanoma will die within 10 years from diagnosis and treatment. As found in the Collaborative Ocular Melanoma Study, for large melanomas the 10-year rates of death secondary to metastasis are 45% in pre-enucleation radiation and 40% and in the enucleation alone treatment groups (10).

It is usually secondary to distant metastases, and the risk is greatest in larger tumors. Though at presentation only 1-3 % of patients have detectable metastases. Overt metastases are fatal and if untreated median survival time is 2-6 months (15, 16). If treated survival time prolongs only up to 12-15 months (17).

Study	Small Size	Medium Size	Large Size
Meta-analysis 1966-1988 [a]	<3mm height <10mm diameter	10-15 mm diameter	>15 mm diameter
	<10 mm diameter	10-15 mm diameter	>15 mm diameter or >5 mm height
	<11 mm diameter	11-15 mm diameter	
	< 300mm^2	<15 mm diameter	
COMS	1,5-2,4 mm height	2,5-10 mm height[b]	>10 apical height
	5-16 mm diameter	<16 mm diameter	>16 mm diameter

[a] Included 8 studies with overlapping size criteria
[b] Changed November 1990 3,1 to 8,0 mm.

Table 1. Definition of size in choroidal melanomas*

---

* Cancer Control 2004 H.Lee Moffitt Cancer Center and Research Institute, Inc.

Commonly accepted clinical risk factors are larger size of the tumor, anterior location, proximity to the foveal avascular zone, advanced patient age and histopathology (Table 1). Especially the character of specific vascular abnormalities such as vascular networks, closed loops, and parallel-with-cross-linking microcirculation-related patterns appear to predict tumors more likely to metastasize (18).

	Small Size Melanoma Mortality	Medium Size Melanoma Mortality	Large Size Melanoma Mortality
Meta analysis	16%	32%	53%
5-year all cause (COMS)	16 %	19% [a] 18% [b]	43% [a] 38% [b]
5-year tumor related (COMS)	1%	11% [a] 9% [b]	28% [a] 26% [b]
(Helsinky Study) [a]		All sizes	
4 year tumor related mortality		31%	
15 year tumor related mortality		45%	
25 year tumor related mortality		49%	
35 year tumor related mortality		52%	

[a] enucleation alone
[b] enucleation with preoperative radiation

Table 2. Mortality rates of choroidal melanoma*

5. Treatment

Treatment modalities for choroidal melanoma are brachytherapy,The Collaborative Ocular Melanoma Study (COMS) is a multicenter investigation designed to evaluate therapeutic interventions for patients who have choroidal melanoma. This study aimed to find out which one of the treatment modalities would prolong the remaining lifetime and which of them would have better prognosis for vision overall. There are several treatment modalities:

a) Observation

If the diagnosis is not definite, the lesion should be followed with fundus photography and ultrasound. Factors that differentiate a choroidal melanoma from choroidal nevi are

---

* Cancer Control 2004 H.Lee Moffitt Cancer Center and Research Institute, Inc.

thickness (>2mm), subretinal fluid, symptoms, orange pigment and a lesion margin that is touching to optic disc.

Observation as a management choice is a situation where:

1. The ophthalmologist has detected a presumably melanocytic choroidal tumor that is either a relatively large but benign choroidal nevus or a small but malignant choroidal melanoma,
2. That he or she has informed the patient of the findings and differential diagnosis,
3. That he or she has recommended comprehensive reevaluation of the suspicious tumor on a periodic basis (at intervals to be determined on a case-by-case basis by the ophthalmologist, depending on his or her level of concern about the lesion's "prior probability" of being a true malignant melanoma), and
4. That he or she had indicated to the patient that some form of intervention is likely to be recommended when a particular threshold of change in the lesion has been identified (19).

b) Transpupillary Thermotherapy

In the mid-1990s the initial observations of Transpupillary Thermotherapy (TTT) for small choroidal melanoma reported successful with minimal side effects (20), but its popularity later waned following documented recurrences (21, 22).

In TTT light in the infrared range (810 nm) is delivered trough a modified slit-lamp. The long wavelenght passes through ocular tissues and it is absorbed by melanin which is found in high concentration in choroidal melanomas. The tumor is heated up to 60°C and causes tissue necrosis. It is preferred when the lesion is under 2 mm thick but a growth in size is documented. It has also been used for tumors up to 4 mm in thickness (23-25), preferably coupled with brachytherapy treating the tumor base. In 1998 Shields et al. reported the results of the largest published case series of TTT for choroidal melanoma with 100 patients. After a mean of three treatment sessions and 14 months of follow-up, tumor control was successful in 94 of 100 eyes. The remaining 6 eyes were classified as treatment failures. Four of these eyes showed partial or no response to thermotherapy, thus requiring plaque radiotherapy or enucleation and two eyes showed recurrence, but subsequently controlled with additional thermotherapy. The most frequent ocular side-effects in that series included vascular obstruction in 23% and retinal traction in 20% of patients, which occurred within a mean time interval of 4–5 months after TTT.

TTT offers great advantages over enucleation or radiation. Because light can be focused easyly, TTT causes minimal callateral damage and therefore it does not cause cataract, optic neuropathy or retinopathy and visual outcome following TTT may be outstanding.

c) Charged particle Irradiation and Plaque Brachytherapy

Radiotherapy may be a vision-sparing alternative to enucleation for patients with choroidal melanoma. The most commonly used forms of radiotherapy are ophthalmic plaque brachytherapy and charged-particle (external beam) radiotherapy.

External beam irradiation of melanomas with charged particles, protons or helium nuclei, has been performed since 1975.

Plaque radiotherapy or charged-particle radiation is particularly recommended for medium or small sized uveal melanoma which are not suitable to TTT. In CMOS study eyes of patients with tumors from 2.5 mm to 10 mm in apical height and basal diameter of 16 mm or less are treated with a radioactive plaque if randomized to radiation.

The tumor control rate after plaque or charged-particle radiotherapy appears to be similar but charged-particle irradiation may produce worse anterior-segment complications than plaque radiotherapy (26, 27). Currently ^{125}I radiation therapy is considered excellent for intraocular tumors because since it lacks alpha or beta rays, its penetrance allows the treatment of large tumors and the seeds are commercially available and can be reused. Only 125I is used in CMOS study.

The local recurrence rate of melanomas treated with ^{125}I plaques is 4% (28). After all forms of radiotherapy many patients experience sight-limiting side effects due to optic neuritis and an average of 16.3% of patients treated with radiotherapy subsequently require enucleation because of tumor regrowth or uncontrollable neovascular glaucoma.

d) Enucleation

Until the 1980's, the standard treatment of choroidal melanoma was the removal of the eye by enucleation (29). Enucleation is still performed for large uveal melanoma when there is no hope of regaining useful vision but based on the published literature, it seems that enucleation carries the same survival prognosis as each of the conservative treatment modalities. According to CMOS study mortality rates following ^{125}I brachytherapy does not differ from those following enucleation through 12 years follow-up time.

6. Reference

[1] Braun RD, Dewhirst MW, Hatchell DL. Quantification of erythrocyte flow in the choroid of the albino rat. Am J Physiol. 1997 Mar;272(3 Pt 2):H1444-53.

[2] Egan KM, Seddon JM, Glynn RJ, Gragoudas ES, Albert DM. Epidemiologic aspects of uveal melanoma. Surv Ophthalmol. 1988 Jan-Feb;32(4):239-51.

[3] Wilkes SR, Robertson DM, Kurland LT, Campbell RJ. Incidence of uveal malignant melanoma in the resident population of Rochester and Olmsted County, Minnesota. Am J Ophthalmol. 1979 May;87(5):639-41.

[4] Flocks M, Gerende JH, Zimmerman LE. The size and shape of malignant melanomas of the choroid and ciliary body in relation to prognosis and histologic characteristics; a statistical study of 210 tumors. Trans Am Acad Ophthalmol Otolaryngol. 1955 Nov-Dec;59(6):740-58.

[5] Ganley JP, Comstock GW. Benign nevi and malignant melanomas of the choroid. Am J Ophthalmol. 1973 Jul;76(1):19-25.

[6] Seddon JM, MacLaughlin DT, Albert DM, Gragoudas ES, Ference M, 3rd. Uveal melanomas presenting during pregnancy and the investigation of oestrogen receptors in melanomas. Br J Ophthalmol. 1982 Nov;66(11):695-704.

[7] Singh AD, Bergman L, Seregard S. Uveal melanoma: epidemiologic aspects. Ophthalmol Clin North Am. 2005 Mar;18(1):75-84, viii.

[8] Velazquez N, Jones IS. Ocular and oculodermal melanocytosis associated with uveal melanoma. Ophthalmology. 1983 Dec;90(12):1472-6.

[9] Singh AD, De Potter P, Fijal BA, et al. Lifetime prevalence of uveal melanoma in white patients with oculo(dermal) melanocytosis. Ophthalmology. 1998 Jan;105(1):195-8.

[10] Accuracy of diagnosis of choroidal melanomas in the Collaborative Ocular Melanoma Study. COMS report no. 1. Arch Ophthalmol. 1990 Sep;108(9):1268-73.

[11] Schaling DF, Oosterhuis JA, Jager MJ, Kakebeeke-Kemme H, Pauwels EK. Possibilities and limitations of radioimmunoscintigraphy and conventional diagnostic modalities in choroidal melanoma. Br J Ophthalmol. 1994 Apr;78(4):244-8.

[12] Augsburger JJ, Shields JA, Folberg R, et al. Fine needle aspiration biopsy in the diagnosis of intraocular cancer. Cytologic-histologic correlations. Ophthalmology. 1985 Jan;92(1):39-49.

[13] Karcioglu ZA, Gordon RA, Karcioglu GL. Tumor seeding in ocular fine needle aspiration biopsy. Ophthalmology. 1985 Dec;92(12):1763-7.

[14] Jensen OA. Malignant melanomas of the human uvea: 25-year follow-up of cases in Denmark, 1943--1952. Acta Ophthalmol (Copenh). 1982 Apr;60(2):161-82.

[15] Woll E, Bedikian A, Legha SS. Uveal melanoma: natural history and treatment options for metastatic disease. Melanoma Res. 1999 Dec;9(6):575-81.

[16] Rajpal S, Moore R, Karakousis CP. Survival in metastatic ocular melanoma. Cancer. 1983 Jul 15;52(2):334-6.

[17] Pyrhonen S, Hahka-Kemppinen M, Muhonen T, et al. Chemoimmunotherapy with bleomycin, vincristine, lomustine, dacarbazine (BOLD), and human leukocyte interferon for metastatic uveal melanoma. Cancer. 2002 Dec 1;95(11):2366-72.

[18] Folberg R, Rummelt V, Parys-Van Ginderdeuren R, et al. The prognostic value of tumor blood vessel morphology in primary uveal melanoma. Ophthalmology. 1993 Sep;100(9):1389-98.

[19] Augsburger JJ. Is observation really appropriate for small choroidal melanomas. Trans Am Ophthalmol Soc. 1993;91:147-68; discussion 69-75.

[20] Oosterhuis JA, Journee-de Korver HG, Kakebeeke-Kemme HM, Bleeker JC. Transpupillary thermotherapy in choroidal melanomas. Arch Ophthalmol. 1995 Mar;113(3):315-21.

[21] Aaberg TM, Jr., Bergstrom CS, Hickner ZJ, Lynn MJ. Long-term results of primary transpupillary thermal therapy for the treatment of choroidal malignant melanoma. Br J Ophthalmol. 2008 Jun;92(6):741-6.

[22] Pan Y, Diddie K, Lim JI. Primary transpupillary thermotherapy for small choroidal melanomas. Br J Ophthalmol. 2008 Jun;92(6):747-50.

[23] Oosterhuis JA, Journee-de Korver HG, Keunen JE. Transpupillary thermotherapy: results in 50 patients with choroidal melanoma. Arch Ophthalmol. 1998 Feb; 116(2):157-62.

[24] Shields CL, Shields JA, Perez N, Singh AD, Cater J. Primary transpupillary thermotherapy for small choroidal melanoma in 256 consecutive cases: outcomes and limitations. Ophthalmology. 2002 Feb;109(2):225-34.

[25] Shields CL, Shields JA. Transpupillary thermotherapy for choroidal melanoma. Curr Opin Ophthalmol. 1999 Jun;10(3):197-203.

[26] De Potter P. [Choroidal melanoma: current therapeutic approaches]. J Fr Ophtalmol. 2002 Feb;25(2):203-11.

[27] Char DH, Quivey JM, Castro JR, Kroll S, Phillips T. Helium ions versus iodine 125 brachytherapy in the management of uveal melanoma. A prospective, randomized, dynamically balanced trial. Ophthalmology. 1993 Oct;100(10):1547-54.

[28] Wilson MW, Hungerford JL. Comparison of episcleral plaque and proton beam radiation therapy for the treatment of choroidal melanoma. Ophthalmology. 1999 Aug;106(8):1579-87.

[29] Singh AD, Rennie IG, Kivela T, Seregard S, Grossniklaus H. The Zimmerman-McLean-Foster hypothesis: 25 years later. Br J Ophthalmol. 2004 Jul;88(7):962-7.

10

Expression of Tumour Associated Transcripts in Malignant Melanoma Metastases - with Methodological Aspects

Malin Farnebäck[1], Annika Håkansson[2],
Leif Håkansson[3], Bertil Gustafsson[4] and Bertil Kågedal[1]
[1]Department of Clinical and Experimental Medicine, Division of Clinical Chemistry,
[2]Division of Diagnostics and Clinical Services, Skåne University Hospital
SE 205 02 Malmö
[3]Division of Oncology, Faculty of Health Sciences, Linköping University
SE-581 85 Linköping
[4]Division of Pathology and Cytology, Faculty of Health Sciences, Linköping University
SE-581 85 Linköping
Sweden

1. Introduction

Several melanoma antigens, recognized by autologous cytotoxic T lymphocytes, have been identified (Boon and van der Bruggen, 1996). The antigens can be divided into two separate groups, (a) antigens associated with pigment formation such as tyrosinase (Wölfel et al., 1994), tyrosinase related protein (TRP)-1 (Wang et al., 1995), TRP-2 (Wang et al., 1996), MART-1/Melan-A (Coulie et al., 1994; Kawakami et al., 1994a) and gp100/Pmel 17 (Kawakami et al., 1994b) present in normal as well as malignant cells of melanocytic lineage, and (b) tumour associated antigens of the MAGE-, BAGE- and GAGE-families that are found in many different malignant cells (Brasseur et al., 1995). These antigens are presented on the cell surface by HLA class I molecules and are important in the immune surveillance of tumour cells and several of these antigens have been utilized in vaccination studies (Parmiani et al., 2002).

In addition to being investigated for their role in the immune response, mRNAs of these antigens, especially tyrosinase, have been used for detection of circulating melanoma cells in blood (Brownbridge et al., 2001; de Vries et al., 1999; Hoon et al., 1995; Johansson et al., 2000; Reynolds et al., 2003; Smith et al., 1991). In this context there are great variations in the results (for a review see (Keilholz et al., 1997)) and the usefulness of this technique is disputed (Hanekom et al., 1999; Mellado et al., 1999; Osella Abate et al., 2000). The variations may be due to several factors, e.g. differences in the methods used and in the selection of participating patients. Low concentrations of the transcripts in the tumours would be reflected in a low detection rate of melanoma cells in blood and high transcript concentrations would result in a higher probability of detecting cells present in blood.

Several of these antigens have earlier been studied by immunohistochemical and conventional RT-PCR methods. A great heterogeneity in the frequency of expression of tyrosinase, MART-1/Melan-A, and gp100/Pmel 17 protein in different melanocytic lesions and melanoma cell lines has been shown (Cormier et al., 1998; de Vries et al., 1997; Sarantou et al., 1997). Similarly, loss of mRNA expression of one or more of the antigens tyrosinase TRP-1, TRP-2, MART-1/Melan-A, and gp100/Pmel 17 was found in 26 % of primary and metastatic tumours (Sarantou, et al., 1997). In addition, Dalerba et al. (Dalerba et al., 1998) found a variable mRNA expression of tyrosinase, MART-1/Melan-A, MAGE-A1, MAGE-A2, MAGE-A3, BAGE and GAGE between multiple in-transit and lymph-node metastases. However, the above mentioned studies did not provide quantitative information. Thus, better understanding of mRNA levels and the factors influencing the expression of these antigens is needed.

We have therefore determined the mRNA concentrations of tyrosinase, TRP-1, TRP-2, MART-1/Melan-A, MAGE-A3, MAGE-A12, S-100 and G_{D2} synthase in sections of snap frozen melanoma metastases from treated and untreated patients. Furthermore, we have compared two different methods, use of section area and use of housekeeping genes for normalization of the expression data for differences in starting amounts of tissue. In addition, we have investigated the influence of tumour-infiltrating lymphocytes on the expression of these antigens.

2. Material and methods

2.1 Tumour material

Melanoma metastases from 7 women and 21 men with regional and systemic disease were investigated. The median age of the patients was 50 years (range 26 to 82 years) and treatment for metastatic disease was given to 15 of the patients before removal of the metastases. Recurrences were cytologically verified by fine needle aspiration biopsy before start of treatment. One metastasis from each patient was studied. In patients with systemic disease easily resectable metastases were chosen. In patients with regional disease, non-necrotic biopsies were randomly chosen by the pathologist. Only sections of good technical quality were included in the study. Thus, sections that were either crackled or damaged, or contained large necrotic areas, or mainly contained lymph node remnants were excluded. The study was approved by the ethical committee at the University Hospital in Linköping, Sweden.

The treatment schedule was cisplatinum 30 mg/m^2 i.v., dacarbazine (DTIC) 250 mg/m^2 i.v. day 1-3 and interferon-α2b 10 million IU s.c. three times weekly. The duration of each cycle was 28 days.

The tumours were snap frozen after resection and stored at -70°C until further processed. Three parallel sections (7 μm) were cut from each metastasis and two of them were immediately transferred to 500 μl of lysis buffer (100 mM Tris-HCl pH 7.6, 500 mM LiCl, 10 mM EDTA, 5 mM DTT, 1% SDS) and homogenized using a Mikro-Dismembrator S (B. Braun Biotech International GmbH, Melsungen Germany). The third section was used for conventional light microscopy studies.

2.2 Analysis of mRNA expression

The lysate was added to 100 μl GenoPrep mRNA Beads (GenoVision , Oslo, Norway) and the mixture was incubated on a rotating mixer for 10 min. The magnetic beads were immobilized using a Dynal MPC-S device (Dynal Biotech, Oslo, Norway) and washed twice in 1 ml 10 mM Tris-HCl, pH 7.6, containing 150 mM LiCl, 1 mM EDTA, and 0.1 % SDS and then twice in 1 ml 10 mM Tris-HCl, pH 7.6, containing 150 mM LiCl, and 1 mM EDTA. mRNA was released from the magnetic beads in 20 µl RNase-free water by incubation at 70°C for 2 min. First strand cDNA was synthesized using random hexamers and Moloney Murine Leukemia Virus reverse transcriptase as described earlier (Johansson, et al., 2000).

Oligonucleotide	Sequence	Conc. (nM)
Tyrosinase FP	ATGGATAAAGCTGCCAATTTCA	100
Tyrosinase RP	GGCATCCGCTATCCCAGTA	100
Tyrosinase Probe	CTTTAGAAATACACTGGAAGGATTTGCTAGTCCAC	50
TRP-1 FP	TCATGAGGGACCAGCTTTTC	100
TRP-1 RP	TCTTGCAACATTTCCTGCAT	100
TRP-1 Probe	CACATGGCACAGGTACCACCACCT	50
TRP-2 FP	GGAAAGAGATCTCCAGCGAC	100
TRP-2 RP	ATCACACTCGTTCCTCCCA	100
TRP-2 Probe	TGCTTTGCCCTACTGGAACTTTGCC	50
MART-1/Melan-A FP	GCCACTCTTACACCACGGC	100
MART-1/Melan-A RP	TCCCAGGATCACTGTCAGGA	100
MART-1/Melan-A Probe	GCCGATCCCAGCGGCCTCTT	100
S-100 FP	CCATTTCTTAGAGGAAATCAAAGAG	100
S-100 RP	ATTCGCCGTCTCCATCAT	100
S-100 Probe	TGTCCAGTGTTTCCATGACTTTGTCCA	100
G_{D2} synthase FP	CCAGGGAGCCCAGTACAAC	100
G_{D2} synthase RP	GCCGTGAAGACGAAGTCG	100
G_{D2} synthase Probe	AACCAGCCCTTGCCGAAGGGC	200
MAGE-A3 FP	TGAGGAGGCAAGGTTCTGA	100
MAGE-A3 RP	ATGGAGACCCACTGGCAG	100
MAGE-A3 Probe	TCTGGTCCTCCAGGTCAGCCTGT	100
MAGE-A12 FP	GTGAGGAGGCAAGGTTCTG	100
MAGE-A12 RP	GGCATGATGACTCTGGTCAG	100
MAGE-A12 Probe	TCCTGCCCACACTCCTACCTGCT	50

Table 1. Sequences and concentrations of primers and probes used in real-time PCR for melanoma transcripts

Transcript	Forward primer	Reverse primer
Tyrosinase	TTGGCAGATTGTCTGTAGCC	AGGCATTGTGCATGCTGCTT
TRP-1	AAAGCTTTGGTGAAGTGGATTT	AGACCACTCGCCATTGAGA
TRP-2	CTACAGGGCCATAGATTTCTC	GTTGTAGTCATCCAAGCTATCAC
MART-1/Melan-A	GACTCTCATTAAGGAAGGTGTCC	TTGTTAAGGCACATTGAGTGC
S-100	GGGAGACAAGCACAAGCTGAAG	TTCAAAGAACTCGTGGCAGGCAGT
G_{D2} synthase	CCAGGGAGCCCAGTACAAC	GCCGTGAAGACGAAGTCG
MAGE-A3	TGAGGAGGCAAGGTTCTGA	ATGGAGACCCACTGGCAG
MAGE-A12	GAGGTCAGAGAACAGCGAGATT	CCGCAGGGTGACTTCC

Table 2. Primers used for synthesis of calibrators

The cDNA was diluted 1:10 before further analysis. From these samples 2.5 µl was analyzed in triplicates by PCR in a total volume of 25 µl (Johansson, et al., 2000).

The mRNAs of tyrosinase, TRP-1, TRP-2, MART-1/Melan-A, MAGE-A3, MAGE-A12, S-100, and G_{D2} synthase were analyzed by real-time PCR using the ABI Prism 7700 Sequence Detector System (Applied Biosystems, Foster City, California, USA). All transcripts were analyzed using the same protocol, 1 x TaqMan PCR Buffer (Applied Biosystems), 5 mM $MgCl_2$ (Applied Biosystems), 200 µM dNTPs (Amersham Biosciences, Uppsala, Sweden), and 0.025 U/µl AmpliTaq Gold (Applied Biosystems) (Johansson, et al., 2000) with the respective primer and probe concentration (Table 1). The oligonucleotides were bought from Scandinavian Gene Synthesis (Köping, Sweden). Their sequences are shown in Table 1.

For each transcript, a specific cDNA calibrator was synthesized using primers located outside the analytical primers (Table 2). The PCR product was quantified by limiting dilution and Poisson distribution as described earlier (Johansson et al., 2002). The calibrators were analyzed in ten-fold dilutions from 100 000 to 10 transcripts/µl in each PCR run.

Three different housekeeping genes, hypoxanthine ribosyl transferase (HPRT), β-glucuronidase (GUS) and β₂-microglobulin (B2M), were amplified using Pre-Developed Assay Reagents from Applied Biosystems. Serial dilutions of cDNA from IMR-32 neuroblastoma cells were used as calibrators. To be able to combine the three housekeeping genes to one normalization factor the expression data of each housekeeping gene need to be at the same level as the others. As the three housekeeping genes differed in their level of expression (Kågedal et al., 2007), a relative expression of each housekeeping gene was defined as the percentage expression of the individual metastasis compared with the mean of all metastases for each housekeeping gene. The mean of the relative expression of the three housekeeping genes was used for normalization. The calculation of the normalization factor (NF) is described by the following equation:

$$NF_i = \left(\frac{x_{iHPRT}}{\bar{x}_{HPRT}} \cdot 100 + \frac{x_{iGUS}}{\bar{x}_{GUS}} \cdot 100 + \frac{x_{iB2M}}{\bar{x}_{B2M}} \cdot 100 \right) \Big/ 3 \tag{1}$$

where x_i is the expression of the respective housekeeping gene in the individual sample and $\bar{x}$ is the respective mean expression.

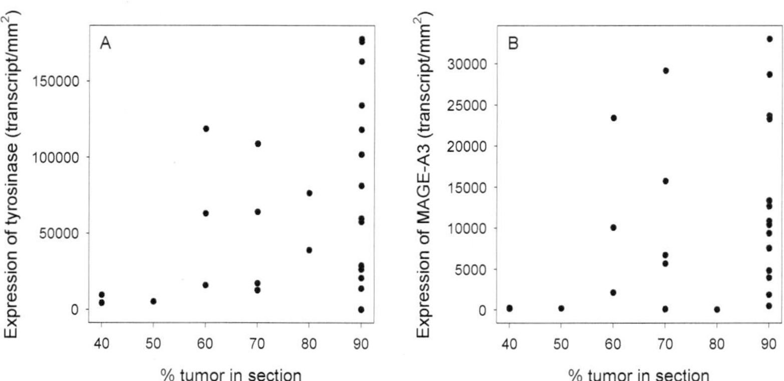

Fig. 1. Expression of tyrosinase (A) and TRP-1 (B) plotted against the tumour content of tissue section of melanoma metastases. The amounts of transcript are given normalized to the area of the respective section

2.3 Staining of sections and evaluation of tumour cells and lymphocytes

The sections used for microscopy were stained with hematoxylin and eosin and mounted in Mountex (Histolab products AB, Göteborg, Sweden). The amounts of tumour-infiltrating lymphocytes were semi-quantitatively scored as <5%, 5-10%, 10-15%, 15-20% and >20%. Metastases scored as <5% were considered to contain low amounts of such cells. The amounts of tumour in the sections were also semi-quantitatively scored to the nearest decile. The scores were made by two independent observers (AH, BG). The sections were also photographed and the area of the sections was measured using the shareware NIH Image 1.63 (http://rsb.info.nih.gov/nih-image/download.html).

2.4 Statistics

Correlations were evaluated using Pearson's correlation coefficient. The Mann-Whitney U-test was used to compare expression of melanoma associated antigens in sections with different amounts of tumour-infiltrating cells and in metastases from untreated and treated patients.

3. Results

The present study is based on analysis of melanoma associated transcripts in 7 μm thick tissue sections from frozen melanoma metastases. Histological analysis of parallel section was performed and biopsies with necrotic areas and lymph node remnants of more than 30 per cent of the section area were not included. The amount of tumour cells was scored and found to vary between 40 per cent and more than 90 per cent of the section area.

	[a]Transcripts/mm^2				[b]Transcripts/HKG			
	Mean	SD	Median	Range	Mean	SD	Median	Range
Tyrosinase	61 000	56 000	48 000	7-180 000	32 000	24 000	25 000	9-94 000
TRP-1	28 000	57 000	1 600	0-210 000	11 000	17 000	1 300	0-59 000
TRP-2	65 000	100 000	16 000	150-410 000	40 000	65 000	12 000	130-260 000
MART-1/Melan-A	120 000	120 000	77 000	520-450 000	63 000	54 000	45 000	360-200 000
S-100	91 000	123 000	45 000	960-530 000	46 000	63 000	27 000	6 800-310 000
G$_{D2}$ synthase	560	670	410	13-2 900	280	410	150	22-2 200
MAGE-A3	10 000	10 000	8 500	36-33 000	4 800	4 400	4 300	36-21 000
MAGE-A12	4 300	5 000	2 100	0-18 000	1 900	2 200	1 400	0-9 800

[a]The results were normalized to the area of the sections.
[b]The results were normalized to the mean expression of the housekeeping genes (HKG) HPRT, GUS and B2M.

Table 3. Expression of melanoma-associated antigens in metastatic lesions

No significant correlations were found between any transcript concentration and the per cent tumour in the sections. This is illustrated in Fig. 1 for tyrosinase and MAGE-A3.
To account for differences in the amounts of starting material, the results of the mRNA analysis were normalized to the tissue section areas measured in parallel sections. The areas

of the tumour sections varied between 7 and 124 mm^2. For comparison the mean of three housekeeping genes was also used in order to normalize the transcript expression data.

For each transcript, there was a large variation between the metastases. Also the mean levels of the different transcripts varied greatly. The pigment-related transcripts (tyrosinase, TRP-1, TRP-2, and MART-1/Melan-A) and that of S-100 had the highest concentrations and widest range (Table 3). For TRP-1 and to some extent for TRP-2, the median was low compared to the mean, which was due to a very low expression in a high proportion of the metastases (Fig. 2). MAGE-A3 and MAGE-A12 were expressed at a somewhat narrower range, whereas G_{D2} synthase was expressed at even lower levels.

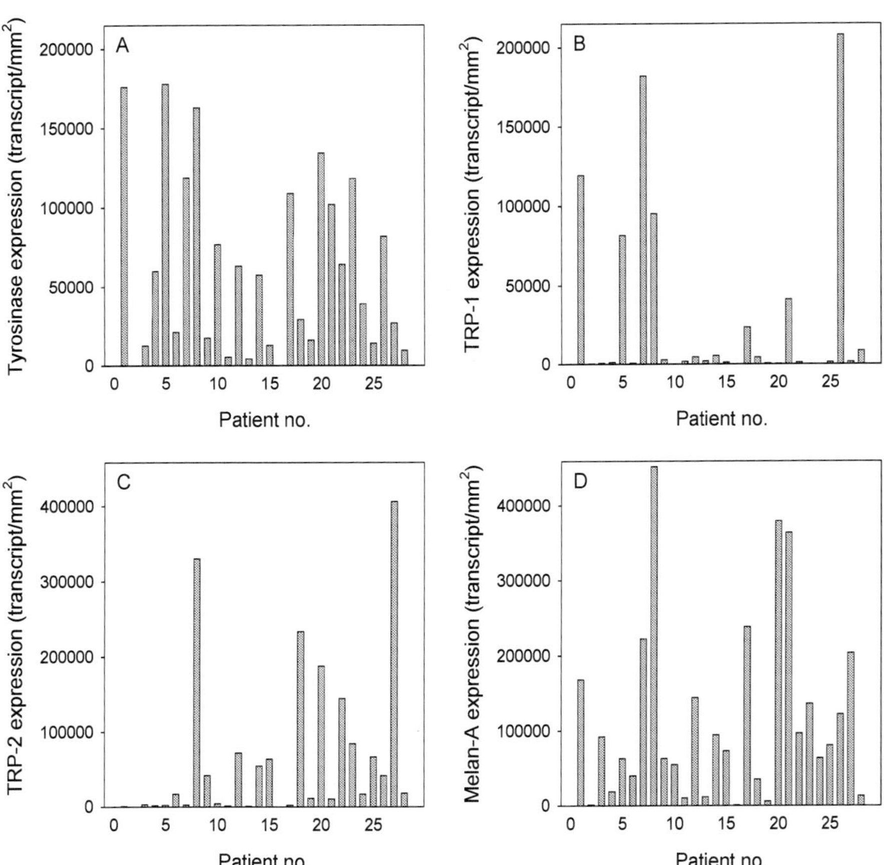

Fig. 2. Expression of (A) tyrosinase, (B) TPR-1, (C) TRP-2, and (D) MART-1/Melan-A mRNAs in frozen sections from malignant melanoma metastases (n=28). The results are given normalized to the area of parallel tissue sections

When housekeeping genes were used for normalization, there was a tendency to less variation of the data, c.f. range of the data (Table 3). Fig. 3 shows the comparison of the two ways of normalization for tyrosinase and MAGE-A3 data of the metastases containing 90 % tumour. It can be seen that some of the highest expressing metastases were equalized when housekeeping genes were used for normalization. Thus, there were transpositions in the orders regarding the amounts of transcripts depending on normalization. There were significant correlations ($p < 0.05$) for all transcripts when normalized by the two methods, but there were great variations around the regression line (data not shown).

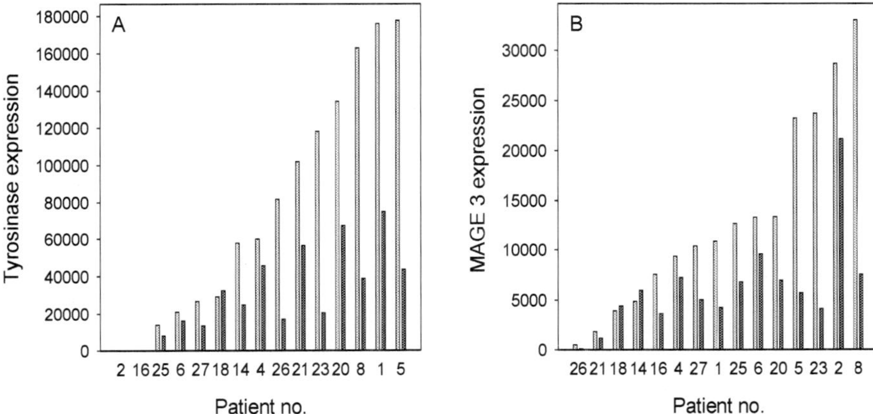

Fig. 3. Comparison of the two methods used for normalization of mRNA data, exemplified by (A) tyrosinase and (B) MAGE-A3 expression. The results normalized to area of the section (gray bars) and to the expression of the three housekeeping genes (black bars) are shown for the metastases containing 90% tumour. The metastases were sorted by the results normalized to area for each transcript

The correlations between the expressions of the different transcripts were examined. Among the pigment-related transcripts a strong correlation was found between tyrosinase and MART-1/Melan-A ($p < 0.001$, $R = 0.67$, Fig. 4A). Weaker correlations ($p < 0.01$, $R = 0.57$ and $R = 0.49$ respectively) were found between the two pairs tyrosinase–TRP-1 and TPR-2–MART-1/Melan-A (data not shown). However, the appearance of these weaker correlations was mainly due to high expressions of these antigens in a few sections. The MAGE-antigens MAGE-A3 and MAGE-A12 also correlated strongly with each other ($p < 0.001$, $R = 0.76$, Fig. 4B). Interestingly when biopsies from treated and untreated patients were analyzed separately, MAGE-A3 was significantly correlated with tyrosinase and MART-1/Melan-A in the sections from the treated patients (Fig. 5, $p < 0.01$, $R = 0.66$ and 0.71 respectively).

When the total material was analyzed, the occurrence of tumour infiltrating lymphocytes did not seem to influence the expression of the genes (12 tumours contained low and 16 contained high amounts of tumour infiltrating lymphocytes). However, if only metastases from untreated patients were analyzed, there was a significantly lower ($p < 0.05$) expression of MART-1/Melan-A and S-100 in the metastases containing high amount of tumour-infiltrating lymphocytes (n=5 and n=8 for low and high respectively, data not shown). These differences were not present in the treated patients.

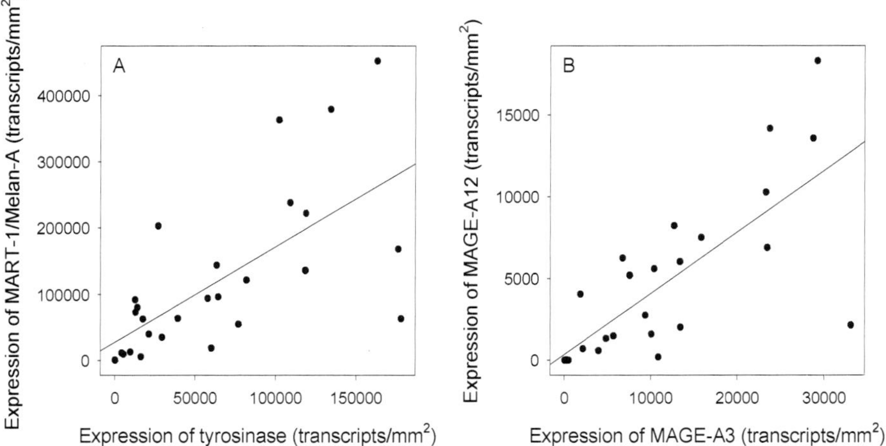

Fig. 4. Correlations between (A) tyrosinase and MART-1/Melan-A expression, and between (B) MAGE-A3 and MAGE-A12 expression in melanoma metastases. The expression data were normalized to the section area

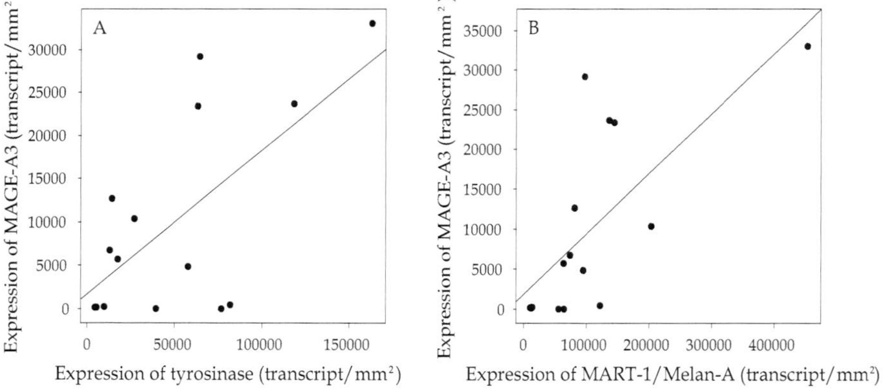

Fig. 5. Correlations of MAGE-A3 with (A) tyrosinase and (B) MART-1/Melan-A in treated patients (n=15). The expression data were normalized to the section area to account for differences in starting amount

The influence of treatment on the mRNA expression was also investigated (Table 4). A significant effect was obtained in TRP-2 expression, where the treated tumours (n=15) showed an increased expression ($p < 0.05$) as compared with the untreated tumours (n=13). The G_{D2} synthase expression on the other hand was decreased in the treated group ($p < 0.05$). With all other transcripts, no significant differences were found.

As the tumour-infiltrating lymphocytes could be of importance for the expression of the antigens, we substratified the sections according to low or high infiltration of tumour-infiltrating lymphocytes (<5% was used as cut-off) before comparing data from untreated and treated patients (Table 4). No difference in TRP-2 expression was found in any of the groups. With G_{D2} synthase, the decrease in the treated patients remained in the metastases containing high amounts of tumour-infiltrating lymphocytes. For the other genes the only difference found was in tyrosinase expression, which was decreased in metastases from treated patients, but only in metastases containing low amounts of tumour-infiltrating lymphocytes. In table 4 the results are also given normalized by housekeeping genes. In addition to the differences found when normalized by area, increased expression of tyrosinase, MART-1/Melan-A, and S-100 in treated patients were found in the metastases containing high amounts of tumour-infiltrating lymphocytes.

	All metastases[a]		Tumour-infiltrating lymphocytes low[b]		Tumour-infiltrating lymphocytes high[c]	
	Tr/mm²	Tr/HKG	Tr/mm²	Tr/HKG	Tr/mm²	Tr/HKG
Tyrosinase	NS[d]	NS	↓ p=0.010	↓ p=0.030	NS	↑ p=0.050
TRP-1	NS	NS	NS	NS	NS	NS
TRP-2	↑ p=0.019	↑ p=0.003	NS	↑ p=0.048	NS	NS
MART-1/Melan-A	NS	NS	NS	NS	NS	↑ p=0.021
S-100	NS	NS	NS	NS	NS	↑ p=0.003
G_{D2} synthase	↓ p=0.010	↓ p=0.065	NS	NS	↓ p=0.007	↓ p=0.028
MAGE-A3	NS	NS	NS	NS	NS	NS
MAGE-A12	NS	NS	NS	NS	NS	NS

[a]The material comprised of 13 metastases from untreated patients and 15 metastases from treated patients. The results were normalized to the area of each section or to the mean expression of three housekeeping genes (HKG) as indicated.
[b]Metastases containing <5% tumour-infiltrating lymphocytes, 5 metastases from untreated patients and 7 metastases from treated patients.
[c]Metastases containing ≥5% tumour-infiltrating lymphocytes, 8 metastases from untreated patients and 8 metastases from treated patients.
[d]NS = not significant. Significant increases and decreases in the treated patients compared with untreated patients are indicated by arrows.

Table 4. Changes in the expression of melanoma associated transcripts in relation to treatment

4. Discussion

In gene expression studies the expression of specific transcripts is generally normalized to the expression of a housekeeping gene (Vandesompele et al., 2002). The rationale for simultaneous analysis of housekeeping genes is to compensate for different amounts of tissue taken to analysis, and for variations in the analytical process, e.g. degradation of mRNA, incomplete extraction etc. Usually housekeeping genes are chosen among genes of fundamental importance for cell metabolism and thus are supposed to be equally expressed in all cell types. However, there is no guarantee that they are adequate for normalization of transcripts in tumour studies as the metabolic and proliferative rates of tumours usually vary considerably with no relation to the expression of specific transcripts. Furthermore, tumour biopsies are usually heterogeneous partly due to the presence of cell types other than tumour cells, e.g. connective tissue and inflammatory cells. Housekeeping gene transcripts derived from such cells will of course limit the value of normalization of the selected tumour cell transcripts, i.e. as a measurement of the amount of tumour cells taken to analysis. In addition, housekeeping genes might vary between different cell types and also between tumours (Lee et al., 2002; Vandesompele, et al., 2002), not necessarily in relation with the occurrence of tumour specific transcripts. Therefore, in the present study on the expression of melanoma associated transcripts, we have reported the transcript data normalized by the area of parallel tissue sections with defined thickness (7 μm).

Based on histological examination, necrotic tumours and tumours with lymph node remnants of more than 30 per cent of the tissue section area were excluded from this material. The percentage of the tissues section areas comprised by tumour was also determined in this analysis and no correlation was found between expression of transcripts and the amount of tumour cells. This shows that the dominating source of variation of expression of tumour associated transcripts is due to individual variation between different tumour cell populations. In the present material of melanoma metastases we found that the housekeeping genes HPRT, GUS and B2M varied greatly between melanoma metastases, and in several cases with a large discrepancy between the genes when normalized to the area of the tissue sections (unpublished results). There can be several reasons for this variation besides variation in the composition of the biopsies analyzed. Housekeeping genes might be modulated by cytokines produced by inflammatory cells or by agents used in the treatment of the tumour. However, as housekeeping genes are usually used in these type of studies, we have also analyzed the transcript data normalized to the mean of the three housekeeping genes. Interestingly, a significant correlation between the two methods was found for all transcripts analyzed and the outcome of the statistical analysis when normalized to housekeeping genes was not as different from that obtained when using the section area as might be expected. A significant correlation between tyrosinase–MART-1/Melan-A and MAGE-A3–MAGE-A12 was also found when the transcript expression data were normalized to the housekeeping genes. The effect of tumour infiltrating lymphocytes on MART-1/Melan-A expression found in metastases from untreated patient remained. This was not the case with S-100 expression. Similarly, the differences found in the comparison of metastases from untreated and treated metastases when normalized to the section area were also found when data were normalized to the housekeeping genes. However, when using housekeeping genes, treatment related increases of tyrosinase, MART-1/Melan-A and S100 expression were found in metastases containing tumour-infiltrating lymphocytes. These differences were also seen as weak tendencies, when the section area was used for normalization.

As could be expected a wide variation in the expression of melanoma associated antigens between tumours was found irrespective of the method used for normalization. Similar results have also been reported by others (Ohnmacht et al., 2001; Riker et al., 2000). The difference in mRNA levels between the markers and tumours could be of importance for the detection of circulating melanoma cells in patients. A higher expression of transcript in each melanoma cell would facilitate the detection of transcripts in blood originating from a few circulating tumour cells. We found higher concentrations of the pigment-related transcripts than of the MAGE transcripts. These results could explain why patients are positive for tyrosinase more frequently than for MAGE-A3 in most studies analyzing several different melanoma markers (Berking et al., 1999; Hoon et al., 2000; Hoon, et al., 1995). One exception was reported by Reynolds et al. (Reynolds, et al., 2003), who detected MAGE-A3 mRNA in a slightly higher proportion of the patients than tyrosinase mRNA.

Several mechanisms are likely to be involved in regulation of the expression of melanoma associated transcripts. We found a strong correlation between tyrosinase and

MART-1/Melan-A. This could perhaps be explained by the findings that both tyrosinase (Bentley et al., 1994; Yasumoto et al., 1994) and MART-1/Melan-A (Du et al., 2003) transcription is regulated by the microphtalmia transcription factor (MITF). MITF is also believed to be involved in the regulation of TRP-1 and TRP-2 (Yasumoto et al., 1997), however these two genes have also been reported to be regulated independently of tyrosinase (Fang et al., 2001; Fang and Setaluri, 1999). Thus, other mechanisms may be involved in the regulation of TRP-1 and TRP-2 expression. This may be the reason why the expression of the pigment-related transcripts was not strongly correlated with each other in the metastases studied here. Also the expression of the two MAGE transcripts, MAGE-A3 and MAGE-A12, were strongly correlated with each other in the present study. Eradication of immunogenic tumour cell clones either spontaneously or induced by immunotherapy will change the occurrence of tumour associated antigens. The mRNA concentrations of these antigens are likely to be of importance for the presentation of antigens to the immune system, provided that there is a quantitative relation between mRNA and protein expression. A correlation between mRNA expression and recognition by cytotoxic T lymphocytes has been shown for gp100/Pmel17 (Riker, et al., 2000). Interestingly, there seemed to be a relation between the stage of the patient and the occurrence of tyrosinase and MAGE-A3. The detection rate of tyrosinase mRNA was higher in advanced melanoma whereas the detection rate of MAGE-A3 mRNA was higher in the earlier stages (Reynolds, et al., 2003). Furthermore, down regulation of tyrosinase and TRP-2 has been shown to correlate with a shorter survival (Takeuchi et al., 2003).

Tumour cells have developed several mechanisms for immune escape. One way is a reduced presentation of antigens in HLA class I (Ohnmacht and Marincola, 2000). This can be accomplished either by down regulation of HLA or a decreased expression of the presented antigens. Immunohistochemical studies showed that vaccination with gp100 peptide decreased the expression of gp100 in metastatic lesions (Riker et al., 1999). When vaccination with gp100 was combined with IL-2 treatment, a decrease was also observed in MART-1/Melan-A expression. In contrast to these findings, it was reported that MART-1/Melan-A was expressed in a stable manner, as assessed by immunohistochemistry, in serial fine needle aspirates from melanoma patients undergoing peptide vaccination (Fetsch et al., 2001). However, studies on gene expression from repeated fine needle aspirates showed that gp100, MART-1/Melan-A and TRP-2 decreased after vaccination treatment, but only in the patients responding to treatment (Ohnmacht, et al., 2001). This might be due to differences in the sensitivity of the two methods and might still be compatible with eradication of the antigen positive clones. In the present study, only tyrosinase and G_{D2} synthase expressions were decreased in treated melanomas compared to untreated. However, for tyrosinase this effect was found only in metastases that did not recruit lymphocytes.

Apart from down regulation or selection due to immune mediated anti-tumour reactivity, the expression of melanoma antigens could be modulated by several other factors. The presence of tumour-infiltrating lymphocytes could affect the expression. Activated lymphocytes secrete various types of cytokines, which are involved in regulatory processes. It was shown that interferon-γ up-regulated tyrosinase and MAGE-A3 in 4/10 and 4/18 cell lines (Hofbauer et al., 2001). This might explain why a treatment related down regulation of tyrosinase was found only in tumours with low numbers of tumour infiltrating lymphocytes since interferon-γ produced by a high number of tumour-infiltrating lymphocytes might have up regulated tyrosinase (Hofbauer et al., 2001).

The drugs used for treatment could either modulate the mRNA expression or perhaps select clones with an altered expression. The patients in this study were treated with cisplatinum, DTIC, and interferon-α. Interferons have been shown to give mixed responses in the regulation of melanoma associated antigens in melanoma cultures. Interferon-α up regulated the expression of MAGE-A3 more than 50% in 5 of 18 melanoma cell cultures (Hofbauer et al., 2001). In the remaining cell lines the expression was either not affected or slightly decreased. In our study, however, there was no effect of treatment on the MAGE transcripts, which might be due to a possible up-regulation being counteracted by eradication of MAGE-A3 positive clones. This multi-factorial regulation of antigen expression can also explain why a correlation between MAGE-A3 expression and tyrosinase and MART-1/MelanA expression in the present study was found only in treated patients.

It has also been speculated that some of the studied antigens can contribute to drug resistance. Hence, a selection of highly expressing clones would be expected. Elevated expression of several members of the MAGE and GAGE gene families have been found in paclitaxel resistant cell lines (Duan et al., 2003). Similarly, Pak et al. (Pak et al., 2000) have shown that melanoma cell lines resistant to cisplatinum had elevated levels of TPR-2. The resistance was independent of the expression of the other two transcripts of the tyrosinase family and no correlation was found between the melanin content of the cell lines and resistance. Thus, it was concluded that the protection against cisplatinum cytotoxicity is mediated through TRP-2 rather than through melanin. This observation can explain the treatment-related up-regulation of TRP-2 as the activity of cisplatinum is of importance for the therapeutic effect of the combination treatment given in the present study. TRP-2 positive clones are thus likely to be protected from therapeutic eradication.

Quantitative analysis of melanoma associated transcripts in tumour material is very complex partly because of problems in selection and use of housekeeping genes as discussed above and partly because of the complex regulation of the expression of these transcripts by cytokines produced by tumour infiltrating inflammatory cells and by the modulatory effects of therapeutic drugs. This study demonstrates that after all it is possible by careful analysis of the data to obtain biologically relevant results.

5. Conclusion

Several antigens expressed in malignant melanoma are involved in the immunological surveillance of the tumour. The mRNAs of these antigens, especially tyrosinase, have also been used in the detection of minimal residual disease in the blood of melanoma patients. We have therefore analyzed the expression of tyrosinase, TRP-1, TRP-2, MART-1/Melan-A, MAGE-A3, MAGE-A12, S-100 and G_{D2} synthase by real-time PCR in snap frozen sections from 28 regional and systemic metastases. Treatment with cisplatinum, dacarbazine and interferon-α2b was given to 15 patients before surgery. The transcript concentrations varied widely between individual metastases. However, in general the pigment-related transcripts and that of S-100 were found at higher levels than those of MAGE-A3, MAGE-A12 and G_{D2} synthase. Significant correlations ($p<0.001$) were found between tyrosinase and MART-1/Melan-A and between MAGE-A3 and MAGE-A12. TRP-2 and G_{D2} synthase were both influenced by the treatment, TRP-2 expression was increased in the metastases from treated patients, whereas G_{D2} synthase expression was decreased. Furthermore, a decrease in tyrosinase expression was found in metastases without tumour-infiltrating lymphocytes. In this work normalization by the section area contra normalization by housekeeping genes was also evaluated and similar results were obtained with the two methods.

The regulation of the expression of tumour associated transcripts is complex and multifactorial and different factors could produce counteracting effects. This study, however, demonstrates that by careful analysis of the data it is possible to obtain biologically relevant results.

6. Acknowledgment

We would like to thank Prof. John Carstensen, Oncological Center, Linköping University Hospital for statistical advice.

7. References

Bentley, N. J., Eisen, T., and Goding, C. R. (1994). *Mol Cell Biol* 14, 7996-8006.

Berking, C., Schlupen, E. M., Schrader, A., Atzpodien, J., and Volkenandt, M. (1999). *Arch Dermatol Res* 291, 479-84.

Boon, T., and van der Bruggen, P. (1996). *J Exp Med* 183, 725-9.

Brasseur, F., Rimoldi, D., Lienard, D., Lethe, B., Carrel, S., Arienti, F., Suter, L., Vanwijck, R., Bourlond, A., Humblet, Y., and et al. (1995). *Int J Cancer* 63, 375-80.

Brownbridge, G. G., Gold, J., Edward, M., and MacKie, R. M. (2001). *Br J Dermatol* 144, 279-87.

Cormier, J. N., Hijazi, Y. M., Abati, A., Fetsch, P., Bettinotti, M., Steinberg, S. M., Rosenberg, S. A., and Marincola, F. M. (1998). *Int J Cancer* 75, 517-24.

Coulie, P. G., Brichard, V., Van Pel, A., Wolfel, T., Schneider, J., Traversari, C., Mattei, S., De Plaen, E., Lurquin, C., Szikora, J. P., Renauld, J. C., and Boon, T. (1994). *J Exp Med* 180, 35-42.

Dalerba, P., Ricci, A., Russo, V., Rigatti, D., Nicotra, M. R., Mottolese, M., Bordignon, C., Natali, P. G., and Traversari, C. (1998). *Int J Cancer* 77, 200-4.

de Vries, T. J., Fourkour, A., Punt, C. J., van de Locht, L. T., Wobbes, T., van den Bosch, S., de Rooij, M. J., Mensink, E. J., Ruiter, D. J., and van Muijen, G. N. (1999). *Br J Cancer* 80, 883-91.

de Vries, T. J., Fourkour, A., Wobbes, T., Verkroost, G., Ruiter, D. J., and van Muijen, G. N. (1997). *Cancer Res* 57, 3223-9.

Du, J., Miller, A. J., Widlund, H. R., Horstmann, M. A., Ramaswamy, S., and Fisher, D. E. (2003). *Am J Pathol* 163, 333-43.

Duan, Z., Duan, Y., Lamendola, D. E., Yusuf, R. Z., Naeem, R., Penson, R. T., and Seiden, M. V. (2003). *Clin Cancer Res* 9, 2778-85.

Fang, D., Kute, T., and Setaluri, V. (2001). *Pigment Cell Res* 14, 132-9.

Fang, D., and Setaluri, V. (1999). *Biochem Biophys Res Commun* 256, 657-63.

Fetsch, P. A., Steinberg, S. M., Riker, A. I., Marincola, F. M., and Abati, A. (2001). *Cancer* 93, 409-14.

Hanekom, G. S., Stubbings, H. M., Johnson, C. A., and Kidson, S. H. (1999). *Melanoma Res* 9, 465-73.

Hofbauer, G. F., Geertsen, R., Laine, E., Burg, G., and Dummer, R. (2001). *Melanoma Res* 11, 213-8.

Hoon, D. S., Bostick, P., Kuo, C., Okamoto, T., Wang, H. J., Elashoff, R., and Morton, D. L. (2000). *Cancer Res* 60, 2253-7.

Hoon, D. S., Wang, Y., Dale, P. S., Conrad, A. J., Schmid, P., Garrison, D., Kuo, C., Foshag, L. J., Nizze, A. J., and Morton, D. L. (1995). *J Clin Oncol* 13, 2109-16.

Johansson, M., Takasaki, A., Lenner, L., Årstrand, K., and Kågedal, B. (2002). *Melanoma Res* 12, 193-200.

Johansson, M., Årstrand, K., Håkansson, A., Lindholm, C., and Kågedal, B. (2000). *Melanoma Res* 10, 213-22.

Kawakami, Y., Eliyahu, S., Delgado, C. H., Robbins, P. F., Rivoltini, L., Topalian, S. L., Miki, T., and Rosenberg, S. A. (1994a). *Proc Natl Acad Sci U S A* 91, 3515-9.

Kawakami, Y., Eliyahu, S., Delgado, C. H., Robbins, P. F., Sakaguchi, K., Appella, E., Yannelli, J. R., Adema, G. J., Miki, T., and Rosenberg, S. A. (1994b). *Proc Natl Acad Sci U S A* 91, 6458-62.

Keilholz, U., Willhauck, M., Scheibenbogen, C., de Vries, T. J., and Burchill, S. (1997). *Melanoma Res* 7 Suppl 2, S133-41.

Kågedal, B., Farnebäck, M., Håkansson, A., Gustafsson, B., and Håkansson, L. (2007). *Clin Chem Lab Med* 45, 1481-7.

Lee, P. D., Sladek, R., Greenwood, C. M., and Hudson, T. J. (2002). *Genome Res* 12, 292-7.

Mellado, B., Gutierrez, L., Castel, T., Colomer, D., Fontanillas, M., Castro, J., and Estape, J. (1999). *Clin Cancer Res* 5, 1843-8.

Ohnmacht, G. A., and Marincola, F. M. (2000). *J Cell Physiol* 182, 332-8.

Ohnmacht, G. A., Wang, E., Mocellin, S., Abati, A., Filie, A., Fetsch, P., Riker, A. I., Kammula, U. S., Rosenberg, S. A., and Marincola, F. M. (2001). *J Immunol* 167, 1809-20.

Osella Abate, S., Savoia, P., Cambieri, I., Salomone, B., Quaglino, P., and Bernengo, M. G. (2000). *Melanoma Res* 10, 545-55.

Pak, B. J., Li, Q., Kerbel, R. S., and Ben-David, Y. (2000). *Melanoma Res* 10, 499-505.

Parmiani, G., Castelli, C., Dalerba, P., Mortarini, R., Rivoltini, L., Marincola, F. M., and Anichini, A. (2002). *J Natl Cancer Inst* 94, 805-18.

Reynolds, S. R., Albrecht, J., Shapiro, R. L., Roses, D. F., Harris, M. N., Conrad, A., Zeleniuch-Jacquotte, A., and Bystryn, J. C. (2003). *Clin Cancer Res* 9, 1497-502.

Riker, A., Cormier, J., Panelli, M., Kammula, U., Wang, E., Abati, A., Fetsch, P., Lee, K. H., Steinberg, S., Rosenberg, S., and Marincola, F. (1999). *Surgery* 126, 112-20.

Riker, A. I., Kammula, U. S., Panelli, M. C., Wang, E., Ohnmacht, G. A., Steinberg, S. M., Rosenberg, S. A., and Marincola, F. M. (2000). *Int J Cancer* 86, 818-26.

Sarantou, T., Chi, D. D., Garrison, D. A., Conrad, A. J., Schmid, P., Morton, D. L., and Hoon, D. S. (1997). *Cancer Res* 57, 1371-6.

Smith, B., Selby, P., Southgate, J., Pittman, K., Bradley, C., and Blair, G. E. (1991). *Lancet* 338, 1227-9.

Takeuchi, H., Kuo, C., Morton, D. L., Wang, H. J., and Hoon, D. S. (2003). *Cancer Res* 63, 441-8.

Vandesompele, J., De Preter, K., Pattyn, F., Poppe, B., Van Roy, N., De Paepe, A., and Speleman, F. (2002). *Genome Biol* 3, RESEARCH0034.

Wang, R. F., Appella, E., Kawakami, Y., Kang, X., and Rosenberg, S. A. (1996). *J Exp Med* 184, 2207-16.

Wang, R. F., Robbins, P. F., Kawakami, Y., Kang, X. Q., and Rosenberg, S. A. (1995). *J Exp Med* 181, 799-804.

Wölfel, T., Van Pel, A., Brichard, V., Schneider, J., Seliger, B., Meyer zum Büschenfelde, K. H., and Boon, T. (1994). *Eur J Immunol* 24, 759-64.

Yasumoto, K., Yokoyama, K., Shibata, K., Tomita, Y., and Shibahara, S. (1994). *Mol Cell Biol* 14, 8058-70.

Yasumoto, K., Yokoyama, K., Takahashi, K., Tomita, Y., and Shibahara, S. (1997). *J Biol Chem* 272, 503-9.

11

Epigenetics: A Possible Link Between Stress and Melanocyte Malignant Transformation

Fernanda Molognoni and Miriam Galvonas Jasiulionis
Pharmacology Department, Universidade Federal de São Paulo, São Paulo
Brazil

1. Introduction

Melanoma incidence has been growing fast, however the only efficient available treatment is the surgical excision of the affected area when the tumor is detected early. Once diagnosed with metastatic melanoma, most patients have an overall surviving time of 2 years (Howell et al., 2009). Melanoma aggressive nature has encouraged many researchers to study possible molecular alterations behind disease development and progression. During many years the focus of studies on melanoma field was genetic alterations. Despite their importance in familial cases, mutation accumulation does not well explain sporadic tumor cases that can take many years to develop. In the past decades, growing attention has been given to the participation of epigenetic alterations, together with mutations, in the aetiology of cancer. Epigenetic marks control gene expression without altering the primary DNA sequence and are potentially reversible by epigenetic drugs. In a different way of mutations, epigenetic marks are plastic and can be influenced by environmental changes. Therefore, aberrant epigenetic patterns could explain the relationship between cancer and environment injury, since chronic injury is one of the causes for increased cancer risk (Bjornsson et al., 2004). In melanoma specifically, UV radiation and inflammation are considered as risk factors and epigenetic mechanisms could be the link between environmental insult and tumor formation and progression (Autier et al., 2011; Gallagner et al., 2010). The epigenetic mechanisms include DNA methylation, histone modifications, nucleosome remodeling and micro-RNAs (miRNAs). Collectively these mechanisms regulate the genetic information accessibility, promoting in this way the cellular diversity. In the next sections, the importance of epigenetics in melanoma will be discussed, as well their possible relation with environmental injuries.

2. Epigenetics and cancer

Cancer disease is complex and involves many factors including aberrant epigenetic alterations. Epigenetic is the study of hereditable patterns of gene expression that do not involve modifications in the primary DNA sequence. These heritable marks are established during embryonic development and stably maintained through cellular division (Reik, 2007). While the genome is the same in each cell type of an individual, the epigenome differs from tissue to tissue and is essential to maintain cellular identity (Mikkelsen et al., 2007). Therefore, its disruption could lead to inappropriate gene expression contributing to diseases such as cancer (Egger et al., 2004). Epigenetic mechanisms comprise DNA methylation, histone modifications, chromatin remodeling and RNA associated silencing by micro-RNAs (miRNAs). These mechanisms work together to regulate the functioning of the genome.

2.1 DNA methylation in cancer

DNA methylation is the most studied epigenetic mechanism, is generally linked to stable gene expression inactivation and normally occurs in mammals by the covalent modification of the CpG dinucleotide (cytosine to 5-methylcytosine). CpG distribution is not random in mammal genome. There are regions with high CpG frequency called CpG islands. Generally, these islands are located at 5' end of about 60% of human genes. Although some of these islands (about 6%) become methylated in a tissue-specific manner during development or in differentiated tissues, they are commonly unmethylated in normal cells (Straussman et al., 2009). One of the hallmarks of cancer cells is the presence of an aberrant DNA methylation pattern, which is characterized by specific DNA hypermethylation of tumor suppressor gene promoters and global DNA hypomethylation compared to normal cells. The hypermethylation of tumor suppressor promoters is associated with loss of their expression. Global DNA hypomethylation can contribute to genomic instability because it is largely a consequence of DNA methylation loss in non-coding DNA (like repetitive DNA sequences) and transposable elements (Rodriguez et al., 2006). Besides that, DNA hypomethylation can also cause oncogene activation (Jun et al., 2009).

2.2 Histone modifications in cancer

Posttranslational histone modifications, such as acetylation and methylation of lysine residues, have also a crucial role in controlling gene expression (Smith & Shilatifard, 2010.). Unlike DNA methylation, histone modifications can lead to either activation or inactivation. Overall, lysine acetylation is linked to gene activation whereas lysine methylation can be a marker for both, gene activation in the case of H3K4 trimethylation or repression in the case of H3K27 and H3K9 trimethylation. Histone posttranslational modification patterns and enzymes catalyzing the addition or removal of histone marks have been found altered in cancer, as well proteins that are specifically recruited by these modifications, such as polycomb group proteins, DNA methylltransferases (DNMTs) and nucleosome remodeling factors (Sharma et al., 2010). Non-covalent mechanisms, such as nucleosome remodeling, also contribute to regulate the gene activity (Svejstrup, 2010). In addition to their role as a basic organization for DNA packaging, nucleosome positioning regulates gene expression by altering DNA accessibility to transcriptional factors (Jiang & Pugh, 2009). The role of such mechanism in cancer is not well understood; nevertheless, recent data have been shown that nucleosome remodeling machinery seems to work together with histone modifications and DNA methylation in tumor-specific gene silencing (Morey et al., 2008).

2.3 Micro-RNAs in cancer

Another mechanism recently considered as epigenetic is RNA associated silencing by micro-RNAs. Micro-RNAs (miRNAs) are small non-coding RNAs that regulate gene expression through posttranscriptional silencing of target genes (Peter, 2010). Micro-RNAs are expressed in a tissue specific manner and can control many important biological processes including cell proliferation, apoptosis and differentiation. They can function as tumor suppressors or oncogenes, depending on their target genes (Peter, 2010). There is a growing number of miRNAs found aberrantly expressed in cancer cells and this abnormal expression seems to be tumor-specific (Lu et al., 2005). Moreover, miRNA expression can be regulated by many processes, including epigenetic mechanisms, such as DNA methylation and histone modifications (Deng et al., 2008).

Besides their individual roles, epigenetic mechanisms interact with each other to determine gene expression status and this interaction is crucial to promote properly chromatin architecture and gene activity during development and to maintain cellular identity after cell commitment process (Cerda & Bergman, 2009). Consequently, it has been shown that aberrant changes in epigenetic marks can compromise cell fate and participate in the early phases of cell malignant transformation (Feinberg et al., 2006). Different of mutations, these modifications can be reversible by chemical components and/or by environment and this reversible nature led to the development of a promising field: "The epigenetic therapy". In this way, this book chapter proposes to discuss what is known about the epigenome of melanoma, the emerging relation among stress, epigenetics and melanoma and the perspectives regarding epigenetic therapies to treat this metastatic disease.

3. Epigenetics and melanoma

The importance of epigenetic mechanisms in cancer formation and progression has been growing in the past decades. Despite of this, there are less published studies about abnormal epigenetic marks in melanoma than in any other cancer type. Additionally, most of the studies in literature refer to tumor suppressor genes silenced by DNA hypermethylation and few of them focus on posttranslational histone modifications, nucleosome remodeling and miRNAs. In the next sections, data concerning the epigenetic marks mentioned before will be discussed in melanoma.

3.1 The methylome of melanoma
3.1.1 Tumor suppressor genes silenced by DNA hypermethylation in melanoma

Melanoma development, as other tumors, is accompanied by disruption of cellular DNA methylation homeostasis, resulting in both hypermethylation of tumor suppressor promoters and genome wide hypomethylation (Molognoni et al., 2011; Soengas et al., 2001; Tenemura et al., 2009; Van Doorn et al., 2005).

Aberrant CpG island hypermethylation is a common event in melanoma and an important mechanism to shut off tumor suppressor genes (TSGs) involved in all key pathways of tumor development and progression, including cell cycle regulation, cell signaling, differentiation, DNA repair, apoptosis, invasion and immune system recognition (Sigalloti et al., 2010). Hypermethylation patterns are tumor-specific and it is still unclear why some DNA regions become hypermethylated, whereas others remain unmethylated. Most of the studies in the field of melanoma epigenetics describe hypermethylation of tumor suppressor genes. The great interest in this topic has an explanation: the considerable prognostic, diagnostic and therapeutic value of these studies. Because of that, some authors have been described the CpG island methylator phenotype (CIMP), which refers to the coordinated inactivation of tumor supressor and tumor-related genes in a determined type of cancer (Toyota et al., 1999). In addition, these epigenetic changes would create a distinct CIMP pattern that could be associated to the disease stage, recurrence and patient survival (Tanemura et al., 2009). At least 60 tumor suppressor genes have been identified to date as silenced by DNA hypermethylation in melanoma (Table 1). Some of them will be discussed in more details. A well-studied example of DNA hypermethylation in melanoma is *CDKN2A* locus. This locus encodes two proteins which are cell cycle regulators through pRB and p53 pathways (p16^{INK4A} and p14^{ARF}, respectively). Aberrant DNA hypermethylation at *CDKN2A* locus can independently affect p16^{INK4A} and p14^{ARF}, which are methylated in 27% and 57% of metastatic melanoma samples, respectively (Freedberg et al., 2008). In addition, *CDKN2A* locus is one of the well-known cases in which genetic alterations can cooperate with DNA methylation to promote gene inactivation (Freedberg et al., 2008; Gonzalgo et al., 1997). In this way, gene deletion can eliminate one allele and DNA hypermethylation silence the remaining one. This cooperation might be responsible for the concomitant inactivation of p16^{INK4A} and p14^{ARF} in a significant percentage of metastatic melanoma. Another important tumor suppressor which expression is lost by DNA hypermethylation in melanomas is *APAF-1*, a cell death effector that mediates p53-dependent apoptosis (Soengas et al., 2001). Then, the successfully shut off of *CDKN2A* locus and *APAF-1* by DNA hypermethylation and/or mutations could be a way utilized by melanoma cells to evade the growth arrest triggered by p53, once p53 is rarely mutated in melanomas (Soussi & Beroud, 2001). *PTEN* is another important gene which activity loss by DNA hypermethylation has been reported to contribute to the melanoma development (Mirmohammadsadegh et al., 2006). *PTEN* gene encodes a phosphatase that degrades PI3K products and its function loss can cause accumulation of PI3K messenger lipids, which in turn increase AKT phosphorylation and activity, leading to apoptosis decrease (Lian et al., 2005). Mirmohammadsadegh and co-workers (2006) observed an increase in *PTEN* CpG island methylation in primary, metastatic melanoma and serum from melanoma patients. Moreover, metastatic disease showed the higher DNA methylation percentage compared to primary tumor.

Besides the classical examples, there are other genes that have been found hypermethylated in melanomas such as *RAR-β2*, *SOCS1* and *SOCS2*. *RAR-β2*, which mediates growth arrest, apoptosis and differentiation triggered by retinoic acid (RA), has been found hypermethylated in 70% of melanoma lesions (Hoon et al., 2004). Interestingly, *RAR-β2* promoter hypermethylation is found with similar frequency in primary and metastatic melanoma lesions, suggesting that this hypermethylation process might be an early event in melanoma disease (Hoon et al., 2004). *SOCS*'s family genes have been implicated in the regulation of signal transduction by a variety of cytokines (Fujimoto & Naka, 2003). Moreover, *SOCS1* restoration suppressed both growth rate and anchorage independent growth of cells in which *SOCS1* was silenced by promoter methylation (Yoshikawa et al., 2001). One study using 20 melanoma cell lines and 40 freshly isolated advanced stage melanoma tumors showed around 90% and 80% of DNA methylation in *SOCS1* and *SOCS2* promoter, respectively (Liu et al., 2008). This methylation percentage was similar in melanoma cell lines and freshly isolated tumors. In addition, at the same work, *RAR-β2* was found with 60% of methylation both in cell lines and freshly isolated advanced stage melanoma tumors. Summarizing there are many tumor suppressor genes silenced by promoter hypermethylation in melanoma and it will be necessary to continue looking for other key genes to provide novel targets for diagnosis and therapy.

3.1.2 Aberrant DNA hypomethylation in melanoma

Global DNA hypomethylation found in cancer cells is largely a consequence of DNA methylation loss in repetitive elements, which in turn, as mentioned before, could contribute to genomic instability and transposon elements activation (Portela & Esteller, 2010). A clear case of repetitive element hypomethylation in cancer is the LINE family member LINE-1,

Pathway	Gene	Common Name	References
Apoptosis	DAPK1	Death- associated protein 1	Hoon et al., 2004
	HSPB6	Heat shock protein, alpha crystalin related, B6	Koga et al., 2009
	HSPB8	Heath shock 22 kDa protein 8	Sharma et al., 2006
	HSP11	Heat shock protein H11	Sharma et al., 2006
	RASSF1A	Ras association domain family protein 1A	Spugnardi et al., 2003
	TNFRSF10C	Tumor necrosis factor receptor superfamily member 10C	Liu et al., 2008
	TNFRSF10D	Tumor necrosis factor receptor superfamily member 10D	Liu et al., 2008
	APAF-1	Apoptotic protease activating factor 1	Soengas et al., 2001
Cell cycle	CDKN1C	Cyclin-dependent kinase inhibitor 1C	Muthusamy et al., 2006
	CDKN2A	Cyclin-dependent kinase inhibitor 2A	Freedberg et al., 2008
	TSPY	Testis specific protein, Y linked	Gallagher et al., 2005
Cell fate determination	MIB2	mindbomb homolog 2	Takeuchi et al., 2006
	APC	Adenomatous polyposis coli gene	Worm et al., 2004
	WIF1	Wnt inhibitory factor 1	Tenemura et al., 2009
Chromatin remodeling	NPM2	Nucleophosmin/nucleoplasmin 2	Koga et al., 2009
Degradation of misfold proteins	DERL3	Der1 like domain family member 3	Furuta et al., 2006
Differentiation	GDF15	Growth differentiation factor 15	Muthusamy et al., 2006
	HOXB13	homeobox B13	Muthusamy et al., 2006
DNA repair	MGMT	O-6-methylguanine-DNA methyltransferase	Hoon et al., 2004
Drug metabolism	CYP1B1	Cytochrome P450, family 1, subfamily B, polypeptide 1	Muthusamy et al., 2006
	DNAJC15	DnaJ (Hsp40) homolog, subfamily C, member 15	Muthusamy et al., 2006
Extracellular matrix	COL1A2	Collagen, type I, alpha 2	Koga et al., 2009
	MFAP2	Microfibrillar-associated protein 2	Muthusamy et al., 2006
inflammation	PTGS2	Prostaglandin-endoperoxide synthase 2	Muthusamy et al., 2006
metastasis	CDH1	E-cadherin	Tellez et al., 2009
	CDH8	Cadherin 8, type 2	Muthusamy et al., 2006
	CDH13	Cadherin 13, H-cadherin	Tellez et al., 2009
	SERPINB5	Serpin peptidase inhibitor, clade B, member 5	Denk et al., 2007
	LOX	Lysyl oxidase	Liu et al., 2008
	THBD	Thrombomodulin	Liu et al., 2008
Proliferation	WFDC1	WAP four-disulfide core domain 1	Liu et al., 2008
Signaling	ERa	Estrogen receptor α	Mori et al., 2006
	PGRβ	Progesterone receptor β	Tellez et al., 2009
	PTEN	Phosphatase and tensin homolog	Mirmohammadsadegh et al., 2006
	3-OST-2	Heparan sulfate (glucosamine) 3-O-sulfotransferase 2	Furuta et al., 2006
	RARRES1	Retinoic acid receptor responder 1	Bonazzi et al., 2009
	RARβ2	Retinoic acd receptor β2	Hoon et al., 2004
	RIL	Reversion-induced LIM	Tellez et al., 2009
	SOCS1	Supressor of cytokin signaling 1	Liu et al., 2008
	SOCS2	Supressor of cytokine signaling 2	Liu et al., 2008
	SOCS3	Supressor of cytokine signaling 3	Tokita et al., 2007
Transcription	HAND1	Heart and neural crest derivatives expressed 1	Furuta et al., 2004
	OLIG2	Oligodendrocyte lineage transcription factor 2	Tellez et al., 2009
	NKX2-3	Homeobox protein Nkx-2.3	Tellez et al., 2009
	PAX2	Paired box 2	Tellez et al., 2009
	PAX7	Paired box 7	Tellez et al., 2009
	GATA4	GATA binding protein 4	Atsushi et al., 2009
To be determined	BST2	Bone marrow stromal cell antigen 2	Muthusamy et al., 2006
	LXN	Latexin	Muthusamy et al., 2006
	QPCT	Glutaminyl-peptide cyclotransferase	Muthusamy et al., 2006

Table 1. Genes found hypermethylated in melanoma

which has been shown hypomethylated in a wide range of cancers (Portela & Esteller, 2010). Tellez and co-workers (2009) showed 75% of hypomethylation in LINE-1 repetitive sequence when they analyzed 16 melanoma cell lines by pyrosequencing. Additionally, DNA hypomethylation at specific promoters can activate expression of oncogenes and induce loss of imprinting (Herman & Baylin, 2003). In melanoma, a group of cancer-testis antigens and other genes considered as oncogenes have been shown to be hypomethylated (Howell et al., 2009). Melanoma antigen (*MAGE*) genes, for example, are normally only expressed by male germline cells. In somatic cells, their expression is silenced by promoter hypermethylation. Nevertheless, in malignant melanoma, aberrant expression of MAGE genes occurs and is associated with DNA hypomethylation (De Smet et al., 1996; Sigalotti et al., 2002). Recent data suggest that re-expression of MAGE genes in melanoma might contribute to malignant phenotype and interfere with therapy response (Simpson et al., 2005). Other genes found hypomethylated in melanoma were *MASPIN*, a serine protease inhibitor (Wada et al., 2005) and *TIMP1*, a metalloprotease inhibitor (Ricca et al., 2009). While the significance of *MASPIN* expression in melanoma formation and progression requires further investigation, *TIMP1* expression in melanoma cells seems to be an early event and promotes *anoikis* resistance (Ricca et al., 2009).

Comparatively to tumor suppressor epigenetic silencing little is known about the role of hypomethylation in melanoma development. More studies are necessary to find new target genes and repetitive sequences regulated by hypomethylation and their possible role in melanocyte malignant transformation.

3.2 Histone modifications in melanoma

The study of histone modifications is more complex than DNA methylation, since there are many possible combinations of histone marks. Additionally, there is the requirement of chromatin immunoprecipitation approaches with specific antibodies for each histone modification and the need of large amounts of starting DNA, which is difficult to obtain from patients' tumor samples. Summarizing, these factors restrict the number of studies about histone modifications in melanoma. Nevertheless, these problems might be solved by the new generation of high-throughput technologies and whole genome amplification protocols. Besides the limited data about histone modifications in melanoma, some studies have revealed changes in the expression of histone modifying enzymes, as well as aberrant changes in the level of global histone modifications in this type of cancer (Richards & Medrano, 2008; Molognoni et al., 2011).

3.2.1 Histone acetylation in melanoma

Generally, available studies have shown a global reduction of monoacetylated H4K16 in many types of cancer (Portela & Esteller, 2010). Loss of acetylation is mediated by histone deacetylases (HDACs), which have been found to be over-expressed or mutated in different types of tumors (Portela & Esteller 2010). It is important to remember that histone deacetylation is linked to inhibition of transcription and histone acetylation with transcription activation. In melanoma, until now there are non-specific studies addressing the global status of histone acetylation. On the other hand, there are some works showing that histone deacetylase inhibitors can re-activate genes that are silenced in melanoma (Sigalotti et al., 2010). These genes are involved in important processes, such as apoptosis (i.e. *BAX, BCL-X*), cell cycle (i.e.*CDKN1A, CDKN2A*), and DNA repair (*RAD 50*) (Munshi et al., 2006; Valentini et al., 2007; Zhang et al., 2004). Therefore, HDAC inhibitors are currently being studied as treatment against the development of malignant melanoma. Apart the global loss of histone acetylation and HDACs overexpression, histone acetyltransferases (HATs) have been shown altered in cancer cells as well by translocation, mutations, deletions and overexpression and have been implicated in the development of various tumors (Lafon-Hughes et al., 2008). Moreover, HATs and HDACs are commonly found in multi-subunit complexes where their activities and substrate specificities may be altered by cofactors and vice versa (Sadoul et al., 2007). The HATs Tip60 and HBO1, for example, are present in a complex with the melanoma tumor suppressors ING3 and ING4, respectively. Such complexes, important to regulate cell cycle, apoptosis and DNA repair, as well important p53 cofactors, are diminished in melanoma (Li et al., 2008, Wang et al., 2007). Besides their role in control tumor growth, Tip60 and other HATs (GCN5 and PCAF) can stabilize the transcription factor c-Myc, considered as a melanoma oncoprotein (Frank et al., 2003; Patel et al., 2004, Schlagbauer-Wadl et al., 1999). Furthermore, the HATs CBP and p300 have been shown associated with microphthalmia-associated transcription factor (MITF), a melanocyte lineage survival oncogene that has been related as overexpressed in melanoma and associated with decreased survival in patients with metastatic melanoma (Garraway et al., 2005; Price et al., 1998; Sato et al., 1997).

3.2.2 Histone methylation in melanoma

In addition to acetylation status, studies have demonstrated a possible role of aberrant histone methylation in melanoma. Melanoma cells were found to express elevated levels of the H3K27 histone methyltransferase EZH2 (McHugh et al., 2007). Moreover, in highly metastatic human melanoma cell line A375, there is a decrease in JARID1b histone demethylase (known by KDM5B as well) expression. The ectopic expression of JARID1b also resulted in cell cycle arrest in G1/S phase, accompanied by decreased cellular proliferation and DNA replication (Roesch et al., 2006). These are preliminary data that need confirmation in large series of melanoma tissues to define the role of histone methylation in melanoma biology. We are far from a clear comprehension of the melanoma histone code profile and further investigations will certainly open new avenues in the understanding of melanoma formation.

3.3 MicroRNAs in melanoma

Like mentioned before, microRNAs (miRNAs) regulate gene expression and are involved in the modulation of important cellular processes related with cancer, like apoptosis and cell proliferation (Peter, 2010). In this way, alterations in their expression might promote tumorigenesis. The study of miRNAs in tumor cells comprises a new scientific field and little is known about their roles in melanoma formation and development. The approach used at most available works is the hybridization of small RNA fractions isolated from cultured cells or tissue samples to specialized miRNA microarrays (Mueller & Bosserhoff, 2010). Many examples of miRNAs found de-regulated in melanoma cells were identified by comparing normal human melanocytes and/or benign nevi with melanoma cell lines or tumor tissue samples (Mueller & Bosserhoff, 2010). In this way, two important miRNAs found de-regulated in melanoma were described, miR-137 and miR-182, both of them regulating *MITF*, an important gene in melanoma genesis. MiR-137 was found down-regulated in melanoma cell lines, which resulted in *MITF* over-expression (Bemis et al.,

2008). In opposite way, miR-182 was shown to be over-expressed in melanoma, which contributed to metastatic potential by repressing *MITF* and *FOXO3* (Segura et al., 2009). MiR-182 seems to be involved in melanoma progression since it has been found over-expressed with the evolution of the disease, from primary to metastatic stages. These conflicted alterations might be related to the complex regulation of *MITF* in melanoma, which has been found up-regulated at the beginning phases of tumorigenesis and down-regulated in cells that acquired invasive and metastatic characteristics (Levy et al., 2006). Additionally, Muller and co-workers (2008) showed down-regulation of miRNA let-7 in melanomas. Let-7 regulates β3-integrin and according to these authors its down-regulation might be responsible for the over-expression of β3-integrin in melanomas.

The use of specialized miRNA microarrays approach limited the analysis to already known miRNAs, restraining the discovery of new miRNAs important in melanocyte transformation. To over cross this limitation, Stark and co-workers (2010) employed next-generation sequencing technology together with microarray profile for studying miRNAs in melanoblasts, melanocytes and melanomas. They identified, with this huge study, 279 novel miRNAs candidates to be important at the progression of the disease. With this work they showed that less-differentiated cell type (melanoblasts) expressed the highest number of miRNAs, whereas the most differentiated cell type, the melanocytes, expressed the fewest miRNAs species. Melanoma cell lines presented an intermediated number of expressed miRNAs. This data is in contrast with what has been shown for other types of cancer. Generally, miRNA global expression is up-regulated during differentiation process and down-regulated when partial de-differentiation occurs during malignant transformation (Lu et al., 2005; Wienholds & Plasterk, 2005). Therefore, the control of miRNA expression during melanocytic lineage commitment might be different from the other types of cells. The miRNAs studies in cancer are attracting many researchers nowadays, nevertheless more studies are necessary to define "melanoma-miRNAs", as well their importance in disease establishment and progression.

4. Microenvironment and melanoma progression

In the human skin, melanocytes reside in the epidermis and interact both with keratinocytes (cell-cell interaction) and the basement membrane (cell-extracellular matrix interaction). The growth and differentiation of melanocytes are tightly regulated by these interactions, which are mediated by adhesion molecules, such as cadherins (Tang et al., 1994) and integrins (Haass et al., 2005), and by soluble factors (Imokawa, 2004). Cell adhesion complexes, the cytoskeleton and the nucleus are linked and changes in the extracellular environment may affect the gene expression. In this way, it is now known that changes in this microenvironment can result in the disruption of melanocyte homeostasis and melanoma development (Haass & Herlyn, 2005; Li et al., 2001; van Kempen et al, 2005), although the molecular mechanisms involved are not completely elucidated.

Epigenetics has provided new insights about the interaction between genome and cellular environment. Since alterations in the skin microenvironment (i.e. ultraviolet radiation, inflammation, cutaneous wounding) seem to be critical factors for malignant transformation (Edwards et al, 1989; Tucker & Goldstein, 2003; van Kempen et al, 2007; von Thaler et al, 2010) and epigenetic abnormalities may substantially contribute to stress-induced pathologies (Johnstone & Baylin, 2010), a better understanding of epigenetic mechanisms underlying melanoma genesis may reveal the causal relationship between stress and cancer.

In addition, the comprehension of the epigenetics of melanoma could lead to the identification of epigenetic marks resulting in aberrant gene expression patterns related to initiation and progression of this tumor type and also contribute to the development of new therapeutic approaches, the epigenetic drugs, for this malignant tumor.

5. Experimental models of melanoma genesis

Experimental models both of murine and human cancers have contributed to a better comprehension of tumor biology and provided tools to develop new cancer therapies. In the case of melanoma, a variety of *in vitro* and *in vivo* models has been utilized, but is important to consider the advantages and drawbacks of each model (for review, see Becker et al, 2010; Santiago-Walker et al, 2009). Some models may be more suitable for answering a specific scientific question than others. Several human melanoma cell lines, mainly from metastatic tumors, have provided important information about gene expression profile, genetic abnormalities and biological phenotype of melanoma. However, many of these cell lines are maintained in culture for long time and, consequently, may accumulate additional alterations, not necessarily involved in the acquisition of malignant or metastatic phenotype. These cells have been utilized in xeno-transplantation models to analyze the aggressive behavior of melanoma, but are not suitable, for example, to study the role of immunological components in tumor progression. In the other way, murine syngeneic transplantation models have shown as a good option to study melanoma immunology and test new immunotherapeutic approaches. Genetically modified animals, in which oncogenes are super-expressed or tumor suppressor genes are silenced, have been used to study the role of specific genes in the genesis of melanoma (Larue & Beermann, 2007).

As mentioned before, cellular microenvironment is crucial for maintaining the normal function of melanocytes. In this way, some models were established in order to recapitulate, as closely as possible, the microenvironment context of the skin (Khavari, 2006). Two-dimensional melanocyte cultures (with or without keratinocytes), multicellular tumor spheroids and, specially, three-dimensional skin reconstructs (although without vascular and lymphatic components) have shown excellent ways to mimic skin environment in patient' lesions and can complement the data coming from murine melanoma models.

Even considering their limitations, mainly regarding the localization of melanocytes in the skin (Khavari, 2006), it has been proved that mouse melanoma models may substantially contribute to better understand the molecular mechanisms underlying the melanoma genesis and also to the evaluation of new drugs and therapies (Becker et al., 2010).

A linear model of melanocyte malignant transformation associated with sustained stress condition was recently established by our group (Oba-Shinjo et al, 2006). In this model, the murine lineage of non-tumorigenic melanocytes, melan-a (Bennett et al, 1987), was submitted to sequential cycles of anchorage impediment (blockade of cell-extracellular matrix interactions), which initially led to evident morphological and gene expression alterations and later to the acquisition of a full malignant phenotype (Molognoni et al, 2011). Melan-a melanocytes subjected to 1, 2, 3 and 4 deadhesion blockades were named respectively 1C, 2C, 3C and 4C cell lines, are non-tumorigenic and correspond to intermediate phases of malignant transformation or pre-malignant melanocytes. Different melanoma cell lines were established after submitting the spheroids obtained after 4C cell line deadhesion to limiting dilution. All clones randomly selected showed to be tumorigenic when subcutaneously transplanted into syngeneic mice. Both non-metastatic (for example,

4C3-, 4C11-, a1, a2, a3) and metastatic (Tm1, Tm4, Tm5) melanoma cell lines were obtained by this process. Some metastatic melanoma lineages (4C3+ and 4C11+) were also established from non-metastatic cell lines (4C3- and 4C11-, respectively) after spontaneously loss of p53 (Figure 1).

Different expression profile of E- and N-cadherin was observed in the transition phases from melan-a to 4C and also from 4C11- to 4C11+ cell lines (unpublished data), suggesting first the onset of epithelial to mesenchymal transition (EMT) and later mesenchymal to epithelial transition (MET). This data is reinforced by high expression of the key EMT regulator, Snail1, in 4C and 4C11- cell lines (unpublished data). Beta-1 integrins, important class of adhesion molecules involved in cell-extracellular matrix interactions, present their expression increased at the cell surface in metastatic melanoma cell lines. Additionally, strong evidences point β1-integrin as target of aberrant N-glycosylation along melanoma genesis (unpublished data). In our model, even with the limitations of a mouse model and a culture system, sustained stress led to significant alterations both in cell-cell (cadherins) and cell-ECM (β1-integrin) adhesion molecules, which have already been well described as proteins consistently involved in the loss of human melanocyte homeostasis.

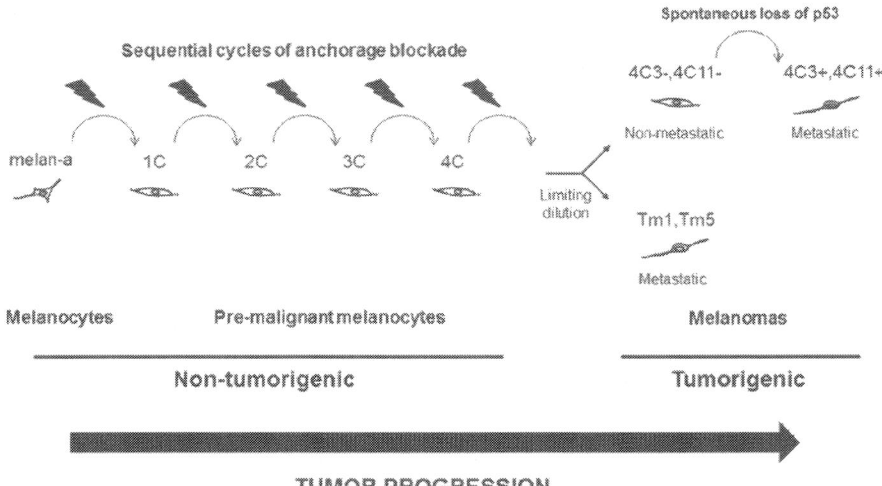

Fig. 1. Model of melanocyte malignant transformation associated with sustained stress condition

No treatment with carcinogenic agent or insertion of oncogene was utilized in our model, the only stimulus applied on non-tumorigenic melan-a melanocytes leading to malignant transformation was a sustained alteration in the microenvironment, the sequential cycles of anchorage blockade (Figure 1). As discussed before, the epigenetics seems to be a crucial link between environment and disease. In fact, alterations in the global level both of DNA methylation and histone marks were detected after few hours of melanocyte anchorage impediment. A global DNA hypermethylation was accompanied by increased mRNA and protein levels of Dnmt1, 3a and 3b (Campos et al., 2007). Regarding histone marks, elevated levels of the activation mark H3K4me3 and silencing mark H3K9me3 was observed in melan-a melanocytes maintained in suspension for 24 hours. Elevated levels of the histone deacetylase Sirt1 was also noted during melanocyte deadhesion (unpublished data). Recently, Kashiwagi and colleagues (2011) described the association of Sirt1 and Dnmt3b in chromatin regions resistant to nuclease, suggesting that Dnmt3b is preferentially recruited into hypoacetylated and condensed chromatin. Interestingly, co-immunoprecipitation assays revealed Sirt1-Dnmt3b interaction in melan-a melanocytes maintained in suspension, but not in adhered melanocytes (unpublished data). It is important to note that deadhered melanocytes also presented global DNA hypermethylation. These data suggest that the sustained stressful condition of anchorage blockade result in significant changes in the chromatin structure, which may have an important impact in the cell fate.

Comparing some epigenetic marks along melanoma genesis, in our model, an interesting pattern came up in which intermediate phases of malignant transformation, represented by the pre-malignant 4C melanocytes and non-metastatic 4C11- melanoma cell line, showed epigenetic marks characterizing an open chromatin state. Among some of these identified marks are increased levels of the activation histone mark H3K4me3, the histone methyltransferase *MLL1* (responsible for methylating H3K4), the chromatin remodelling factor *Chd1* (that recognizes the H3K4me3 histone mark), and the stress-related protein and histone deacetylase Sirt1 (that deacetylates the H4K16ac histone mark and many other non-histone proteins) (Molognoni et al., 2011). Regarding DNA methylation, a progressive global DNA hypomethylation along melanoma genesis and a drastic reduction in the expression of the methyl-binding protein MeCP2 since pre-malignant 4C melanocytes occurs. These results suggest that a decrease in MeCP2, protein that recognizes methylated CpGs and is implicated in gene repression, takes place before global DNA hypomethylation. Dnmt1 expression is increased since pre-malignant 4C melanocytes to metastatic melanoma cells while only metastatic melanoma cells present elevated levels of Dnmt3a and no significant difference in the expression of Dnmt3b is observed along melanocyte malignant transformation (Molognoni et al., 2011).

An open and highly accessible chromatin is a hallmark of stem cells and essential for their ability to give rise to any cell type (plurypotency). *Chd1* expression was showed to be required to maintain the open chromatin state of pluripotent mouse embryonic stem cells and also for somatic cell reprogramming to the pluripotent state (Gaspar-Maia et al., 2009). *Chd1* seems to promote the disassembly of nucleosomes at promoter regions, resulting in active transcription and open chromatin (Persson & Erkwall, 2010). Another molecular alteration that corroborates with the hypothesis that a less differentiated phenotype is acquired in the beginning of melan-a melanocyte malignant transformation is the increase in Sirt1 expression, which is related with pluripotent state. Recently, Calvanese and coworkers (2010) demonstrated that Sirt1 down-regulation is necessary for human embryonic stem cell differentiation. Low levels of Sirt1 allow the expression of key developmental genes, which are epigenetically silenced in first phases of embryogenesis. In this way, Sirt1 has been considered a regulator of stem cell pluripotency and differentiation. The elevated expression of Snail1, a major transcription factor regulating EMT (Barrallo-Gimeno & Nieto, 2005), also reinforces the acquisition of a less differentiated state by pre-malignant 4C melanocytes and non-metastatic 4C11- melanoma cells, which present a mesenchymal phenotype, different to melan-a melanocytes and metastatic 4C11+ melanoma cells that express low levels of Snail1 and a epithelial phenotype (unpublished result). Finally, the acquisition of tumorigenic properties (transition 4C to 4C11- cell lines) was characterized by the augment of silencing histone marks H3K9me3 and H3K27me3, whereas the acquisition of metastatic properties was accompanied by elevated expression of Dnmt3a, the highest grade of global DNA hypomethylation, and loss of Sirt1, Mll1, H3K4me3 mark, Chd1 and Snail1 (Molognoni et al., 2011). Besides that, a higher number of coding genes and miRNAs has their expression up-regulated in the tumorigenic cell lines 4C11- and 4C11+ after treatment with epigenetic drugs than in non-tumorigenic melan-a and 4C melanocytes (Molognoni et al., 2011), suggesting a higher number of genes and miRNAs aberrantly silenced by abnormal epigenetic marks.

In our model, it is possible that sustained stress condition (cycles of anchorage blockade) have led melan-a melanocytes to acquire early epigenetic marks conferring an open chromatin state and a less differentiated state in order to adapt the cells to the injury conditions and permit, later, the epigenetic reprogramming resulting in an incorrect differentiated state characterized by a full malignant phenotype (Figure 2).

A great number of genes were identified as having their expression abnormally regulated by aberrant epigenetic marks in our melanoma genesis model (unpublished data). Among them, Tissue Inhibitor of Metalloprotease-1 (Timp1) was described as presenting its promoter progressively demethylated along melanoma genesis and its expression increased since the early steps of melanocyte malignant transformation (Ricca et al., 2009). Apart its well-known function as a metalloprotease inhibitor, this protein regulates many other processes, such as cell proliferation and apoptosis (Chirco et al., 2006; Li et al., 1999). Our group showed that the expression of Timp1 confers *anoikis* resistance along melanocyte malignant transformation and also favors metastatic process (Ricca et al., 2009). Other examples of genes, which aberrant expression along melanoma genesis seems to be regulated by epigenetic alterations, are *Snail1*, *Chd1*, *p14^ARF*, *p16^INK4A*, *Cdkn2b*, *Cbs*, *Itga4*, *Xist*, *Vav1*, *Serpine1*, among others (unpublished data). Although these data came from a murine melanoma model, according to Melanoma Molecular Map Project (available online at http://www.mmmp.org/MMMP/) consistent parallel was observed in the expression of these genes in human melanoma samples. This analysis might provide novel epigenetic markers related to prognosis, diagnosis and response to treatment.

6. Oxidative stress and epigenetic reprogramming

As mentioned before, stress conditions (i.e., inflammation, UV radiation) have been implicated in the genesis of different pathologies, including cancer. Recently, Johnstone and Baylin (2010) pointed the emergent link between chronic stress and epigenetic alterations and its association with abnormal cell expansion, cellular dysfunction, changes in cell fate in cell renewal systems. They proposed that heritable epigenetic changes caused by stress could result in the evolution of abnormal cell states that contribute to disease.

In our model, in which the malignant phenotype was achieved after submitting non-tumorigenic melanocytes to a sustained stress condition, significant alterations were identified in the global DNA methylation level, histone marks and expression of different components of the epigenetic machinery (for example, Dnmts, HDACs, HATs, EZh2, MeCP2, Chd1, Sirt1). Abnormal epigenetic marks seems to profoundly impact in the expression of both coding genes and microRNAs, since different number of coding genes and microRNAs was re-expressed along melanoma genesis after treatment with the epigenetic drugs (Molognoni et al., 2011). These data strongly suggest a role of aberrant epigenetic marks in the initiation and progression of melanoma.

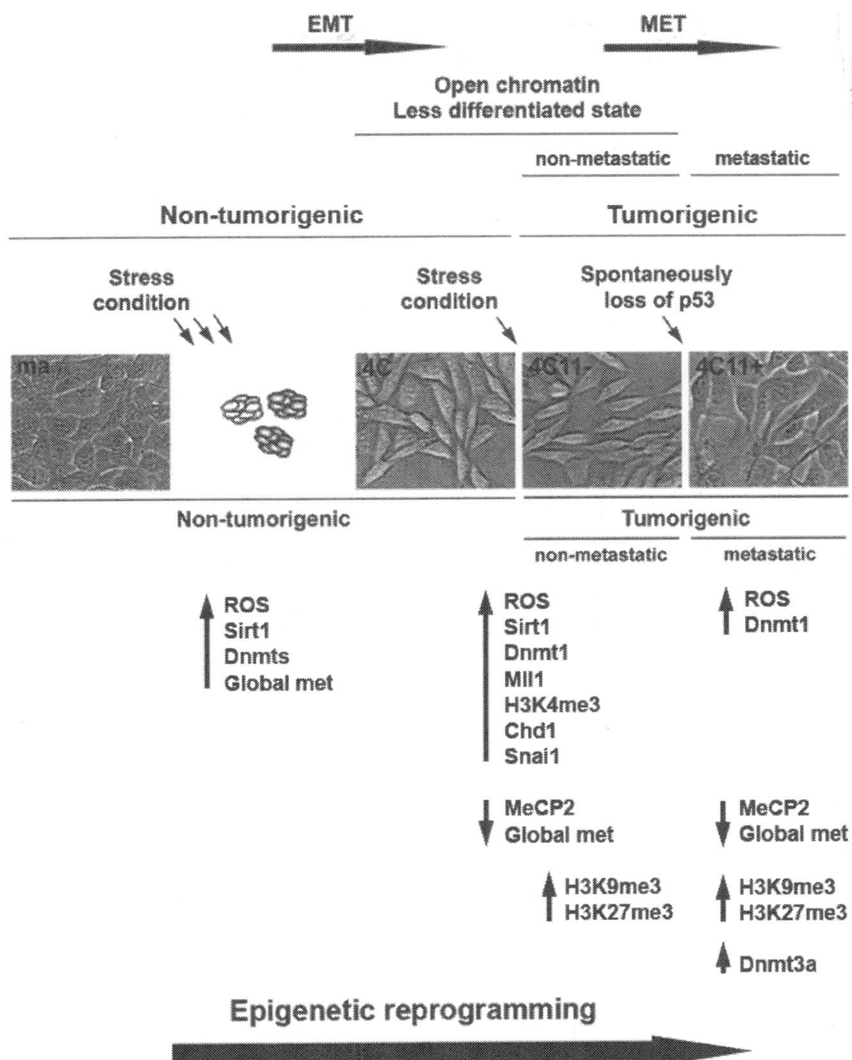

Fig. 2. Epigenetic reprogramming along murine melanocyte malignant transformation associated with sustained stress

The anchorage impediment, the driving force for malignant transformation in our model, was accompanied by global DNA hypermethylation and increased levels of DNA methyltransferases (Dnmts) (Campos et al., 2007) (Figure 2). In addition, elevated production of reactive oxygen species (ROS), such as superoxide anion and hydrogen peroxide, and nitric oxide characterized oxidative stress in this condition (Campos et al., 2007; Melo et al., 2011). Reinforcing the association between epigenetic and stress hypothesized by Johnstone and Baylin (2010) and Hitchler and Domann (2007), inhibiting oxidative stress by scavenging superoxide anion abrogated epigenetic alterations observed during the anchorage blockade (Campos et al., 2007). Moreover, melan-a melanocytes treated with the demethylating agent 5-aza-2`-deoxycytidine (Molognoni et al., 2011) or with the eNOS inhibitor L-NAME (Melo et al., 2011) before each deadhesion cycles do not transform. ROS-activated signaling pathways regulating Dnmts protein levels are still unknown and are under investigation in our laboratory. These data indicate that abnormal epigenetic patterns seems to be one of the initial events in the melanocyte malignant transformation related to microenvironment changes characterized by sustained oxidative stress.

Overall, the mechanisms underlying the regulation of epigenetic marks by oxidative stress still need to be elucidated. An instigating study by O'Hagan and coworkers (2008) showed the recruitment of the stress-related protein SIRT1 to double-strand DNA breaks induced in an exogenous promoter construct of the E-cadherin CpG island, which is frequently aberrantly DNA hypermethylated in epithelial cancers. DNA damage caused by oxidative stress induces the dissociation of Sirt1 from repetitive sequences and a functionally diverse set of genes and its re-localization to DNA breaks to promote repair, resulting in transcriptional changes that parallel with those in the aging (Oberdoerffer et al., 2008).

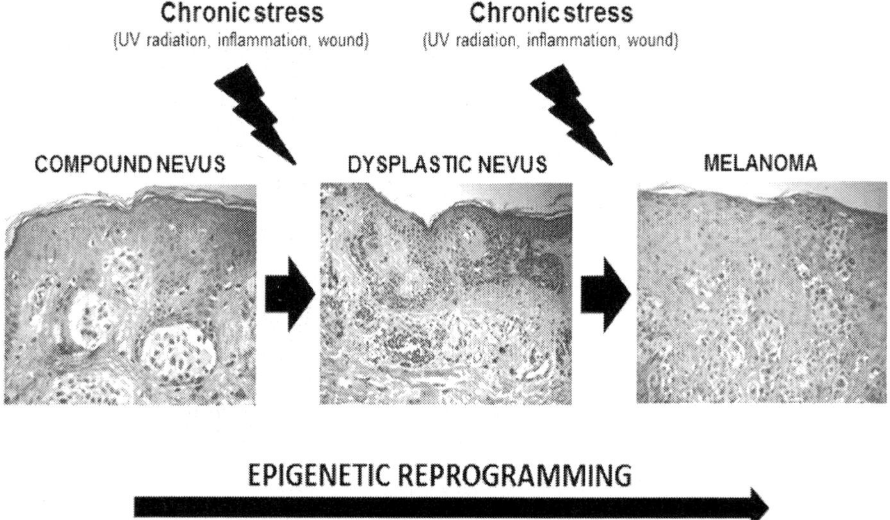

Fig. 3. Epigenetic reprogramming as a key contributor to human melanocyte malignant transformation associated with chronic stress.

O'Hagan and coworkers (2008) showed that, at the damage site, SIRT1 recruited epigenetic machinery components, such as EZH2 and DNMTs. Most cells had their DNA repaired, but a small number of cells presented the exogenous E-cadherin promoter silenced by heritable epigenetic marks. A similar event may be occurring in our malignant transformation model, since double-strand breaks, revealed by increased levels of γ-H2AX, and elevated levels of Sirt1 (unpublished data) were detected during the melanocyte anchorage blockade.

It is important to reinforce that ultraviolet radiation, a known environment factor predisposing to melanoma development (Autier & Dore, 1998; MacKie, 2006), and even inflammation, observed mainly in the early phases of melanoma genesis (Van Kempen et al., 2005), induces ROS generation. In this way, we can hypothesize that increases in ROS levels, caused for example by chronic inflammation, aging and UV radiation, might be responsible for aberrant epigenetic marks as a result of fails in the repair of primary DNA damage. It is easy to suppose that melanoma development associated with sustained exposition to these conditions may be related to oxidative stress and, possibly, to progressive epigenetic alterations (Figure 3).

7. Clinical applications

Melanoma is one of the most aggressive and radio- and chemo-resistant tumor types. In this way, the understanding of epigenetic mechanisms involved with both initiation and progression of melanoma could provide new avenues to identify diagnosis and prognosis markers and also develop novel therapeutic approaches.

7.1 Epigenetic tumor markers

Aberrant DNA methylation marks have some advantages to be used as tumor markers. One of these advantages is that DNA methylation is a stable and heritable mark. Additionally, DNA is less prone to degradation than RNA and can be easily obtained from patients' samples, such as sputum, serum and urine samples (Herman & Baylin, 2003). Highly sensitive techniques for detecting and quantifying DNA methylation are currently available, as methylation-specific polymerase chain reaction (Cottrell & Laird, 2003) and bisulfite treatment followed by DNA sequencing.

Aberrant epigenetic marks can be used to assess clinical outcomes or response to therapies. Both abnormally hypermethylated and hypomehtylated genes can be used as tumor markers in clinical application for early detection of disease, tumor progression, metastatic potential and response to therapeutic agents. Different epigenetic biomarkers have been described as presenting clinical relevance in different tumor types, such as gliomas, neuroblastomas, leukemias, prostate, bladder, lung, and colorectal cancer (Taby & Issa, 2010). However, very few data are available concerning both diagnosis/prognosis markers and the predictive value of markers in response to therapy in melanoma (Howell et al., 2009; Schinke et al., 2010). A promising predictive marker of melanoma progression was that reported by Mori and coworkers (2006), in which estrogen receptor A (*ER-A*) methylation was showed as a poor prognostic factor for melanoma patients. Recently, Shinojima and colleagues (2010) identified zygote arrest 1 (*ZAR1*) gene, responsible for oocyte-to-embryo transition, as frequently aberrant methylated in melanoma surgical specimens and melanoma cell lines, but not in normal human epidermal melanocyte cell lines or melanocytic nevi, suggesting *ZAR1* methylation as an early diagnostic marker for malignant melanoma. The methylation of circulating *RASSF1A* DNA showed to be less frequent in responder melanoma patients compared to non-responders to biochemotherapy (Mori et al., 2005).

7.2 Epigenetic therapy

Since epigenetic marks are potentially reversible by pharmacologic drugs, a better understanding of epigenetic alterations in melanoma may be valuable to establish novel therapeutic regimes in the treatment of patients with advanced melanoma. There are two classes of drugs approved by the US Food and Drug Administration (FDA) for cancer treatment that affect epigenetic marks: demethylating agents and histone deacetylase inhibitors (HDACi). Demethylating agents, as 5-azacytidine (Fenaux et al, 2009) and decitabine (Kantarjian et al., 2007), are nucleoside analogues that induce passive DNA demethylation through irreversible colavent bond with Dnmts (Issa, 2009). These DNA methylation inhibitors have been shown effective in a variety of non-solid tumors, such as acute myeloid leukemia and myelodysplastic syndrome, but the earlier clinical trials using decitabine as the only drug for solid tumors, including melanoma, have been disappointing (Abele et al., 1987; Schwartamman et al., 2000). Apart the unsuccessful results obtained by the treatment of solid tumors with demethylating agents, a promising use of this drugs relies on combined therapies, for examples with immunotherapy and chemotherapy. For melanoma, decitabine treatment seems to potentiate the effect of IL-2 therapy (Gollob et al., 2006) and overcome the resistance to interferon-induced apoptosis (Reu et al., 2006) in humans.

HDAC inhibitors target the catalytic domain of HDACs, blocking their substrate recognition (Xu et al., 2007). Short-chain fatty acids (such as valproic acid and sodium butyrate), hydroxamic acids (such as trichostatin A and vorinostat), benzamides (such as entinostat) and cyclic peptides (such as romidepsin) are different classes of HDACs. Among them, vorinostat and romidepsin were approved by the US FDA for the treatment of lymphoma (Mann et al., 2007). In melanomas and other tumor types, a number of genes involved in growth and survival have been described as up-regulated after HDAC inhibitors (Boyle et al., 2005; Minucci & Pelicci, 2006). Several HDAC inhibitors are under clinical trials in other cancer types, but the results have also indicated low activity in solid tumors (Prince et al., 2009). Experimental data from combined treatment of the SIRT1/2 inhibitor suramin and the xanthine derivative pentoxifylline showed synergistic inhibition of antitumor and antimetastatic activity in murine B16F10 melanoma cells (Dua et al., 2007). Valproic acid was showed to induce dose-dependent growth arrest, apoptosis, and sensitization to cisplatin and ectoposide in M14 human melanoma cells (Valentini et al., 2007).

An important aspect that needs to be considered about the use of epigenetic drugs in clinical practice is that they lack specificity and then may induce the reactivation of normally silenced sequences, such as imprinted genes, repetitive sequences and even pro-metastatic genes. Although this possibility exists, until now no clinical data support these concerns. Drugs selectively targeting specific genes are been investigated and may provide a promising future in the cancer therapy.

8. Conclusions

Since environmental factors, in special UV radiation, are important risk factors contributing to melanoma formation, and epigenetic changes may vary according to environment alterations, it is imposed to suppose the role of aberrant epigenetic marks induced by stress conditions in the genesis of melanoma. Epigenetics has emerged as a promising field in developing novel and efficient drugs against cancer. In this way, efforts should be done in order to determine not only genes which aberrant expression as a consequence of abnormal epigenetic marks, but also clarify the molecular pathways involved in deregulation of epigenetic machinery in response of stress conditions. This knowledge may bring new insights concerning chronic stress, epigenetic alterations and melanoma genesis, and also may provide novel targets to drug development and epigenetic marks with value in diagnosis, prognosis and response to treatment.

9. Acknowledgments

We express our thanks for all integrands of our laboratory whose have been working hardly and enthusiastically. We thank Dr. Gilles Landman (Pathology Department, Universidade Federal de São Paulo) for kindly providing the photomicrographs from figure 3. We also acknowledge the financial support from Fundação de Amparo à Pesquisa do Estado de São Paulo (FAPESP, grants 08/50366-3 and 06/61293-1).

10. References

Abele R, Clavel M, Dodion P, Bruntsch U, Gundersen S, Smyth J, Renard J, van Glabbeke M & Pinedo HM (1987). The EORTC Early Clinical Trials Cooperative Group experience with 5-aza-2'-deoxycytidine (NSC 127716) in patients with colo-rectal, head and neck, renal carcinomas and malignant melanomas. *Eur. J. Cancer Clin. Oncol.* 23: 1921-1924

Autier P, & Dore JF (1998). Influence of sun exposures during childhood and during adulthood on melanoma risk. EPIMEL and EORTC Melanoma Cooperative Group. European Organisation for Research and Treatment of Cancer. *Int. J. Cancer* 77: 533-537

Autier P, Doré JF, Eggermont AM, & Coebergh JW (2011). Epidemiological evidence that UVA radiation is involved in the genesis of cutaneous melanoma. *Curr. Opin. Oncol.* 23(2): 189-196

Barrallo-Gimeno A, & Nieto MA (2005). The Snail genes as inducers of cell movement and survival: implications in development and cancer. Development 132(14): 3151-3561

Becker JC, Houben R, Schrama D, Voigt H, Ugurel S, & Reisfeld RA (2009). Mouse models for melanoma: a personal perspective. *Exp. Dermatol.* 19: 157-164

Bemis LT, Chen R, Amato CM, Classen EH, Robinson SE, Coffey DG, Erickson PF, Shellman YG, & Robinson WA (2008). MicroRNA-137 targets microphthalmia-associated transcription factor in melanoma cell lines. *Cancer Res.* 68(5): 1362-1368

Bennett DC, Cooper PJ, & Hart IR (1987). A line of non-tumorigenic mouse melanocytes, syngeneic with the B16 melanoma and requiring a tumor promoter for growth. *Int. J. Cancer* 39: 414-418

Bjornsson HT, Fallin MD, & Feinberg AP (2004). An integrated epigenetic and genetic approach to common human disease. Trends Genet. 20(8): 350-358

Bonazzi VF, Irwin D, & Hayward NK (2009). Identification of candidate tumor suppressor genes inactivated by promoter methylation in melanoma. *Genes Chromosomes Cancer* 48(1): 10-21

Boyle GM, Marlyn AC, & Parsons PG (2005). Histone deacetylase inhibitors and malignant melanoma. *Pigment Cell Res.* 18(3): 160-166

Calvanese V, Lara E, Suárez-Alvarez B, Abu Dawud R, Vázquez-Chantada M, Martínez-Chantar ML, Embade N, López-Nieva P, Horrillo A, Hmadcha A, Soria B, Piazzolla D, Herranz D, Serrano M, Mato JM, Andrews PW, López-Larrea C, Esteller M, & Fraga MF (2010). Sirtuin 1 regulation of developmental genes during differentiation of stem cells. *Proc. Natl. Acad. Sci. USA* 107:13736-13741

Cedar H, & Bergman Y (2009). Linking DNA methylation and histone modification: patterns and paradigms. *Nat. Rev. Genet.* 10(5):295-304

Chirco R, Liu XW, Jung KK, & Kim HR (2006). Novel functions of Timps in cell signaling. *Cancer Metastasis Rev.* 25, 99–113

Cottrell SE, &Laird PW (2003). Sensitive detection of DNA methylation. *Ann. N. Y. Acad. Sci.* 983: 120-130

De Smet C, De Backer O, Faraoni I, Lurquin C, Brasseur F, & Boon T (1996). The activation of human gene MAGE-1 in tumor cells is correlated with genome-wide demethylation. *Proc. Natl. Acad. Sci. USA* 93(14): 7149-7153

Deng S, Calin GA, Croce CM, Coukos G, & Zhang L (2008). Mechanisms of microRNA deregulation in human cancer. *Cell Cycle* 7(17): 2643-2646

Denk AE, Bettstetter M, Wild PJ, Hoek K, Bataille F, Dietmaier W, & Bosserhoff AK (2007). Loss of maspin expression contributes to a more invasive potential in malignant melanoma. *Pigment Cell Res.* 20(2): 112-119

Dua P, Ingle A, & Gude RP (2007). Suramin augments the antitumor and antimetastatic activity of pentoxifylline in B16F10 melanoma. *Int. J. Cancer* 121(7): 1600-1608

Edwards MJ, Hirsch RM, Broadwater JR, Netscher DT, & Ames FC (1989). Squamous cell carcinoma arising in previously burned or irradiated skin. *Arch. Surg.* 124: 115-117

Egger G, Liang G, Aparicio A, & Jones PA (2004). Epigenetics in human disease and prospects for epigenetic therapy. *Nature* 429(6990): 457-463

Fenaux P, Mufti GJ, Hellstrom-Lindberg E, Santini V, Finelli C, Giagounidis A, Schoch R, Gattermann N, Sanz G, List A, Gore SD, Seymour JF, Bennett JM, Byrd J, Backstrom J, Zimmerman L, McKenzie D, Beach C, Silverman LR; & International Vidaza High-Risk MDS Survival Study Group (2009). Efficacy of azacitidine compared with that of conventional care regimens in the treatment of higher-risk myelodysplastic syndromes: a randomised, open-label, phase III study. *Lancet Oncol.* 10: 223-232

Frank SR, Parisi T, Taubert S, Fernandez P, Fuchs M, Chan HM, Livingston DM, & Amati B (2003). MYC recruits the TIP60 histone acetyltransferase complex to chromatin. *EMBO Rep.* 4(6): 575-580

Freedberg DE, Rigas SH, Russak J, Gai W, Kaplow M, Osman I, Turner F, Randerson-Moor JA, Houghton A, Busam K, Timothy Bishop D, Bastian BC, Newton-Bishop JA, & Polsky D (2008). Frequent p16-independent inactivation of p14ARF in human melanoma. *J. Natl. Cancer Inst.* 100(11): 784-795

Fujimoto M, & Naka T (2003). Regulation of cytokine signaling by SOCS family molecules. Trends Immunol. 24(12): 659-666

Furuta J, Nobeyama Y, Umebayashi Y, Otsuka F, Kikuchi K, & Ushijima T (2006). Silencing of Peroxiredoxin 2 and aberrant methylation of 33 CpG islands in putative promoter regions in human malignant melanomas. *Cancer Res* 66(12): 6080-6086

Gallagher WM, Bergin OE, Rafferty M, Kelly ZD, Nolan IM, Fox EJ, Culhane AC, McArdle L, Fraga MF, Hughes L, Currid CA, O'Mahony F, Byrne A, Murphy AA, Moss C, McDonnell S, Stallings RL, Plumb JA, Esteller M, Brown R, Dervan PA, & Easty DJ (2005). Multiple markers for melanoma progression regulated by DNA methylation: insights from transcriptomic studies. *Carcinogenesis* 26(11): 1856-1867

Gallagher RP, Lee TK, Bajdik CD, & Borugian M (2010). Ultraviolet radiation. *Chronic Dis. Can.* 1: 51-68

Garraway LA, Widlund HR, Rubin MA, Getz G, Berger AJ, Ramaswamy S, Beroukhim R, Milner DA, Granter SR, Du J, Lee C, Wagner SN, Li C, Golub TR, Rimm DL, Meyerson ML, Fisher DE, & Sellers WR (2005). Integrative genomic analyses identify MITF as a lineage survival oncogene amplified in malignant melanoma. *Nature* 436(7047): 117-122

Gaspar-Maia A, Alajem A, Polesso F, Sridharan R, Mason MJ, Heidersbach A, Ramalho-Santos J, McManus MT, Plath K, Meshorer E, & Ramalho-Santos M (2009). Chd1 regulates open chromatin and pluripotency of embryonic stem cells. *Nature* 460(7257):863-868

Gollob JA, Sciambi CJ, Peterson BL, Richmond T, Thoreson M, Moran K, Dressman HK, Jelinek J, & Issa JP (2006). Phase I trial of sequential low-dose 5-aza-2'-deoxycytidine plus high-dose intravenous bolus interleukin-2 in patients with melanoma or renal cell carcinoma. Clin. Cancer Res. 12: 4619-4627

Gonzalgo ML, Bender CM, You EH, Glendening JM, Flores JF, Walker GJ, Hayward NK, Jones PA, & Fountain JW (1997). Low frequency of p16/CDKN2A methylation in sporadic melanoma: comparative approaches for methylation analysis of primary tumors. *Cancer Res.* 57(23): 5336-5347

Haass NK, & Herlyn M (2005). Normal human melanocyte homeostasis as a paradigm for understanding melanoma. *J. Investig. Dermatol. Symp. Proc.* 10: 153-163

Haass NK, Smalley KS, Li L, & Herlyn M (2005). Adhesion, migration and communication in melanocytes and melanoma. *Pigment Cell Res.* 18: 150-159

Herman JG, & Baylin SB (2003). Gene silencing in cancer in association with promoter hypermethylation. *N. Engl. J. Med.* 349: 2042-2054

Hitchler MJ, & Domann FE (2007). An epigenetic perspective on the free radical theory of development. *Free Rad. Biol. Med.* 43: 1023-1036

Hoon DS, Spugnardi M, Kuo C, Huang SK, Morton DL, & Taback B (2004). Profiling epigenetic inactivation of tumor suppressor genes in tumors and plasma from cutaneous melanoma patients. *Oncogene* 23(22): 4014-4022

Howell PM, Liu S, Ren S, Behlen C, Fodstad O, & Riker AI (2009). Epigenetics in human melanoma. *Cancer Control* 16(3): 200-218

Imokawa G (2004). Autocrine and paracrine regulation of melanocytes in human skin and in pigmentary disorders. *Pigment Cell Res.* 17: 96-110

Issa JP, & Kantarjian HM (2009). Targeting DNA methylation. *Clin. Cancer Res.* 15: 3938-3946

Jiang C, & Pugh BF (2009). Nucleosome positioning and gene regulation: advances through genomics. *Nat. Rev. Genet.* 10(3): 161-172

Johnstone SE, & Baylin SB (2010). Stress and the epigenetic landscape: a link to the pathobiology of human diseases? *Nat. Rev. Genet.* 11: 806-812

Jun HJ, Woolfenden S, Coven S, Lane K, Bronson R, Housman D, & Charest A (2009). Epigenetic regulation of c-ROS receptor tyrosine kinase expression in malignant gliomas. *Cancer Res.* 69(6): 2180-2184

Kantarjian H, Oki Y, Garcia-Manero G, Huang X, O'Brien S, Cortes J, Faderl S, Bueso-Ramos C, Ravandi F, Estrov Z, Ferrajoli A, Wierda W, Shan J, Davis J, Giles F, Saba HI, & Issa JP (2007). Results of a randomized study of 3 schedules of low-dose decitabine in higher-risk myelodysplastic syndrome and chronic myelomonocytic leukemia. *Blood* 109(1): 52-57

Kashiwagi K, Nimura K, & Kaneda Y (2011). DNA methyltransferase 3b preferentially associates with condensed chromatin. Nucleic Acids Res. 39(3): 874-888

Khavari PA (2006). Modelling cancer in human skin tissue. *Nat. Rev. Cancer* 6: 270-280

Koga Y, Pelizzola M, Cheng E, Krauthammer M, Sznol M, Ariyan S, Narayan D, Molinaro AM, Halaban R, & Weissman SM (2009). Genome-wide screen of promoter methylation identifies novel markers in melanoma. *Genome Res.* 19(8): 146214-70

Lafon-Hughes L, Di Tomaso MV, Méndez-Acuña L, & Martínez-López W (2008). Chromatin-remodelling mechanisms in cancer. *Mutat. Res.* 658(3): 191-214

Larue L, & Beermann F (2007). Cutaneous melanoma in genetically modified animals. *Pigment Cell Res.* 20: 485-497

Levy C, Khaled M, & Fisher DE (2006). MITF: master regulator of melanocyte development and melanoma oncogene. Trends Mol. Med. 12(9): 406-414

Li G, Fridman R, & Kim HR (1999). Tissue inhibitor of metalloproteinase-1 inhibits apoptosis of human breast epithelial cells. *Cancer Res.* 59, 6267–6275

Li G, Schaider H, Satyamoorthy K, Hanakawa Y, Hashimoto K, & Herlyn M (2001). Downregulation of E-cadherin and desmoglein 1 by autocrine hepatocyte growth factor during melanoma development. *Oncogene* 20: 8125-8135

Lian Z, & Di Cristofano A (2005). Class reunion: PTEN joins the nuclear crew. *Oncogene* 24(50): 7394-7400

Liu S, Ren S, Howell P, Fodstad O, & Riker AI (2008). Identification of novel epigenetically modified genes in human melanoma via promoter methylation gene profiling. *Pigment Cell Melanoma Res.* 21(5): 545-558

Lu C, Tej SS, Luo S, Haudenschild CD, Meyers BC, & Green PJ (2005). Elucidation of the small RNA component of the transcriptome. *Science* 309(5740): 1567-1569

Lu J, Getz G, Miska EA, Alvarez-Saavedra E, Lamb J, Peck D, Sweet-Cordero A, Ebert BL, Mak RH, Ferrando AA, Downing JR, Jacks T, Horvitz HR, & Golub TR (2005). MicroRNA expression profiles classify human cancers. *Nature* 435(7043): 834-838

MacKie RM (2006). Long-term health risk to the skin of ultraviolet radiation. *Prog. Biophys. Mol. Biol.* 92: 92-96

Mann BS, Johnson JR, Cohen MH, Justice R, & Pazdur R (2007). FDA approval summary: vorinostatfor treatment of advanced primary cutaneous T-cell lymphoma. *Oncologist* 12: 1247-1252

McHugh JB, Fullen DR, Ma L, Kleer CG, & Su LD (2007). Expression of polycomb group protein EZH2 in nevi and melanoma. *J. Cutan. Pathol.* 34(8): 597-600

Melo FH, Molognoni F, Morais AS, Toricelli M, Mouro MG, Higa EM, Lopes JD, & Jasiulionis MG (2011). Endothelial nitric oxide synthase uncoupling as a key mediator of melanocyte malignant transformation associated with sustained stress conditions. *Free Radic. Biol. Med.* (mar 14), epub ahead of print

Mikkelsen TS, Ku M, Jaffe DB, Issac B, Lieberman E, Giannoukos G, Alvarez P, Brockman W, Kim TK, Koche RP, Lee W, Mendenhall E, O'Donovan A, Presser A, Russ C, Xie X, Meissner A, Wernig M, Jaenisch R, Nusbaum C, Lander ES, & Bernstein BE (2007). Genome-wide maps of chromatin state in pluripotent and lineage-committed cells. Nature 448(7153): 553-560

Minucci S, & Pelicci PG (2006). Histone deacetylase inhibitors and the promise of epigenetic (and more) treatments for cancer. *Nat. Rev. Cancer* 6(1): 38-51

Mirmohammadsadegh A, Marini A, Nambiar S, Hassan M, Tannapfel A, Ruzicka T, & Hengge UR (2006). Epigenetic silencing of the PTEN gene in melanoma. *Cancer Res.* 66(13): 6546-6552

Molognoni F, Cruz AT, Meliso FM, Morais AS, Souza CF, Xander P, Bischof JM, Costa FF, Soares MB, Liang G, Jones PA, & Jasiulionis MG (2011). Epigenetic reprogramming as a key contributor to melanocyte malignant transformation. *Epigenetics* 6(4): epub ahead of print

Morey L, Brenner C, Fazi F, Villa R, Gutierrez A, Buschbeck M, Nervi C, Minucci S, Fuks F, & Di Croce L (2008). MBD3, a component of the NuRD complex, facilitateschromatin alteration and deposition of epigenetic marks. *Mol. Cell Biol.* 28(19): 5912-5923

Mori T, O'Day SJ, Umetani N, Martinez SR, Kitago M, Koyanagi K, Kuo C, Takeshima TL, Milford R, Wang HJ, Vu VD, Nguyen SL, & Hoon DS (2005). Predictive utility of circulating methylated DNA in serum of melanoma patients receiving biochemotherapy. *J. Clin Oncol.* 23(36):9351-9358

Mori T, Martinez SR, O'Day SJ, Morton DL, Umetani N, Kitago M, Tanemura A, Nguyen SL, Tran AN, Wang HJ, & Hoon DS (2006) Estrogen receptor-alpha methylation predicts melanoma progression. *Cancer Res.* 66(13): 6692-6698

Mueller DW, & Bosserhoff AK (2010). The evolving concept of 'melano-miRs' microRNAs in melanomagenesis. Pigment Cell Melanoma Res. 23(5): 620-626

Müller DW, & Bosserhoff AK (2008). Integrin beta 3 expression is regulated by let-7a miRNA in malignant melanoma. *Oncogene* 27(52): 6698-6706

Munshi A, Tanaka T, Hobbs ML, Tucker SL, Richon VM, & Meyn RE (2006). Vorinostat, a histone deacetylase inhibitor, enhances the response of human tumor cells to ionizing radiation through prolongation of gamma-H2AX foci. *Mol. Cancer Ther.* 5(8): 1967-1974

Murr R, Loizou JI, Yang YG, Cuenin C, Li H, Wang ZQ, & Herceg Z (2005). Histone acetylation by Trrap-Tip60 modulates loading of repair proteins and repair of DNA double-strand breaks. *Nat. Cell Biol.* 8(1): 91-99

Muthusamy V, Duraisamy S, Bradbury CM, Hobbs C, Curley DP, Nelson B, & Bosenberg M (2006). Epigenetic silencing of novel tumor suppressors in malignant melanoma. *Cancer Res.* 66(23): 11187-11193

Oba-Shinjo SM, Correa M, Ricca TI, Molognoni F, Pinhal MA, Neves IA, Marie SK, Sampaio LO, Nader HB, Chammas R, & Jasiulionis MG (2006). Melanocyte transformation associated with substrate adhesion impediment. *Neoplasia* 8(3): 231-241

Oberdoerffer P, Michan S, McVay M, Mostoslavsky R, Vann J, Park S, Hartlerode A, Stegmuller J, Hafner A, Loerch P, Wright SM, Mills KD, Bonni A, Yankner BA, Scully R, Prolla TA, Alt FW, & Sinclair DA (2008). SIRT1 redistribution on chromatin promotes genomic stability but alters gene expression during aging. *Cell* 135: 907-918

O'Hagan HM, Mohammad HP, & Baylin SB (2008). Double Strand Breaks Can Initiate Gene silencing and SIRT1-dependent onset of DNA methylation in an exogenous promoter CpG island. *PLoS Genet.* 4(8): e1000155

Patel JH, Du Y, Ard PG, Phillips C, Carella B, Chen CJ, Rakowski C, Chatterjee C, Lieberman PM, Lane WS, Blobel GA, & McMahon SB (2004). The c-MYC oncoprotein is a substrate of the acetyltransferases hGCN5/PCAF and TIP60. *Mol. Cell Biol.* 24(24): 10826-10834

Persson J, & Erkwall K (2010) Chd1 remodelers maintain open chromatin and regulate the epigenetics of differentiation. *Exp. Cell Res.* 316(8): 1316-1323

Peter ME (2010). Targeting of mRNAs by multiple miRNAs: the next step. Oncogene 29(15): 2161-2164

Portela A, & Esteller M (2010). Epigenetic modifications and human disease. *Nat. Biotechnol.* 28(10): 1057-1068

Price ER, Ding HF, Badalian T, Bhattacharya S, Takemoto C, Yao TP, Hemesath TJ, & Fisher DE (1998). Lineage-specific signaling in melanocytes. C-kit stimulation recruits p300/CBP to microphthalmia. *J. Biol. Chem.* 273(29): 17983-1796

Prince HM, Bishton MJ, & Harrison SJ (2009). Clinical studies of histone deacetylase inhibitors. *Clin. Cancer Res.* 15: 3958-3969

Reik W (2007). Stability and flexibility of epigenetic gene regulation in mammalian development. *Nature* 447(7143): 425-432

Reu FJ, Bae SI, Cherkassky L, Leaman DW, Lindner D, Beaulieu N, MacLeod AR, & Borden EC (2006). Overcoming resistance to interferon-induced apoptosis of renal carcinoma and melanoma cells by DNA demethylation. *J. Clin. Oncol.* 24(23): 3771-3779

Ricca TI, Liang G, Suenaga AP, Han SW, Jones PA, & Jasiulionis MG (2009). Tissue inhibitor of metalloproteinase 1 expression associated with gene demethylation confers anoikis resistance in early phases of melanocyte malignant transformation. *Transl. Oncol.* 2(4): 329-340

Richards WH, & Medrano EE (2008). Epigenetic marks in melanoma. Pigment Cell Melanoma Res. 22: 14-29

Riker AI, Enkemann SA, Fodstad O, Liu S, Ren S, Morris C, Xi Y, Howell P, Metge B, Samant RS, Shevde LA, Li W, Eschrich S, Daud A, Ju J, & Matta J (2008). The gene expression profiles of primary and metastatic melanoma yields a transition point of tumor progression and metastasis. *BMC Med. Genomics* 1: 13

Rodriguez J, Frigola J, Vendrell E, Risques RA, Fraga MF, Morales C, Moreno V, Esteller M, Capellà G, Ribas M, & Peinado MA (2006). Chromosomal instability correlates with genome-wide DNA demethylation in human primary colorectal cancers. *Cancer Res.* 66(17): 8462-8468

Roesch A, Becker B, Schneider-Brachert W, Hagen I, Landthaler M, & Vogt T (2006). Re-expression of the retinoblastoma-binding protein 2-homolog 1 reveals tumor-suppressive functions in highly metastatic melanoma cells. *J. Invest. Dermatol.* 126(8): 1850-1859

Sadoul K, Boyault C, Pabion M, & Khochbin S (2007). Regulation of protein turnover byacetyltransferases and deacetylases. *Biochimie* 90(2): 306-312

Santiago-Walker A, Li L, Haass NK, & Herlyn M (2009). Melanocytes: From morphology to application. *Skin Pharmacol. Physiol.* 22: 114-121

Sato S, Roberts K, Gambino G, Cook A, Kouzarides T, & Goding CR (1997). CBP/p300 as a co-factor for the Microphthalmia transcription factor. *Oncogene* 14(25): 3083-3092

Schinke C, Mo Y, Yu Y, Amiri K, Sosman J, Greally J, & Verma A (2010). Aberrant DNA methylation in malignant melanoma. *Melanoma Res.* 20: 253-265

Schlagbauer-Wadl H, Griffioen M, van Elsas A, Schrier PI, Pustelnik T, Eichler HG, Wolff K, Pehamberger H, & Jansen B (1999). Influence of increased c-Myc expression on the growth characteristics of human melanoma. *J. Invest. Dermatol.* 112(3): 332-336

Schwartsmann G, Schunemann H, Gorini CN, Filho AF, Garbino C, Sabini G, Muse I, DiLeone L, & Mans DR (2000). A phase I trial of cisplatin plus decitabine, a new DNA-hypomethylating agent, in patients with advanced solid tumors and a follow-up early phase II evaluation in patients with inoperable non-small cell lung cancer. javascript:AL_get(this, 'jour', 'Invest New Drugs.'); *Invest. New Drugs* 18(1):83-91

Segura MF, Hanniford D, Menendez S, Reavie L, Zou X, Alvarez-Diaz S, Zakrzewski J, Blochin E, Rose A, Bogunovic D, Polsky D, Wei J, Lee P, Belitskaya-Levy I, Bhardwaj N, Osman I, & Hernando E (2009). Aberrant miR-182 expression promotes melanoma metastasis by repressing FOXO3 and microphthalmia-associated transcription factor. *Proc. Natl. Acad. Sci. USA* 106(6): 1814-1819

Sharma BK, Smith CC, Laing JM, Rucker DA, Burnett JW, & Aurelian L (2006). Aberrant DNA methylation silences the novel heat shock protein H11 in melanoma but not benign melanocytic lesions. *Dermatology* 213(3): 192-199

Sharma S, Kelly TK, & Jones PA (2010). Epigenetics in cancer. *Carcinogenesis* 31(1): 27-36

Sigalotti L, Coral S, Nardi G, Spessotto A, Cortini E, Cattarossi I, Colizzi F, Altomonte M, & Maio M (2002). Promoter methylation controls the expression of MAGE2, 3 and 4 genes in human cutaneous melanoma. *J. Immunother.* 25(1): 16-26

Sigalotti L, Covre A, Fratta E, Parisi G, Colizzi F, Rizzo A, Danielli R, Nicolay HJ, Coral S, & Maio M (2010). Epigenetics of human cutaneous melanoma: setting the stage for new therapeutic strategies. *J. Transl. Med.* 8: 56

Smith E, & Shilatifard A (2010). The chromatin signaling pathway: diverse mechanisms of recruitment of histone-modifying enzymes and varied biological outcomes. Mol. Cell 40(5): 689-701

Soengas MS, Capodieci P, Polsky D, Mora J, Esteller M, Opitz-Araya X, McCombie R, Herman JG, Gerald WL, Lazebnik YA, Cordón-Cardó C, & Lowe SW (2001). Inactivation of the apoptosis effector Apaf-1 in malignant melanoma. *Nature* 409(6817): 207-211

Soussi T, & Béroud C (2001). Assessing TP53 status in human tumours to evaluate clinical outcome. *Nat. Rev. Cancer* 1(3): 233-240

Spugnardi M, Tommasi S, Dammann R, Pfeifer GP, & Hoon DS (2003). Epigenetic inactivation of RAS association domain family protein 1 (RASSF1A) in malignant cutaneous melanoma. *Cancer Res.* 63(7): 1639-1643

Stark MS, Tyagi S, Nancarrow DJ, Boyle GM, Cook AL, Whiteman DC, Parsons PG, Schmidt C, Sturm RA, & Hayward NK (2010). Characterization of the Melanoma miRNAome by Deep Sequencing. *PLoS One* 5(3): e9685

Straussman R, Nejman D, Roberts D, Steinfeld I, Blum B, Benvenisty N, Simon I,Yakhini Z, & Cedar H (2009). Developmental programming of CpG island methylation profiles in the human genome. *Nat. Struct. Mol. Biol.* 16(5): 564-571

Svejstrup JQ (2010). The interface between transcription and mechanisms maintaining genome integrity. Trends Biochem. Sci. 35(6): 333-338

Taby R, & Issa JP (2010). Cancer epigenetics. *CA Cancer J. Clin.* 60: 376-392

Takeuchi T, Adachi Y, Sonobe H, Furihata M, & Ohtsuki Y (2006). A ubiquitin ligase,skeletrophin, is a negative regulator of melanoma invasion. *Oncogene* 25(53): 7059-7069

Tanemura A, Terando AM, Sim MS, van Hoesel AQ, de Maat MF, Morton DL, & Hoon DS (2009). CpG island methylator phenotype predicts progression of malignant melanoma. *Clin. Cancer Res.* 15(5): 1801-1807

Tang A, Eller MS, Hara M, Yaar M, Hirohashi S, & Gilchrest BA (1994). E-cadherin is the major mediator of human melanocyte adhesion to keratinocytes in vitro. *J. Cell Sci.* 107: 983-992

Tellez CS, Shen L, Estécio MR, Jelinek J, Gershenwald JE, & Issa JP (2009). CpG island methylation profiling in human melanoma cell lines. *Melanoma Res.* 19(3): 146-155

Toyota M, Ahuja N, Suzuki H, Itoh F, Ohe-Toyota M, Imai K, Baylin SB, & Issa JP (1999). Aberrant methylation in gastric cancer associated with the CpG island methylator phenotype. *Cancer Res.* 59(21): 5438-5442

Tucker MA, & Goldstein AM (2003). Melanoma etiology: where are we? Oncogene 22: 3042-3052

Valentini A, Gravina P, Federici G, & Bernardini S (2007). Valproic acid induces apoptosis, p16INK4A upregulation and sensitization to chemotherapy in human melanoma cells. *Cancer Biol. Ther.* 6(2): 185-191

van Doorn R, Gruis NA, Willemze R, van der Velden PA & Tensen CP (2005). Aberrant DNA methylation in cutaneous malignancies. *Semin. Oncol.* 32(5): 479-487

Van Kempen LC, van Muijen GN, & Ruiter DJ (2005). Stromal responses in human primary melanoma of the skin. *Front. Biosci.* 10: 2922-2931

Van Kempen LC, Goos NP, van Muijen, & Ruiter DJ (2007). Melanoma progression in a changing environment. *Eur. J. Cell Biol.* 86: 65-67

Von Thaler AK, Kamenisch Y, & Berneburg M (2010). The role of ultraviolet radiation in melanomagenesis. *Exp. Dermatol.* 19(2): 81-88

Wada K, Maesawa C, Akasaka T, & Masuda T (2004). Aberrant expression of the maspin gene associated with epigenetic modification in melanoma cells. *J. Invest. Dermatol.* 122(3): 805-811

Wang Y, Dai DL, Martinka M, & Li G (2007). Prognostic significance of nuclear ING3 expression in human cutaneous melanoma. *Clin. Cancer Res.* 13(14): 4111-4116

Wienholds E, & Plasterk RH (2005). MicroRNA function in animal development. *FEBS Lett.* 579(26): 5911-5922

Worm J, Christensen C, Grønbaek K, Tulchinsky E, & Guldberg P (2004). Genetic and epigenetic alterations of the APC gene in malignant melanoma. *Oncogene* 23(30): 5215-5226

Xu WS, Parmigiani RB, & Marks PA (2007). Histone deacetylase inhibitors: molecular mechanisms of action. *Oncogene* 26: 5541-5552

Yoshikawa H, Matsubara K, Qian GS, Jackson P, Groopman JD, Manning JE, Harris CC, & Herman JG (2001). SOCS-1, a negative regulator of the JAK/STAT pathway, is silenced by methylation in human hepatocellular carcinoma and shows growth-suppression activity. *Nat. Genet.* 28(1): 29-35

Zhang XD, Gillespie SK, Borrow JM, & Hersey P (2004). The histone deacetylase inhibitor suberic bishydroxamate regulates the expression of multiple apoptotic mediators and induces mitochondria-dependent apoptosis of melanoma cells. *Mol. Cancer Ther.* 3(4): 425-435.

12

Antioxidant Defense and UV-Induced Melanogenesis: Implications for Melanoma Prevention

Uraiwan Panich
Department of Pharmacology, Faculty of Medicine Siriraj Hospital,
Mahidol University
Thailand

1. Introduction

Ultraviolet radiation (UVR) has been implicated as a major environmental factor in the pathogenesis of photoaging and skin cancers including melanoma. Hypermelanosis induced by UVR has been previously suggested to associate with melanomageneis, although the role of UVR in the development of melanoma is complicated since melanogenesis may depend on several factors such as skin type, genetic influence, the extent of sun exposure (e.g., intensity, timing and duration of UVR) and types of moles representing disturbed melanin synthesis (Parvel et al., 2004; Rass & Reichrath, 2008; Tran et al., 2008). Melanin has been well recognized for its photoprotective properties, although melanogenic intermediates can be phototoxic and UVR-dependent elevated melanogenesis could thus be biologically harmful, genotoxic and contributed to melanoma initiation, especially in lightly pigmented individuals (Brenner & Hearing, 2008; Smit et al., 2008; Takeuchi et al., 2004; Yamaguchi et al., 2006). The desire to have fair or tanned skin depends on different cultures. The use of whitening agents has been growing in the Eastern culture, whereas having tanned skin is favorable and attractive in the Western culture that makes artificial tanning products become increasingly popular. Various factors including endocrine and environmental factors, in particular UVR, affect melanogenesis, mainly regulated by tyrosinase in melanocytes and/or melanoma cells, in response to physiological and pathological changes (H.Y. Park et al., 2009; Slominski et al., 2004).

This chapter focuses on the role of UV-induced oxidative stress in association with melanogenesis, which can be modulated by antioxidant defenses. Several studies have supported the relationship between UVR-mediated melanogenesis and oxidative stress, which takes place when there is increased production of reactive oxygen species (ROS) and/or reactive nitrogen species (RNS) as well as antioxidant network impairment (Baldea et al., 2009; H.T. Wang et al., 2010). Therefore, improving antioxidant defense capacity to cope with oxidative insults may be beneficial in attenuation of abnormal production of melanin that could have a biological significance for the skin in protecting against photodamage. Whereas hyperpigmentation mediated by UV irradiation could reflect a sign of defensive response of the skin to stress, alteration in melanin synthesis may be implicated in skin damage and probably melanomagenesis, particularly in individuals with fair skin. Therefore, understanding the mechanisms by which antioxidants may modulate UVR-induced melanogenesis is of significance in order to develop effective antimelanogenic agents, which may be therapeutically useful for melanoma prevention.

2. UV-induced melanogenesis and melanomagenesis

Recently, the incidence of various diseases and disorders of the skin related to solar radiation continues to grow. Acute and chronic exposure of the skin to UVR can induce various cellular and biological changes including sunburn cell formation, DNA damage, loss of cell homeostasis and function, abnormal pigmentation, immunosuppression and inflammation responsible for several skin problems, particularly photoaging and skin cancers including non-melanoma and melanoma, the most aggressive type of skin cancer (Afaq & Mukhtar, 2001; Scharffetter-Kochanek et al., 2000). Skin can be exposed to both UVB (290-320 nm) and UVA (320-400 nm) radiation exhibiting various detrimental effects on the skin by triggering cellular and molecular responses that are responsible for damage of epidermis composed of keratinocytes, melanocytes and Langerhans cells as well as dermis consisting of fibroblasts and other skin components, especially extracellular matrix including collagen and elastin (Pinnell, 2003). The acute effects of UVR cause keratinocyte toxicity or sunburn, DNA damage and altered melanin synthesis. The chronic effects of UVR result in accumulation of degraded collagen and abnormal elastin that could contribute to photoaging as well as mutagenesis leading to photocarcinogenesis including melanomagenesis (von Thaler et al., 2010). UVB radiation is considered as the "burning ray" and makes up 4-5% of UV light reaching to the earth and more than 90% of solar radiation that reaches us is UVA. UVA reaches the earth's surface to the greater extent than UVB and the longer wavelength of UVA makes it penetrate deeper through the epidermal layer, reaching the dermis, whereas UVB, which has a shorter wavelength, is more energetic and mutagenic than UVA (Bennett, 2008). The biological effects of UVB and UVA on the skin are different. UVB radiation preferentially results in direct DNA damage, which happens when DNA directly absorbs the UVB photon, to produce DNA photoproducts, typically cyclobutane pyrimidine dimers (CPD) and 6,4-photoproducts implicated in genotoxicity (Seite et al., 2010). However, UVA has no direct influence on DNA as the absorption of UVA photons by chromophores in the skin cells can induce generation of ROS, e.g., singlet oxygen and hydrogen peroxide (H_2O_2), which in turn damages DNA through formation of mutagenic oxidative DNA products such as 8-hydroxydeoxyguanosine (8-OHdG), single-strand breaks in DNA and DNA-protein crosslinks (Pfeifer et al., 2005). Fortunately, the cells including melanocytes have many DNA repair systems including nucleotide excision repair (NER), a vital repair mechanism for photodamaged skin, that remove various types of DNA lesions induced by UVR. However, when the repair mechanisms are not capable of restoring genomic integrity, mutations can occur and lead to the development of skin cancer (Gaddameedhi et al., 2010).

Experimental and epidemiological studies have indicated that UVB capable of generating photoproducts might be the primary cause for non-melanoma skin cancer and UVA-mediated oxidative damage may be a possible risk factor of malignant melanoma (Bennett, 2008; Rass & Reichrath, 2008). In addition, UVA-dependent indirect DNA damage via oxidative stress in melanocytes has been postulated to be involved in the development of malignant melanoma via different mechanisms (Pavel et al., 2004). UVA radiation was observed to contribute more to the generation of photoproducts-related oxidative damage of DNA including CPD than UVB (Besaratinia et al., 2005). The ROS/RNS primarily generated by UVA radiation can cause direct deleterious chemical modifications to cellular components including lipids, proteins and, especially DNA, which can eventually initiate melanomagenesis (Cotter et al., 2007). A disturbance in the antioxidant network and an accumulation of oxidative products were also demonstrated in skin tissues of melanoma skin cancer and in melanocytes from atypical nevi (Sander et al., 2003; Smit et al., 2008). Moreover, the presence of high levels of RNS, in particular nitric oxide (NO), and nitrosative products in cutaneous melanoma has been observed to be correlated with poor prognosis of patients and contributed to melanoma invasiveness (Chin & Deen, 2010). Thus, excessive ROS/RNS-mediated imbalanced redox state and oxidative damage to the biomolecules of melanocytes might play a role in the pathogenesis of malignant melanoma by disturbing cellular machinery that further impairs cellular homeostasis and function involving differentiation, proliferation and malignant transformation of melanocytes (Campos et al., 2007; Kadekaro et al., 2005). Ultimately, UVR can initiate melanomagenesis via various pathways including mutagenicity of DNA photoproducts and interference in cell signaling that subsequently affects melanocyte apoptosis, proliferation, differentiation and functions including the regulation of melanogenesis (von Thaler et al., 2010; Wittgen & van Kempen, 2007). It has been proposed that UVR-dependent disrupted synthesis of melanin, known to be photoprotective or phototoxic, is regarded as an indirect effect of UVR responsible for melanomagenesis, although the connection between melanin production and the development of melanoma is poorly understood. UVR-mediated abnormality of melanogenic responses may result in cytotoxicity and mutagenicity, particularly in lightly pigmented melanocytes, that could contribute to malignant transformation of melanocytes (Baldea et al., 2009; Marrot et al., 2005; Riley, 2003; Slominski et al, 2004). Development of melanoma could also be associated with aggravation of melanogenesis in the melanocytes having disrupted melanosomes leading to leakage of melanin, which can further damage the cells through oxidative products (Gidanian et al., 2008; Sarangarajan & Apte, 2006). The melanin was demonstrated to significantly augment process of UVA-generated ROS and oxidative DNA damage probably responsible for melanomagenesis in Xeroderma pigmentosum patients, which exhibited impaired NER (H.T. Wang et al., 2010). Higher levels of oxidative DNA products including 8-OHdG induced by UVA exposure also correlated to the melanin contents in the human melanoma cells (Kvam & Tyrrell, 1999). Furthermore, alteration in melanogenic mechanisms in congenital melanocytic nevi was suggested to be accountable for melanoma promotion via aggravation of oxidative stress in melanocytes (Dessars et al., 2009). Hence, attenuation of abnormal melanin production, which could yield damaging effect on the skin, may have a dermatological significance for individuals with high melanoma risk. Targeting strategy for prevention of UVR-induced melanomagenesis therefore may include development of effective antimelanogenic agents and elucidating the antioxidant mechanisms in regulation of melanogenesis is of importance.

3. Melanogenesis and oxidative stress

3.1 Melanin synthesis: The role of UVR

Skin color is attributed to the type, amount and distribution of melanin in the skin. Besides the influence of melanin on the skin color, it also plays a pivotal role in protecting the skin against harmful UVR (Westerhof, 2006). Melanocytes located at the epidermis-dermis junction are dendritic cells with dendrites extending outward from the cell body and the dendritic processes of differentiated melanocytes are interspersed between neighbouring keratinocytes, forming the so-called epidermal melanin unit (Fig. 1). The melanogenic process takes place within melanosome, which are specialized membrane-bound cytoplasmic organelles, in melanocytes. Melanocytes synthesize melanin in melanosome before passing the melanosomes to the surrounding keratinocytes (Seiberg, 2001).

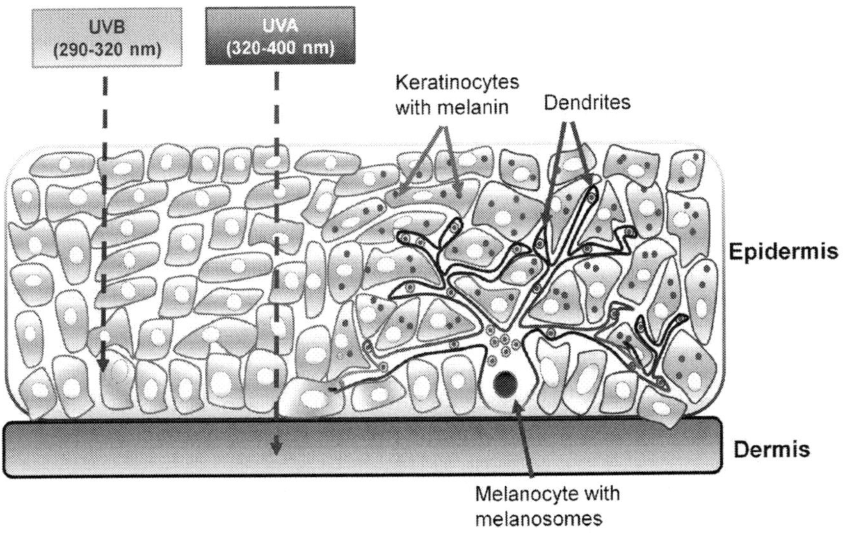

Fig. 1. Epidermal melanin unit

Melanin is synthesized by tyrosinase, a copper-containing metalloglycoprotein and the rate-limiting enzyme, capable of utilizing L-tyrosine, dihydroxyphenylalanine (L-DOPA) and 5,6-dihydroxyindole as substrates. In addition, other enzymes including the tyrosinase related proteins (TRP-1) and dopachrome tautomerase, also known as TRP-2, are responsible for melanogenesis. Melanogenesis is based on the enzymatic conversion of the amino acid tyrosine, through a series of intermediates, to melanin pigments (Ando et al., 2007). Firstly, L-tyrosine is hydroxylated to form L-DOPA. Subsequently, L-DOPA is oxidized to L-DOPAquinone, which will be further processed into either eumelanin (black or brown pigment) or pheomelanin (yellow or red pigment) (Costin & Hearing, 2007). The DOPAquinone produced generally form eumelanin through spontaneous reactions involving cyclization, decarboxylation, oxidation and polymerization. However, TRP-2 can generate 5,6-dihydroxyindole-2-carboxylic acid (DHICA) from DOPAchrome and TRP-1 catalyzes the oxidation of DHICA to indole-5,6-quinone carboxylic acid. In the absence of thiols, DOPAquinone is immediately converted to DOPAchrome and leads to eumelanin production. However, when glutatione (GSH) and cysteine are present, they can react with DOAPquinone intermediates to divert melanin pigment synthesis from eumelanin to pheomelanin through cysteinylDOPA (Ito & Wakamatsu, 2008) (Fig. 2). Besides enzymatic reactions, melanogenic pathway also involves non-enzymatic reactions by evolution of o-quinones, generated enzymatically by the action of tyrosinase, to produce several unstable intermediates, which polymerize to render melanins. A series of both enzymatic and non-enzymatic reactions in eumelanin and pheomelanin synthesis has been observed to subsequently result in H_2O_2 formation (Munoz-Munoz et al., 2009).

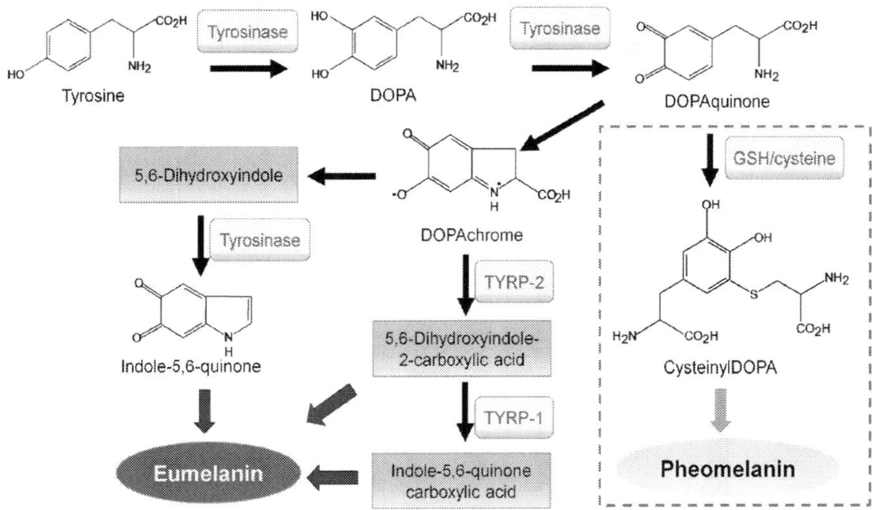

Fig. 2. Melanin synthesis pathway

Generally, variations of the skin or hair color are attributed to the composition of the mixed type of pheomelanin and eumelanin. Disturbance in melanin production can cause esthetic problems including skin hypopigmentary disorders, such as vitiligo, and hyperpigmentary disorders, such as melasma, freckles and postinflammatory hyperpigmentation, that may affect the quality of life of the patients (Halder & Nootheti, 2003). Environmental factors (e.g., UVR and drugs) and endogenous factors (e.g., hormone and age) can mediate the stimulation of melanin production through various signal pathways, which influence tyrosinase regulation. UV can aggravate melanin production in melanocytes either by directly affecting melanocytes or inducing keratinocytes to release signal molecules such as α-melanocyte-stimulating hormone (α-MSH), prostaglandin E_2 (PGE$_2$), adenocorticotropic hormone (ACTH) and endotholin-1, which can upregulate tyrosinase mRNA (Abdel-Malek et al., 1995; H.Y. Park et al., 2009). Important signaling pathways controlling melanogenesis include melanocortin-1 receptor (MC1R), microphthalmia-associated transcription factor (MITF), cyclic 3'-5'-cyclic adenosine monophosphate (cAMP), mitogen-activated protein kinases (MAPK) and adenyl cyclase. In particular, MC1R-MITF signaling is critical to melanocyte viability and function. Binding of melanogenic proteins or signal molecules, especially α-MSH, to MC1R in melanocytes leads to MITF induction, which subsequently activates transcription of the tyrosinase gene involved in melanin synthesis (Cui et al., 2007).

The roles of UV-mediated oxidative stress implicated in melanogenesis in relation to melanoma are the primary focus of this chapter. An increase in pigmentation is a hallmark of biological response of melanocytes to UVR. Immediate responses to UVR mediated preferentially by UVA include the tanning, which occurs as a result of photooxidation of melanin, increased dendrite formation and subsequent induction of melanosome transfer from melanocytes to keratinocytes (Maeda & Hatao, 2004). For the delayed response, pigmentation can be generated by both UVB and UVA radiation and correlated to proliferation of melanocytes, increased transfer of melanosomes to keratinocytes and elevated synthesis of melanin. An induction of melanogenesis in response to UVR also depends on different melanocyte cell types, e.g., lightly-pigmented or darkly-pigmented cells (Kadekaro et al., 2003). Melanogenesis has long been recognized to serve as a major defense mechanism to protect the skin against damaging effects of UVR as both eumelanin and pheomelanin can absorb UVR and have antioxidant properties capable of limiting the penetration of UVR into the skin (Meredith & Sarna, 2006). Detrimental effects of UVR on DNA damage and the repair mechanisms could interfere with cellular signals and subsequently stimulate melanogenic response (Eller et al., 1996). Nevertheless, the protective roles of melanin against UVR-mediated skin damage are controversial. It was previously demonstrated that exposures of UVA-mediated skin pigmentation, which occurred as a result of photooxidation of melanin without increased melanin synthesis, failed to provide photoprotective effect on the skin against UVR including UVB radiation (Miyamura et al., 2011; Ou-Yang et al., 2004). The photoprotective properties of melanin are complex and possibly depend on several factors including type of melanins (eumelanin or pheomelain) and UV rays (UVA or UVB) (Miller & Tsao, 2010; Pfeifer et al., 2005). When eumelanin present in almost every type of human skin serves as a UV filter and ROS scavenger to neutralize the toxic intermediates, pheomelanin prevalent in fair-skinned individuals with red hair has been shown to be a photosensitizer aggravating ROS formation after UVR (Takeuchi et al., 2004). Melanocytes produce varying ratios of eumelanin or pheomelanin that affect skin colors in different human populations and also have an influence involving the interplay between genetic factors and UV exposure on susceptibility to melanomagenesis (Scherer & Kumar, 2010). The possible contribution of oxidative stress to the development of melanoma involve several mechanisms and probably associates with melanogenesis since pheomelanin and eumelanin could lead to photogeneration of ROS and serve as a potential source of H_2O_2 (Nofsinger et al., 2002). As reported by epidemiological studies, incidence of melanoma is different with regard to the variety of ethnicity or skin color (Sneyd & Cox, 2009; Veierod et al., 2003). Researchers have thus been attempting to gain insight into the genetic and biochemical factors responsible for melanomagenesis and postulated that UV exposure and pigmentary characteristics may link to melanoma risk (Barsh & Attardi, 2007). The risk observed to be greater for red-haired women could be attributed to genetic influence and sun exposure. Higher sensitivity of the skin to sun exposure appears to be correlated with red hair, which is more common in fair-skinned populations (Veierod et al., 2003). Previous studies suggested that UVR-mediated stimulation of pheomelanin production in association with redox imbalance in lightly pigmented skin could be accountable for melanomagenesis (Meredith & Sarna, 2006; Pavel et al., 2004; Smit et al., 2008). Moreover, in lightly pigmented melanocytes with increased melanogenesis, UVA radiation was observed to trigger greater DNA and membrane damage. Pheomelanin was regarded as a photosensitizer aggravating UVA-mediated DNA damage and cytotoxicity that would explain higher susceptibility of light-skinned individuals to melanomagenesis induced by UVR (H.Z. Hill & G.J. Hill, 2000; Kvam & Tyrrell, 1999; Wenczl et al., 1998).

3.2 The association of melanogenesis and oxidative stress

The production of melanin, primarily pheomelanin, upon UVR results in continuous generation of ROS including H_2O_2, hydroxyl radicals and superoxide radical ($O_2^{\bullet-}$) in melanocytes (Lin & Fisher, 2007; Mastore et al., 2005). In addition, oxidative intermediates including reactive quinones, which are cytotoxic to proteins and DNA in the cells, are generated during melanogenesis (Ito & Wakamatsu, 2008; Wenczl et al., 1998). An accumulation of H_2O_2 in normal melanocytes is found to be in direct proportion with the synthesis of melanin. While melanin can yield photoprotective effect, this situation is complex because its antioxidant or pro-oxidant property appears to rely on the redox state in the melanocytes (Sarangarajan & Apte, 2006). When the process of melanin production itself can be a crucial source of ROS, on the other hand, the presence of ROS can give rise to abnormal melanogenesis including overproduction of melanin. Previous studies have reported that enhanced ROS/RNS formation induced by UVR was correlated to elevation of melanogenesis possibly through upregulation of tyrosinase activity, protein and mRNA in melanocytes and/or melanoma cells (Dong et al., 2010; Horikoshi et al., 2000; Mastore et al., 2005; Yap et al., 2010). In addition, UVA-induced upregulation of heme oxygenase-1 (HO-1) mRNA, a known stress-response gene normally expressed under photooxidative stress, has been shown to associate with stimulation of melanin synthesis in melanocytes (Marrot et al., 2005). Formation of H_2O_2 or NO and oxidative damage was also found to mediate the promotion of melanin production in melanocytes through activating α-MSH/MC1R or MITF signaling pathway, which is crucial for melanogenic process (Chou et al., 2010; Dong et al., 2010).

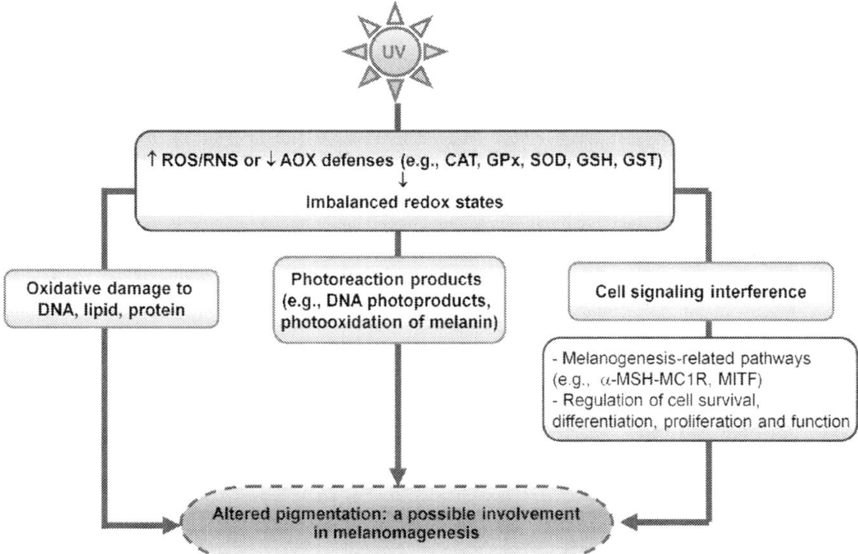

Fig. 3. UVR-induced oxidative stress and alteration in pigmentation

ROS/RNS generation resulting in melanogenesis could occur either as a direct or indirect response of the skin cells to UVR. Directly, UVB and UVA radiation can interact with chromophores and melanin in the melanocytes to generate ROS such as H_2O_2 and $O_2^{\bullet-}$ capable of upregulating tyrosinase to promote melanin formation ((Takeuchi et al., 2004; Xiao et al., 2007). Indirectly, UVB and UVA exposure generates ROS and NO through inflammatory and immune responses of keratinocytes to produce various mediators such as α-MSH, cytokines and growth factors. Furthermore, UVA radiation is suggested to exert an influence on melanogenesis preferentially associated with oxidative stress. Previous *in vitro* and *in vivo* studies have reported that UVR-induced ROS/RNS generation could not only interfere with melanogenesis but also contribute to melanocyte proliferation and transformation, which ultimately leads to melanomagenesis (Horikoshi et al., 2000; Weller, 2003). Fig. 3 shows possible mechanisms by which UVR-induced redox imbalance contributes to altered pigmentation probably involved in melanomagenesis. Thus, antioxidant defenses might play a beneficial role in controlling detrimental effect of excessive melanin induced by oxidant formation.

4. Antioxidant defense system and melanogenesis

During the process of melanogenesis induced by UVR, oxidative insults responsible for melanocyte damage can be generated by various sources including reactive intermediates, particularly H_2O_2, produced during melanogenic process and photochemical reactions of melanin as well as melanin intermediates possessing oxidant properties (Sarangarajan & Apte, 2006). Endogenous antioxidants have been widely recognized to function as an important defense system to prevent skin damage from the hazardous effects of UVR. The abilities of various antioxidants to preserve redox balance could also be crucial for the homeostasis of the skin cells including melanocytes, which are continuously exposed to an oxidative environment (Meyskens et al., 2001). They include enzymatic antioxidants (e.g., superoxide dismutase (SOD), catalase (CAT), glutathione peroxidase (GPx), glutathione reductase and thioredoxin reductase) and non-enzymatic antioxidants or low molecular weight antioxidants (ascorbate or vitamin C, GSH and α-tocopherol) (Hanada et al., 1997; Pinnell, 2003). SOD converts $O_2^{\bullet-}$ into H_2O_2 as well as CAT and GPx degrades H_2O_2 into water. Enzymatic and non-enzymatic antioxidants work in a complex network to maintain a redox balance by several mechanisms such as neutralization of oxidants, inhibition of oxidative damage and regulation of transcription factors involved in cell homeostasis and function (Wood & Schallreuter, 2008). As far as a relationship between UVR-mediated oxidative stress and melanogenesis is concerned, it is significant to understand the photoprotective effects of antioxidant defenses, which may be beneficial for the prevention of melanomagenesis.

4.1 Antioxidant defenses: Their protective role against photooxidative stress

Since UVR-mediated ROS production has been postulated to contribute to enhanced melanogenesis possibly regarded an adaptive response to oxidative stress, eliminating excessive ROS production and/or potentiating the capacity of endogenous antioxidants may be the potential therapeutic strategies for photodamaged skin and, maybe, melanoma development induced by UVR. Major endogenous antioxidants of the skin include GSH, a ubiquitous thiol antioxidant, which potentially maintains redox balance and serves as a substrate for GPx or glutathione-S-transferase (GST), and antioxidant enzymes including CAT and GPx that are primarily involved in the neutralization of H_2O_2, a byproduct of melanogenic process (Campos et al., 2007; Masaki et al., 1998). UVR could result in deficiency in antioxidant defenses in association with melanocyte damage and disturbance of melanin synthesis (Kvam & Dahle, 2003; Maresca et al, 2008). Additionally, phase II detoxification enzymes, e.g., GST and NAD(P)H quinone oxidoreductase (NQO) and γ-glutamylcysteine synthetase (GCS), a rate-limiting enzyme in GSH synthesis, serve as an important antioxidant enzymes of the skin and play a vital role in protection against cell damage by facilitating the elimination of various xenobiotics including chemicals, drugs and pollutants that generate ROS as by-products from the body (Afaq & Mukhtar, 2001; Kokot et al., 2009). Thiol antioxidants, GSH and cysteine involved in a step in pheomelanin synthesis, are capable of protecting melanocytes against unfavorable effects of the reactive species and GSH is also responsible for the conjugation reaction catalyzed by GST to convert a xenobiotic to a non-toxic metabolite (Cotter et al., 2007; Degl'Innocenti et al., 1999; E.S. Park et al., 2007). GST can act as detoxifying antioxidants by catalyzing conjugation reaction of GSH with toxic substrates including quinones and oxidative products as well as by scavenging H_2O_2 occurred during formation of eumelanin and pheomelanin (Meysken et al., 2001). Therefore, detoxification enzymes are essential for the skin in protecting against photooxidative stress. UVR was observed to affect molecular regulation of detoxifying enzymes including GST, NQO and GCS in the skin cells through the transcription factor NF-E2-related factor 2 (Nrf2) (Kannan & Jaiswal, 2006). Nrf2 has been identified to be involved in the human skin adaption to the environmental stress including UVR through the antioxidant response element (ARE), a *cis*-acting enhancer sequence, which transcriptionally regulates the genes encoding phase II enzymes to protect against oxidative damage by maintaining the cellular redox status (Y. Liu et al., 2011; Marrot et al., 2008; Schafer et al., 2010). It has been demonstrated that inhibition of tyrosinase involved in upregulation of GSH detoxification systems including GSH content and GPx and GST activities was able to suppress tumor promotion in mouse skin (Nakamura et al., 2000). Moreover, an influence of GST variations (e.g., GST deficiency) on melanoma risk has been previously discussed (Mossner et al., 2007). Further studies are needed in order to explore whether compounds capable of upregulating various antioxidant defenses including detoxification enzymes could be developed as chemopreventive agents against skin cancers including melanoma.

4.2 Antioxidant defenses: A target for development of antimelanogenic agents

While proper use of sunscreens has been widely recommended to protect against UVR-mediated skin damage leading to a variety of skin disorders including hyperpigmentation, their photoprotective effects could be insufficient when there is overproduction of ROS/RNS. Attempts have thus been made to develop potential antimelanogenic agents from natural and synthetic compounds and to study the mechanisms by which they function. Several depigmenting agents are now available in oral and topical formulations. Kojic acid and arbutin, the well-known tyrosinase inhibitors, are usually used as standard skin whitening agents in several studies for testing candidate compounds and as ingredients in a variety of skin care products (Parvez et al., 2006). In general, agents exhibit depigmenting effects by acting at various levels of melanogenesis. Since tyrosinase is the rate-limiting enzyme for melanin synthesis, it thus has been the main target of drug designers for new depigmenting agents. Tyrosinase inhibitors can serve as competitive inhibitors of tyrosinase or non-competitive inhibitors (such as inhibitors of melanosome transport and inhibitors of non-enzymatic or oxidative reactions in the melanogenic pathway) (Briganti et al., 2003). Moreover, antimelanogenic agents that have traditionally been used for the treatment of hyperpigmentation include melanocytotoxic agents, e.g., hydroquinone and azelaic acid, which can be converted to cytotoxic species (Kasraee, 2002). Nevertheless, based on the findings that oxidative stress, which occurs through increased formation of ROS/RNS, may be implicated in melanogenesis, agents that can remove oxidants or block the oxidative reactions should also have promising depigmenting properties. This gives a new direction for the search of potential depigmenting agents, and explains the connection between oxidative stress and various pigmentation disorders. Antimelanogenic effects of natural antioxidants (Table 1), phytochemicals (Table 2) and botanicals processing antioxidant properties (Table 3) have been intensively explored in a variety of preclinical *in vitro* cell culture and animal models as well as clinical trials (Gomez-Cordoves et al. 2001; Saikia et al. 2006). Phytochemicals including phenolics and essential oils, usually identified as active ingredients in botanicals, are capable of scavenging ROS/RNS and inhibiting cellular oxidative stress and thus might be responsible for the pharmacological effects of the plant extracts (Verschooten et al. 2006; K.H. Wang, 2006).

Natural antioxidants	Antimelanogenic actions
Ascorbic acid and its derivatives e.g., magnesium L-ascorbyl-2-phosphate (VC-PMG), ascorbyl 2-phosphate 6 palmitate (APPS) and tetra-isopalmitoyl ascorbic acid (VC-IP)	Application of VC-PMG cream for 3 months reduced hyperpigmentation in some patients (Kameyama et al., 1996). APPS lotion applied for 4 weeks reduced perifollicular pigmentation in a randomized, single-blinded, placebo-controlled clinical trial (Inui & Itami, 2007). Topical application of VC-IP for 3 weeks suppressed UVB-induced pigmentation in subjects (Ochiai et al., 2006). Their actions may involve inhibitory effects on non-enzymatic or oxidative reactions in the melanogenic pathway (Ando et al., 2007).
Lipoic acid	Suppressed tyrosinase activity, protein and mRNA in B16 melanoma cells (J.H. Kim et al., 2008).
Tocopherol analogues and tocotrienols (e.g., γ- and δ- tocotrienols)	Hydrophilic γ-tocotrienol reduced UV-induced pigmentation in guinea pig skin via inhibition of tyrosinase activity (Kuwabara et al., 2006). Tocotrienols inhibited UVB-induced melanogenesis in different melanoma cells through downregulation of tyrosinase activity and protein (Yap et al., 2010). Their actions may be related to inhibition of oxidative reactions in the melanogeic process and of lipid peroxidation as well as promotion of GSH (Yamamura et al., 2002).
α-Tocopheylferulate (α-tocopherol linked to ferulic acid by an ester bond)	Suppressed tyrosinase activity at the post-translational level possibly via anti-oxidative action in normal human melanocytes (Funasaka et al., 2000).

Table 1. Studies on the antimelanogenic actions of natural antioxidants

Phytochemicals/sources	Antimelanogenic actions
Daidzein derivatives (e.g., 8-hydroxydaidzein)	Exhibited antityrosinase effect on B16 melanoma cells. Application of 8-hydroxydaidzein cream for 2 months provided whitening activity in human volunteers (Tai et al., 2009).
Gallic acid	Inhibited tyrosinase activity possibly via reduction of ROS formation and elevation of GSH/GSSG ratio in B16 melanoma cells (Y. J. Kim, 2007)
Hydroxycinnamic acids (e.g., caffeic acid, ferulic acid and *p*-coumaric acid) from corn bran	Suppressed tyrosinase activity in B16 melanoma cells via free radical scavenging activity (S.W. Choi et al., 2007).
Luteolin	Suppressed tyrosinase activity via inhibiting ROS formation in B16 melanoma cells (M.Y. Choi et al., 2008).
Origanoside from *Origanum vulgare*	Downregulated tyrosinase activity as well as tyrosinase, MITF and TRP-2 proteins in B16 melanoma cells and reduced pigmentation in mice skin (Liang et al., 2010)
Proanthocyanidins from grape seed	Oral administration reduced UV-induced pigmentation of guinea pig skin. Their actions may involve ROS/RNS scavenging activities as well as inhibition of oxidative damage of lipid and DNA (Yamakoshi et al., 2003).
Quercetin from rose hip (*Rosa canina L.*)	Downregulated tyrosinase activity and protein in B16 melanoma cells (Fujii & Saito, 2009)
Resveratrol from red wine	Downregulated tyrosinase at post-transcriptional level in human melanocytes (Newton et al., 2007)
Polyphenols such as epigallocatechin-3-gallate (EGCG)	Downregulated tyrosinase and MITF proteins in mouse melanocyte cell line (D.S. Kim et al., 2004)
Vanillin and vanillic acid from *Origanum vulgare*	Downregulated melanogenesis-related signaling including MITF, MC1R, tyrosinase, TRP-1 and TRP-2 via inhibiting ROS formation and lipid peroxidation in B16 melanoma cells (Chou et al., 2010)

Table 2. Studies on the antimelanogenic actions of phytochemicals

Since the skin is the body part that is most accessible to UVR, in order to prevent the cells from harm, the antioxidant defenses of the skin continuously respond to elevated levels of ROS and play an important role in prevention of UVR-induced biological response and damage of the skin cells including melanocytes. However, insufficient protection by antioxidant defense against photodamaged skin can happen due to the accumulation of stress or oxidative insults induced by UVR. Moreover, antioxidant defenses might fail to neither prevent melanocyte damage nor abnormal pigmentation in relation of UVR-dependent oxidative damage. Recent studies have indicated the possible involvement of defect of antioxidant defenses in increased melanogenesis. UVA-mediated augmentation of melanogenesis was correlated to depletion of SOD and catalase activities and GSH content as well as aggravation of ROS production in lightly pigmented melanocytes (Baldea et al., 2009; Smit et al., 2008). On the other hand, promotion of antioxidant defenses such as GSH level and GPx activity and decrease in ROS/RNS formation have been found to associate with reduction of melanogenesis by inhibiting tyrosinase activity in cultured melanoma cells and human melanocytes (Benathan, 1997; Y.J. Kim et al., 2008). Thus, exploring antimelanogenic effects of candidate antioxidants and underlying mechanisms involving modulation of antioxidant network could lead to the development of promising depigmenting agents.

Besides abilities of antioxidants to restore redox balance, they have also been found to regulate signaling pathways implicated in the regulation of melanogenesis include α-MSH/MC1R pathway and MITF. Modulation of pigmentation by antioxidants has been proposed to be achieved through regulating MITF activity. Decrease in ROS levels and recovery of antioxidant defenses including GSH correlated with downregulation of MC1R, MITF and other melanogenesis related signaling pathways (e.g., cAMP, PKA or MAPK) that resulted in reduction of tyrosinase activity and melanin content (Chou et al., 2010; Yanase et al., 2001).

Indeed, the roles of antioxidants in mediating melanogenic signaling cascades are complex and further studies are needed in order to verify implication of antioxidant defenses for regulation of melanogenesis. As reported in many studies concerning depigmenting activity of natural antioxidants or phytochemicals/botanicals possessing antioxidant properties (Table 1-3), they possibly provide antimelanogenic effects involving several mechanisms including (a) antioxidative actions or free radical scavenging activities capable of inhibiting non-enzymatic reactions in the melanogenic pathway and suppressing oxidative damage of biomolecules including DNA damage, (b) promotion of antioxidant defense capacity to maintain redox homeostasis (c) inhibition of tyrosinase at cellular or molecular levels and (d) regulation of melanogenic signaling cascades.

In addition, antioxidant combinations are suggested to have higher efficacy than single antioxidant that may be due to synergistic effects of the combined preparation (Bialy et al., 2002). Ascorbic acid is often combined with other antioxidants in several skin care formulations as it can recycle other antioxidants, such as α-tocopherol, from their radical forms and thus plays a vital role in the synergistic effects of antioxidant combinations. Tomato extract rich in carotenoids combined with vitamin C and vitamin E yielded protective effects against UVA-mediated hyperpigmentation and DNA damage in human melanocytes (Smit et al., 2004). An open pilot study reported that oral administration of vitamin C combined with bioflavonoids for 4 weeks improved progressive pigmented purpura (Reinhold et al., 1999). Therefore, a combination of depigmenting compounds that target different steps of melanogenic process and give synergistic effects would yield a greater effect and better outcome.

4.3 Antioxidant defenses: Implications for melanoma prevention

Melanin is crucial for skin homeostasis and its complex biosynthesis has a pivotal impact on the melanocyte biology. As discussed earlier, lightly pigmented melanocytes appear to be

Botanicals/their active ingredients	Antimelanogenic actions
Citrus hassaku fruit/ flavanone glycosides	Inhibited tyrosinase activity in B16 melanoma cells and protected against UVB-induced pigmentation in guinea pig skin via radical scavenging activity (Itoh et al., 2009)
Curcuma longa/curcumin	Inhibited tyrosinase activity as well as melanogenesis-related signaling proteins such as MITF and TRP in B16F10 cells (Jang et al., 2009)
Pomegranate/ellagic acid	Oral administration inhibited UV-induced pigmentation in guinea pig skin (Yoshimura et al., 2005).
Polypodium leucotomos/ hydroxycinnamic acids	Oral administration for 4 months reduced psoralen-UVA-mediated pigmentation and possibly prevented UVA-induced mitochondrial DNA damage of human skin (Middelkamp et al., 2004; Villa et al., 2010).
Pycnogenol® (French pine bark extract)/ proanthrocyanidins and hydroxycinnamic acids	Oral administration for 30 days reduced pigmentation in women with melasma (Ni et al., 2002) and its action in B16 melanoma cells involved the ROS/RNS scavenging activity and upregulation of GSH (Y.J. Kim et al., 2008).
Silymarin (milk thistle or *Silybum marianum* L.)	Downregulated tyrosinase protein in mouse melanocyte cell line (Choo et al., 2009).
Alpinia spp. (e.g., *A. officinarum*)	Downregulated TRP-1 and TRP-2 mRNA and MITF protein in B16 melanoma cells (Matsuda et al., 2009)
Chestnut flowers/gallic acid and flavonoids	Downregulated tyrosinase, TRP-1 and TRP-2 proteins possibly via radical scavenging activity in human melanoma cells (Sapkota et al., 2010)
Oolong tea/polyphenols e.g., EGCG, epicatechin-3-gallate and epicatechin	Oral administration inhibited UVB-induced pigmentation in guinea pig skin by suppression of tyrosinase protein and mRNA (Aoki et al., 2007).

Table 3. Studies on the antimelanogenic actions of botanicals and the possible active ingredients

more susceptible to accumulate DNA damage in UVR-induced tanning, which may be reflected as a protective or stress response of the skin. Melanin in fair skin could be accountable for UVR-induced genotoxicity involving elevated ROS production that may lead to melanocyte transformation (Marrot et al., 2005). A disturbance of redox state, which can be mediated by melanogenesis, may subsequently affect cellular machinery involving differentiation and proliferation of melanocytes and/or melanoma cells. Decreased activities of antioxidant enzymes (e.g., SOD) were observed to associate with melanoma cell proliferation (Bravard et al., 1999). Nevertheless, redox regulation in melanogenesis related to the pathogenesis of melanoma is complex and the modulation of melanocyte and melanoma cell homeostasis by redox states remains controversial. Attenuation of ROS formation or upregulation of antioxidant defenses can either enhance or reduce melanogenesis in melanocytes as well as affect melanoma survival. Melanin is well recognized to have photoprotective properties against UVR-mediated melanocyte damage and could be beneficial for the prevention of melanomagenesis induced by UVR. Signaling pathways required for regulation of melanocyte homeostasis and pigmentation including α–MSH-MC1R and MITF were demonstrated to play an essential role in restoring DNA repair as well as in survival and transformation of melanocytes in response to increased intracellular ROS (Abdel-Malek et al., 2006; F. Liu et al, 2009). H_2O_2 also can cause an attenuation of melanin production and, on the other hand, increased melanogenesis associated with elevated activities of antioxidant enzymes including CAT in darkly pigmented melanocytes is more resistant to harmful effects of UVR (Maresca et al., 2008). Therefore, contribution of UV-mediated oxidative stress involved in disturbed melanin synthesis to the pathogenesis of malignant melanoma is complicated and different cell types of melanocytes and melanoma cells studied need to be taken into account. However, beneficial effects of antioxidants on individuals with melanoma susceptibility and under stress environment against development of melanoma seem warranted. As proposed by previous *in vitro* and *in vivo* studies that antioxidants could be useful as chemopreventive agents, antioxidants (e.g., N-acetylcysteine/NAC) and phytochemicals (e.g., genistein) have been determined to exhibit inhibitory effects on UV-induced melanoma promotion through inhibition of oxidative DNA damage (Cotter et al., 2007; Russo et al., 2006). Oral administration of NAC may yield chemopreventive effects on patients having a high risk for melanoma since it could inhibit UV-induced oxidative stress and GSH depletion in melanocytic nevi (Goodson et al., 2009). Furthermore, phytochemicals (e.g., eugenol from clove oil) and botanicals (e.g., *P. leucotomos*) possessing antimelanogenic properties exhibited photoprotective effects against melanoma development via regulation of signaling cascades involving cell cycle and growth factor (Ghosh et al., 2005; Philip et al., 2009). Possible mechanisms by which augmentation of antioxidant capacity contributes to the protection against melanoma initiation include detoxification of carcinogens and reactive intermediates produced from UVR, inhibition of genotoxicity induced by photochemical reactions in melanogenic process and restoration of redox balance related to signaling cascades involved in cell growth and proliferation (Meyskens et al., 2001). The roles of antioxidants in the inhibition of melanomagenesis yet are controversial as phytochemicals possibly yield anticancer effects on melanoma through increased oxidative stress through aggravation of ROS levels and impairment of antioxidant defense system (e.g., GSH depletion), although they exhibited selective cancer cell toxicity, probably attributed to chemical structures of phytochemicals and differences in redox states and ROS levels between normal cells and cancer cells (Thanasamy et al., 2007).

While applications of sunscreens offer satisfactory effect against sunburn and squamous cell carcinoma, protection against melanoma is more complicated since some studies giving conflicting results on the effect of sunscreens against melanomagenesis (Lin & Fisher, 2007). Additionally, the protective effect of sunscreens against UVR-mediated skin damage appears to be insufficient that may be due to inadequate quantities applied and its ineffectiveness in quenching ROS generated in response to UVR. It is widely recommended that sufficient prevention from deleterious effects of UV radiation is beneficial and thus applying exogenous antioxidants to counteract oxidative stress and/or promote antioxidant defense capacity may offer a potential pharmacological approach for the prevention of skin cancers including melanoma. Moreover, the approach of applying antioxidants cannot be the sole strategy to prevent the adverse effects of UVR. Combined strategies including avoidance of excessive sun exposure, appropriate use of sunscreens and skin care products as well as modification of lifestyle and dietary habits are necessary and may yield benefit for prevention of UV-induced melanomagenesis.

This chapter focuses on the aspect of adverse effect of UVR and it is important to emphasize that the contribution of UV exposure to the development of melanoma depends on several factors. Therefore the benefits of moderate sun exposure, for example, UVB, an essential source of vitamin D, that have a remarkable impact on health should not be ignored.

5. Conclusion

While there is a rising demand for antimelanogenic agents and several promising natural compounds are under intensive development, they remain challenging because there is no entirely satisfactory outcome and many agents cause adverse effects. Since UVA irradiation-mediated disturbance in antioxidant defense system and redox state is postulated to play a vital role in melanogenesis, antioxidant-rich medicinal plants have therefore gained attention for their properties in regulating skin pigmentation. We have reported that a recovery of antioxidant defenses including increased CAT and GPx activity and GSH content by *Alpinia galanga* (AG) and *Curcuma aromatica* (CA) was able to counteract UVA-mediated increased melanogenesis through downregulation of tyrosinase in human G361 melanoma cells. Terpenoid derivatives including eugenol and curcuminoids identified in the rhizome extracts of AG and CA, respectively, could be active components responsible for their antimelanogenic effects (Panich et al, 2010). Elucidating the protective roles of phytochemicals and botanicals containing antioxidants against UVR-induced disrupted homeostasis including abnormal pigmentation could offer an approach for development of photoprotective agents that may provide not only cosmetic benefits but also promising interventions for melanoma prevention. Moreover, it is crucial to perform the studies of putative antimelanogenic agents using physiologically relevant skin models such as primary human melanocytes as melanocytes and melanoma cells have different redox states and might provide different responses of antioxidant defenses to UVR-mediated oxidative damage.

6. References

Abdel-Malek, Z., Swope, V.B., Suzuki, I., Akcali, C., Harriger, M.D., Boyce, S.T., Urabe, K. & Hearing, V.J. (1995). Mitogenic and melanogenic stimulation of normal human melanocytes by melanotropic peptides. *Proceedings of the National Academy of Sciences of the United States of America*, Vol.92, No.5, (February 1995) pp. 1789-1793, ISSN 0027-8424

Abdel-Malek, Z.A., Kadekaro, A.L., Kavanagh, R.J., Todorovic, A., Koikov, L.N., McNulty, J.C., Jackson, P.J., Millhauser, G.L., Schwemberger, S., Babcock, G., Haskell-Luevano, C. & Knittel, J.J. (2006). Melanoma prevention strategy based on using tetrapeptide alpha-MSH analogs that protect human melanocytes from UV-induced DNA damage and cytotoxicity. *The FASEB Journal*, Vol.20, No.9, (July 2006) pp. 1561-1563, ISSN 0892-6638

Afaq, F. & Mukhtar, H. (2001). Effects of solar radiation on cutaneous detoxification pathways. *Journal of Photochemistry and Photobiology B*, Vol.63, No.1-3, (October 2001) pp. 61-69, ISSN 1011-1344

Ando, H., Kondoh, H., Ichihashi, M. & Hearing, V.J. (2007). Approaches to identify inhibitors of melanin biosynthesis via the quality control of tyrosinase. *Journal of Investigative Dermatology*, Vol.127, No.4, (April 2007) pp. 751-761, ISSN 0022-202X

Aoki, Y., Tanigawa, T., Abe, H. & Fujiwara, Y. (2007). Melanogenesis inhibition by an oolong tea extract in b16 mouse melanoma cells and UV-induced skin pigmentation in brownish guinea pigs. *Bioscience, Biotechnology, and Biochemistry*, Vol.71, No.8, (August 2007) pp. 1879-1885, ISSN 0916-8451

Baldea, I, Mocan, T. & Cosgarea, R. (2009). The role of ultraviolet radiation and tyrosine stimulated melanogenesis in the induction of oxidative stress alterations in fair skin melanocytes. *Experimental Oncology*, Vol.31, No.4, (December 2009) pp. 200-208, ISSN 1812-9269

Barsh, G. & Attardi, L.D. (2007). A healthy tan? *New England Journal of Medicine*, Vol.356, No.21, (May 2007) pp. 2208-2210, ISSN 0028-4793

Benathan, M. (1997). Opposite regulation of tyrosinase and glutathione peroxidase by intracellular thiols in human melanoma cells. *Archives of Dermatological Research*, Vol.289, No.6, (May 1997) pp. 341-346, ISSN 0340-3696

Bennett, D.C. (2008). Ultraviolet wavebands and melanoma initiation. *Pigment Cell & Melanoma Research*, Vol.21, No.5, (October 2008) pp. 520-524, ISSN 1755-1471

Besaratinia, A., Synold, T.W., Chen, H.H., Chang, C., Xi, B., Riggs, A.D. & Pfeifer, G.P. (2005). DNA lesions induced by UV A1 and B radiation in human cells: comparative analyses in the overall genome and in the p53 tumor suppressor gene. *Proceedings of the National Academy of Sciences of the United States of America*, Vol.102, No.29, (July 2005) pp. 10058-10063, ISSN 0027-8424

Bialy, T.L., Rothe, M.J., Grant-Kels, J.M. (2002). Dietary factors in the prevention and treatment of nonmelanoma skin cancer and melanoma. *Dermatologic Surgery*, Vol.28, No.12, (December 2002) pp. 1143-1152, ISSN 1076-0512

Bravard, A., Petridis, F. & Luccioni,C. (1999). Modulation of antioxidant enzymes p21WAF1 and p53 expression during proliferation and differentiation of human melanoma cell lines. *Free Radical Biology and Medicine*, Vol.26, No.7-8, (April 1999) pp. 1027-1033, ISSN 0891-5849

Brenner, M. & Hearing,V.J. (2008). The protective role of melanin against UV damage in human skin. *Photochemistry and Photobiology*, Vol.84, No.3, (May-June 2008) pp. 539-549, ISSN 0031-8655

Briganti, S., Camera, E. & Picardo, M. (2003). Chemical and instrumental approaches to treat hyperpigmentation. *Pigment Cell Research*, Vol.16, No.2, (April 2003) pp. 101-110, ISSN 0893-5785

Campos, A.C., Molognoni, F., Melo, F.H., Galdieri, L.C., Carneiro, C.R., D'Almeida, V., Correa, M. & Jasiulionis, M.G. (2007). Oxidative stress modulates DNA methylation during melanocyte anchorage blockade associated with malignant transformation. *Neoplasia*, Vol.9, No.12, (December 2007) pp. 1111-1121, ISSN 1522-8002

Chin, M.P. & Deen, W.M. (2010). Prediction of nitric oxide concentrations in melanomas. *Nitric Oxide*, Vol.23, No.4, (December 2010) pp. 319-326, ISSN 1089-8603

Choi, M.Y., Song, H.S., Hur, H.S. & Sim, S.S. (2008). Whitening activity of luteolin related to the inhibition of cAMP pathway in alpha-MSH-stimulated B16 melanoma cells. *Archives of Pharmacal Research*, Vol.31, No.9, (September 2008) pp. 1166-1171, ISSN 0253-6269

Choi, S.W., Lee, S.K., Kim, E.O., Oh, J.H., Yoon, K.S., Parris, N., Hicks, K.B. & Moreau, R.A. (2007). Antioxidant and antimelanogenic activities of polyamine conjugates from corn bran and related hydroxycinnamic acids. *Journal of Agricultural and Food Chemistry*, Vol.55, No.10, (May 2007) pp. 3920-3925, ISSN 0021-8561

Choo, S.J., Ryoo, I.J., Kim, Y.H., Xu, G.H., Kim, W.G., Kim, K.H., Moon, S.J., Son, E.D., Bae, K. & Yoo, I.D. (2009). Silymarin inhibits melanin synthesis in melanocyte cells. *Journal of Pharmacy and Pharmacology*, Vol.61, No.5, (May 2009) pp. 663-667, ISSN 0022-3573

Chou, T.H., Ding, H.Y., Hung, W.J. & Liang, C.H. (2010). Antioxidative characteristics and inhibition of alpha-melanocyte-stimulating hormone-stimulated melanogenesis of vanillin and vanillic acid from Origanum vulgare. *Experimental Dermatology*, Vol.19, No.8, (August 2010) pp. 742-750, ISSN 0906-6705

Costin, G.E. & Hearing, V.J. (2007). Human skin pigmentation: melanocytes modulate skin color in response to stress. *The FASEB Journal*, Vol.21, No.4, (April 2007) pp. 976-994, ISSN 0892-6638

Cotter, M.A., Thomas, J., Cassidy, P., Robinette, K., Jenkins, N., Florell, S.R., Leachman, S., Samlowski, W.E. & Grossman, D. (2007). N-acetylcysteine protects melanocytes against oxidative stress/damage and delays onset of ultraviolet-induced melanoma in mice. *Clinical Cancer Research*, Vol.13, No.19, (October 2007) pp. 5952-5958, ISSN 1078-0432

Cui, R., Widlund, H.R., Feige, E., Lin, J.Y., Wilensky, D.L., Igras, V.E., D'Orazio, J., Fung, C.Y., Schanbacher, C.F., Granter, S.R. & Fisher, D.E. (2007). Central role of p53 in the suntan response and pathologic hyperpigmentation. *Cell*, Vol.128, No.5, (March 2007) pp. 853-864, ISSN 0092-8674

Dong, Y., Cao, J., Wang, H., Zhang, J., Zhu, Z., Bai, R., Hao, H., He, X., Fan, R. & Dong, C. (2010). Nitric oxide enhances the sensitivity of alpaca melanocytes to respond to alpha-melanocyte-stimulating hormone by up-regulating melanocortin-1 receptor. *Biochemical and Biophysical Research Communications*, Vol.396, No.4, (June 2010) pp. 849-853, ISSN 0006-291X

Eller, M.S., Ostrom, K. & Gilchrest, B.A. (1996). DNA damage enhances melanogenesis. *Proceedings of the National Academy of Sciences of the United States of America*, Vol.93, No.3, (February 1996) pp. 1087-1092, ISSN 0027-8424

Degl'Innocenti, D., Rosati, F., Iantomasi, T., Vincenzini, M.T., Ramponi, G. (1999). GSH system in relation to redox state in dystrophic skin fibroblasts. *Biochimie*, Vol.81, No.11, (November 1999) pp. 1025-1029, ISSN 0300-9084

Dessars, B., De Raeve, L.E., Morandini, R., Lefort, A., El Housni, H., Ghanem, G.E., Van den Eynde, B.J., Ma, W., Roseeuw, D., Vassart, G., Libert, F. & Heimann, P. (2009). Genotypic and gene expression studies in congenital melanocytic nevi: insight into initial steps of melanotumorigenesis. *Journal of Investigative Dermatology*, Vol.129, No.1, (January 2009) pp. 139-147, ISSN 0022-202X

Fujii, T. & Saito, M. (2009). Inhibitory effect of quercetin isolated from rose hip (Rosa canina L.) against melanogenesis by mouse melanoma cells. *Bioscience, Biotechnology, and Biochemistry*, Vol.73, No.9, (September 2009) pp. 1989-1993, ISSN 0916-8451

Funasaka, Y., Komoto, M., Ichihashi,M. (2000). Depigmenting effect of alpha-tocopheryl ferulate on normal human melanocytes. *Pigment Cell Research*, Vol.13 (Suppl 8), (2000) pp. 170-174, ISSN 0893-5785

Gaddameedhi, S., Kemp, M.G., Reardon, J.T., Shields, J.M., Smith-Roe, S.L., Kaufmann, W.K. & Sancar, A. (2010). Similar nucleotide excision repair capacity in melanocytes and melanoma cells. *Cancer Research*, Vol.70, No.12, (June 2010) pp. 4922-4930, ISSN 0008-5472

Ghosh, R., Nadiminty, N., Fitzpatrick, J.E., Alworth, W.L., Slaga, T.J. & Kumar, A.P. (2005). Eugenol causes melanoma growth suppression through inhibition of E2F1 transcriptional activity. *The Journal of Biological Chemistry*, Vol.280, No.7, (February 2005) pp. 5812-5819, ISSN 0021-9258

Gidanian, S., Mentelle, M., Meyskens, F.L.,Jr. & Farmer, P.J. (2008). Melanosomal damage in normal human melanocytes induced by UVB and metal uptake--a basis for the pro-oxidant state of melanoma. *Photochemistry and Photobiology*, Vol.84, No.3, (May-June 2008) pp. 556-564, ISSN 0031-8655

Gomez-Cordoves, C., Bartolome, B., Vieira, W. & Virador, V.M. (2001). Effects of wine phenolics and sorghum tannins on tyrosinase activity and growth of melanoma cells. *Journal of Agricultural and Food Chemistry*, Vol.49, No.3, (March 2001) pp. 1620-1624, ISSN 0021-8561

Goodson, A.G., Cotter, M.A., Cassidy, P., Wade, M., Florell, S.R., Liu, T., Boucher, K.M. & Grossman, D. (2009). Use of oral N-acetylcysteine for protection of melanocytic nevi against UV-induced oxidative stress: towards a novel paradigm for melanoma chemoprevention. *Clinical Cancer Research*, Vol.15, No.23, (December 2009) pp. 7434-7440, ISSN 1078-0432

Halder, R.M. & Nootheti, P.K. (2003). Ethnic skin disorders overview. *Journal of the American Academy of Dermatology*, Vol.48, No.6 Suppl, (June 2003) pp. S143-S148, ISSN 0190-9622

Hanada, K., Sawamura, D., Tamai, K., Hashimoto, I. & Kobayashi, S. (1997). Photoprotective effect of esterified glutathione against ultraviolet B-induced sunburn cell formation in the hairless mice. *Journal of Investigative Dermatology*, Vol.108, No.5, (May 1997) pp. 727-730, ISSN 0022-202X

Hill, H.Z. & Hill,G.J. (2000). UVA, pheomelanin and the carcinogenesis of melanoma. *Pigment Cell Research*, Vol.13 (Suppl 8), (2000) pp. 140-144, ISSN 0893-5785

Horikoshi, T., Nakahara, M., Kaminaga, H., Sasaki, M., Uchiwa, H. & Miyachi, Y. (2000). Involvement of nitric oxide in UVB-induced pigmentation in guinea pig skin. *Pigment Cell Research*, Vol.13, No. 5, (October 2000) pp. 358-363, ISSN 0893-5785

Inui, S. & Itami, S. (2007). Perifollicular pigmentation is the first target for topical vitamin C derivative ascorbyl 2-phosphate 6-palmitate (APPS): randomized, single-blinded, placebo-controlled study. *The Journal of Dermatology*, Vol.34, No.3, (March 2007) pp. 221-223, ISSN 0385-2407

Ito, S. & Wakamatsu, K. (2008). Chemistry of mixed melanogenesis--pivotal roles of dopaquinone. *Photochemistry and Photobiology*, Vol.84, No.3, (May-June 2008) pp. 582-592, ISSN 0031-8655

Itoh, K., Hirata, N., Masuda, M., Naruto, S., Murata, K., Wakabayashi, K. & Matsuda, H. (2009). Inhibitory effects of Citrus hassaku extract and its flavanone glycosides on melanogenesis. *Biological & Pharmaceutical Bulletin*, Vol.32, No.3, (March 2009) pp. 410-415, ISSN 0918-6158

Jang, J.Y., Lee, J.H., Jeong, S.Y., Chung, K.T., Choi, Y.H. & Choi, B.T. (2009). Partially purified Curcuma longa inhibits alpha-melanocyte-stimulating hormone-stimulated melanogenesis through extracellular signal-regulated kinase or Akt activation-mediated signalling in B16F10 cells. *Experimental Dermatology*, Vol.18, No.8, (August 2009) pp. 689-694, ISSN 0906-6705

Kadekaro, A.L., Kavanagh, R.J., Wakamatsu, K., Ito, S., Pipitone, M.A. & Abdel-Malek,Z.A. (2003). Cutaneous photobiology. The melanocyte vs. the sun: who will win the final round? *Pigment Cell Research*, Vol.16, No.5, (October 2003) pp. 434-447, ISSN 0893-5785

Kadekaro, A.L., Kavanagh, R., Kanto, H., Terzieva, S., Hauser, J., Kobayashi, N., Schwemberger, S., Cornelius, J., Babcock, G., Shertzer, H.G., Scott, G. & Abdel-Malek,Z.A. (2005). alpha-Melanocortin and endothelin-1 activate antiapoptotic pathways and reduce DNA damage in human melanocytes. *Cancer Research*, Vol.65, No.10, (May 2005) pp. 4292-4299, ISSN 0008-5472

Kameyama, K., Sakai, C., Kondoh, S., Yonemoto, K., Nishiyama, S., Tagawa, M., Murata, T., Ohnuma, T., Quigley, J., Dorsky, A., Bucks, D. & Blanock, K. (1996). Inhibitory effect of magnesium L-ascorbyl-2-phosphate (VC-PMG) on melanogenesis in vitro and in vivo. *Journal of the American Academy of Dermatology*, Vol.34, No.1, (January 1996) pp. 29-33, ISSN 0190-9622

Kannan, S. & Jaiswal, A.K. (2006). Low and high dose UVB regulation of transcription factor NF-E2-related factor 2. *Cancer Research*, Vol.66, No.17, (September 2006) pp. 8421-8429, ISSN 0008-5472

Kasraee,B. (2002). Peroxidase-mediated mechanisms are involved in the melanocytotoxic and melanogenesis-inhibiting effects of chemical agents. *Dermatology*, Vol.205, No.4, (2002) pp. 329-339, ISSN 1018-8665

Kim, D.S., Park, S.H., Kwon, S.B., Li, K., Youn, S.W. & Park, K.C. (2004). (-)-Epigallocatechin-3-gallate and hinokitiol reduce melanin synthesis via decreased MITF production. *Archives of Pharmacal Research*, Vol.27, No.3, (March 2004) pp. 334-339, ISSN 0253-6269

Kim, J.H., Sim, G.S., Bae, J.T., Oh, J.Y., Lee, G.S., Lee, D.H., Lee, B.C. & Pyo, H.B. (2008). Synthesis and anti-melanogenic effects of lipoic acid-polyethylene glycol ester. *Journal of Pharmacy and Pharmacology*, Vol.60, No.7, (July 2008) pp. 863-870, ISSN 0022-3573

Kim, Y.J. (2007). Antimelanogenic and antioxidant properties of gallic Acid. *Biological & Pharmaceutical Bulletin*, Vol.30, No.6, (June 2007) pp. 1052-1055, ISSN 0918-6158

Kim, Y.J., Kang, K.S. & Yokozawa, T. (2008). The anti-melanogenic effect of pycnogenol by its anti-oxidative actions. *Food and Chemical Toxicology*, Vol.46, No.7, (July 2008) pp. 2466-2471, ISSN 0278-6915

Kokot, A., Metze, D., Mouchet, N., Galibert, M.D., Schiller, M., Luger, T.A. & Bohm,M. (2009). Alpha-melanocyte-stimulating hormone counteracts the suppressive effect of UVB on Nrf2 and Nrf-dependent gene expression in human skin. *Endocrinology*, Vol.150, No.7, (July 2009) pp. 3197-3206, ISSN 0013-7227

Kuwabara, Y., Watanabe, T., Yasuoka, S., Fukui, K., Takata, J., Karube, Y., Okamoto, Y., Asano, S., Katoh, E., Tsuzuki, T. & Kobayashi, S. (2006). Topical application of gamma-tocopherol derivative prevents UV-induced skin pigmentation. *Biological & Pharmaceutical Bulletin*, Vol.29, No.6, (June 2006) pp. 1175-1179, ISSN 0918-6158

Kvam, E. & Dahle, J. (2003). Pigmented melanocytes are protected against ultraviolet-A-induced membrane damage. *Journal of Investigative Dermatology*, Vol.121, No.3, (September 2003) pp. 564-569, ISSN 0022-202X

Kvam, E. & Tyrrell, R.M. (1999). The role of melanin in the induction of oxidative DNA base damage by ultraviolet A irradiation of DNA or melanoma cells. *Journal of Investigative Dermatology*, Vol.113, No.2, (August 1999) pp. 209-213, ISSN 0022-202X

Liang, C.H., Chou, T.H. & Ding, H.Y. (2010). Inhibition of melanogensis by a novel origanoside from Origanum vulgare. *Journal of Dermatological Science*, Vol.57, No.3, (Mar 2010) pp. 170-177, ISSN 0923-1811

Lin, J.Y. & Fisher, D.E. (2007). Melanocyte biology and skin pigmentation. *Nature*, Vol.445, No.7130, (February 2007) pp. 843-850, ISSN 0028-0836

Liu, Y., Chan, F., Sun, H., Yan, J., Fan, D., Zhao, D., An, J. & Zhou, D. (2011). Resveratrol protects human keratinocytes HaCaT cells from UVA-induced oxidative stress damage by downregulating Keap1 expression. *European Journal of Pharmacology*, Vol.650, No.1, (January 2011) pp. 130-137, ISSN 0014-2999

Liu, F., Fu, Y. & Meyskens, F.L.,Jr. (2009). MiTF regulates cellular response to reactive oxygen species through transcriptional regulation of APE-1/Ref-1. *Journal of Investigative Dermatology*, Vol.129, No.2, (February 2009) pp. 422-431, ISSN 0022-202X

Maeda, K. & Hatao, M. (2004). Involvement of photooxidation of melanogenic precursors in prolonged pigmentation induced by ultraviolet A. *Journal of Investigative Dermatology*, Vol.122, No.2, (February 2004) pp. 503-509, ISSN 0022-202X

Maresca, V., Flori, E., Briganti, S., Mastrofrancesco, A., Fabbri, C., Mileo, A.M., Paggi, M.G. & Picardo, M. (2008). Correlation between melanogenic and catalase activity in in vitro human melanocytes: a synergic strategy against oxidative stress. *Pigment Cell & Melanoma Research*, Vol.21, No.2, (April 2008) pp. 200-205, ISSN 1755-1471

Marrot, L., Belaidi, J.P., Jones, C., Perez, P. & Meunier, J.R. (2005). Molecular responses to stress induced in normal human caucasian melanocytes in culture by exposure to simulated solar UV. *Photochemistry and Photobiology*, Vol.81, No.2, (Mar-April 2005) pp. 367-375, ISSN 0031-8655

Marrot, L., Jones, C., Perez, P. & Meunier, J.R. (2008). The significance of Nrf2 pathway in (photo)-oxidative stress response in melanocytes and keratinocytes of the human epidermis. *Pigment Cell & Melanoma Research*, Vol.21, No.1, (February 2008) pp. 79-88, ISSN 1755-1471

Masaki, H., Okano, Y. & Sakurai, H. (1998). Differential role of catalase and glutathione peroxidase in cultured human fibroblasts under exposure of H2O2 or ultraviolet B light. *Archives of Dermatological Research*, Vol.290, No.3, (March 1998) pp. 113-118, ISSN 0340-3696

Mastore, M., Kohler, L. & Nappi, A.J. (2005). Production and utilization of hydrogen peroxide associated with melanogenesis and tyrosinase-mediated oxidations of DOPA and dopamine. *FEBS Journal*, Vol.272, No.10, (May 2005) pp. 2407-2415, ISSN 1742-464X

Matsuda, H., Nakashima, S., Oda, Y., Nakamura, S. & Yoshikawa, M. (2009). Melanogenesis inhibitors from the rhizomes of Alpinia officinarum in B16 melanoma cells. *Bioorganic & Medicinal Chemistry*, Vol.17, No.16, (August 2009) pp. 6048-6053, ISSN 0968-0896

Meredith, P. & Sarna, T. (2006). The physical and chemical properties of eumelanin. *Pigment Cell Research*, Vol.19, No.6, (December 2006) pp. 572-594, ISSN 0893-5785

Meyskens, F.L.,Jr., Farmer, P. & Fruehauf, J.P. (2001). Redox regulation in human melanocytes and melanoma. *Pigment Cell Research*, Vol.14, No. 3, (June 2001) pp. 148-154, ISSN 0893-5785

Middelkamp-Hup, M.A., Pathak, M.A., Parrado, C., Garcia-Caballero, T., Rius-Diaz, F., Fitzpatrick, T.B. & Gonzalez, S. (2004). Orally administered Polypodium leucotomos extract decreases psoralen-UVA-induced phototoxicity, pigmentation, and damage of human skin. *Journal of the American Academy of Dermatology*, Vol.50, No.1, (January 2004) pp. 41-49, ISSN 0190-9622

Miller, A.J., Tsao, H. (2010). New insights into pigmentary pathways and skin cancer. *British Journal of Dermatology*, Vol.162, No.1 (January 2010) pp. 22-28, ISSN 0007-0963

Miyamura, Y., Coelho, S.G., Schlenz, K., Batzer, J., Smuda, C., Choi, W., Brenner, M., Passeron, T., Zhang, G., Kolbe, L., Wolber, R. & Hearing, V.J. (2011). The deceptive nature of UVA tanning versus the modest protective effects of UVB tanning on human skin. *Pigment Cell & Melanoma Research*, Vol.24, No.1, (February 2011) pp. 136-147, ISSN 1755-1471

Mossner, R., Anders, N., Konig, I.R., Kruger, U., Schmidt, D., Berking, C., Ziegler, A., Brockmoller, J., Kaiser, R., Volkenandt, M., Westphal, G.A. & Reich, K. (2007). Variations of the melanocortin-1 receptor and the glutathione-S transferase T1 and M1 genes in cutaneous malignant melanoma. *Archives of Dermatological Research*, Vol.298, No.8 (January 2007) pp. 371-379, ISSN 0340-3696

Munoz-Munoz, J.L., Garcia-Molina, F., Varon, R., Tudela, J., Garcia-Canovas, F. & Rodriguez-Lopez, J.N. (2009). Generation of hydrogen peroxide in the melanin biosynthesis pathway. *Biochimica et Biophysica Acta*, Vol.1794, No.7, (July 2009) pp. 1017-1029, ISSN 0006-3002

Nakamura, Y., Torikai, K., Ohto, Y., Murakami, A., Tanaka, T., Ohigashi, H. (2000). A simple phenolic antioxidant protocatechuic acid enhances tumor promotion and oxidative stress in female ICR mouse skin: dose-and timing-dependent enhancement and involvement of bioactivation by tyrosinase. *Carcinogenesis*, Vol.21, No.10, (October 2000) pp. 1899-1907, ISSN 0143-3334

Newton, R.A., Cook, A.L., Roberts, D.W., Leonard, J.H. & Sturm, R.A. (2007). Post-transcriptional regulation of melanin biosynthetic enzymes by cAMP and resveratrol in human melanocytes. *Journal of Investigative Dermatology*, Vol.127, No.9, (September 2007) pp. 2216-2227, ISSN 0022-202X

Ni, Z., Mu, Y. & Gulati, O. (2002). Treatment of melasma with Pycnogenol. *Phytotherapy Research*, Vol.16, No.6, (September 2002) pp. 567-571, ISSN 0951-418X

Nofsinger, J.B., Liu, Y. & Simon, J.D. (2002). Aggregation of eumelanin mitigates photogeneration of reactive oxygen species. *Free Radical Biology and Medicine*, Vol.32, No.8, (April 2002) pp. 720-730, ISSN 0891-5849

Ochiai, Y., Kaburagi, S., Obayashi, K., Ujiie, N., Hashimoto, S., Okano, Y., Masaki, H., Ichihashi, M. & Sakurai, H. (2006). A new lipophilic pro-vitamin C, tetra-isopalmitoyl ascorbic acid (VC-IP), prevents UV-induced skin pigmentation through its anti-oxidative properties. *Journal of Dermatological Science*, Vol.44, No.1, (October 2006) pp. 37-44, ISSN 0923-1811

Ou-Yang, H., Stamatas, G. & Kollias, N. (2004). Spectral responses of melanin to ultraviolet A irradiation. . *Journal of Investigative Dermatology*, Vol.122, No.2, (February 2004) pp. 492-496, ISSN 0022-202X

Park, E.S., Kim, S.Y., Na, J.I., Ryu, H.S., Youn, S.W., Kim, D.S., Yun, H.Y. & Park, K.C. (2007). Glutathione prevented dopamine-induced apoptosis of melanocytes and its signaling. *Journal of Dermatological Science*, Vol.47, No.2, (August 2007) pp. 141-149, ISSN 0923-1811

Park, H.Y., Kosmadaki, M., Yaar, M. & Gilchrest, B.A. (2009). Cellular mechanisms regulating human melanogenesis. *Cellular and Molecular Life Sciences*, Vol.66, No.9, (May 2009) pp. 1423-1430, ISSN 1420-682X

Parvez, S., Kang, M., Chung, H.S., Cho, C., Hong, M.C., Shin, M.K. & Bae,H. (2006). Survey and mechanism of skin depigmenting and lightening agents. *Phytotherapy Research*, Vol.20, No.11, (November 2006) pp. 921-934, ISSN 0951-418X

Pavel, S., van Nieuwpoort, F., van der, Meulen H., Out, C., Pizinger, K., Cetkovska, P., Smit, N.P. & Koerten, H.K. (2004). Disturbed melanin synthesis and chronic oxidative stress in dysplastic naevi. *European Journal of Cancer*, Vol.40, No.9, (June 2004) pp. 1423-1430, ISSN 0959-8049

Pfeifer, G.P., You, Y.H. & Besaratinia, A. (2005). Mutations induced by ultraviolet light. *Mutation Research*, Vol.571, No.1-2, (April 2005) pp. 19-31, ISSN 0027-5107

Philips, N., Conte, J., Chen, Y.J., Natrajan, P., Taw, M., Keller, T., Givant, J., Tuason, M., Dulaj, L., Leonardi,D. & Gonzalez, S. (2009). Beneficial regulation of matrixmetalloproteinases and their inhibitors, fibrillar collagens and transforming growth factor-beta by Polypodium leucotomos, directly or in dermal fibroblasts, ultraviolet radiated fibroblasts, and melanoma cells. *Archives of Dermatological Research*, Vol.301, No.7 (August 2007) pp. 487-495, ISSN 0340-3696

Pinnell, S.R. (2003). Cutaneous photodamage, oxidative stress, and topical antioxidant protection. *Journal of the American Academy of Dermatology*, Vol.48, No.1, (January 2003) pp. 1-19, ISSN 0190-9622

Rass, K. & Reichrath, J. (2008). UV damage and DNA repair in malignant melanoma and nonmelanoma skin cancer. *Advances in Experimental Medicine and Biology*, Vol.624, (2008) pp. 162-178, ISSN 0065-2598

Riley, P.A. (2003). Melanogenesis and melanoma. *Pigment Cell Research*, Vol.16, No.5, (October 2003) pp. 548-552, ISSN 0893-5785

Russo, A., Cardile, V., Lombardo, L., Vanella, L. & Acquaviva,R. (2006). Genistin inhibits UV light-induced plasmid DNA damage and cell growth in human melanoma cells. *The Journal of Nutritional Biochemistry*, Vol.17, No.2, (February 2006) pp. 103-108, ISSN 0955-2863

Saikia, A.P., Ryakala, V.K., Sharma, P., Goswami, P. & Bora,U. (2006). Ethnobotany of medicinal plants used by Assamese people for various skin ailments and cosmetics. *Journal of Ethnopharmacology*, Vol.106, No.2, (Jun 2006) pp. 149-157, ISSN 0378-8741

Sander, C.S., Hamm, F., Elsner, P. & Thiele, J.J. (2003). Oxidative stress in malignant melanoma and non-melanoma skin cancer. *British Journal of Dermatology*, Vol.148, No.5 (May 2003) pp. 913-922, ISSN 0007-0963

Sapkota, K., Park, S.E., Kim, J.E., Kim, S., Choi, H.S., Chun, H.S. & Kim, S.J. (2010). Antioxidant and antimelanogenic properties of chestnut flower extract. *Bioscience, Biotechnology, and Biochemistry*, Vol.74, No.8, (August 2010) pp. 1527-1533, ISSN 0916-8451

Sarangarajan, R. & Apte, S.P. (2006). The polymerization of melanin: a poorly understood phenomenon with egregious biological implications. *Melanoma Research*, Vol.16, No.1 (February 2006) pp. 3-10, ISSN 0960-8931

Schafer, M., Dutsch, S., auf dem, Keller U., Navid, F., Schwarz, A., Johnson, D.A., Johnson, J.A. & Werner, S. (2010). Nrf2 establishes a glutathione-mediated gradient of UVB cytoprotection in the epidermis. *Genes & Development*, Vol.24, No.10 (May 2010) pp. 1045-1058, ISSN 0890-9369

Scharffetter-Kochanek, K., Brenneisen, P., Wenk, J., Herrmann, G., Ma, W., Kuhr, L., Meewes, C. & Wlaschek, M. (2000). Photoaging of the skin from phenotype to mechanisms. *Experimental Gerontology*, Vol.35, No.3 (May 2000) pp. 307-316, ISSN 0531-5565

Scherer, D. & Kumar, R. (2010). Genetics of pigmentation in skin cancer--a review. *Mutation Research*, Vol.705, No.2, (October 2010) pp. 141-153, ISSN 0027-5107

Seiberg, M. (2001). Keratinocyte-melanocyte interactions during melanosome transfer. *Pigment Cell Research*, Vol.14, No.4, (August 2001) pp. 236-242, ISSN 0893-5785

Seite, S., Fourtanier, A., Moyal, D. & Young, A.R. (2010). Photodamage to human skin by suberythemal exposure to solar ultraviolet radiation can be attenuated by sunscreens: a review. *British Journal of Dermatology*, Vol.163, No.5 (November 2010) pp. 903-914, ISSN 0007-0963

Slominski, A., Tobin, D.J., Shibahara, S. & Wortsman, J. (2004). Melanin pigmentation in mammalian skin and its hormonal regulation. *Physiology Review*, Vol.84, No.4 (October 2004) pp. 1155-1228, ISSN 0031-9333

Smit, N., Vicanova, J., Cramers, P., Vrolijk, H. & Pavel, S. (2004). The combined effects of extracts containing carotenoids and vitamins E and C on growth and pigmentation of cultured human melanocytes. *Skin Pharmacology and Physiology*, Vol.17, No.5, (September-October 2004) pp. 238-245, ISSN 1660-5527

Smit, N.P., van Nieuwpoort, F.A., Marrot, L., Out, C., Poorthuis, B., van Pelt, H., Meunier, J.R. & Pavel, S. (2008). Increased melanogenesis is a risk factor for oxidative DNA damage--study on cultured melanocytes and atypical nevus cells. *Photochemistry and Photobiology*, Vol.84, No.3, (May-June 2008) pp. 550-555, ISSN 0031-8655

Sneyd, M.J. & Cox,B. (2009). Melanoma in Maori, Asian, and Pacific peoples in New Zealand. *Cancer Epidemiology, Biomarkers & Prevention*, Vol.18, No.6, (June 2009) pp. 1706-1713, ISSN 1055-9965

Tai, S.S., Lin, C.G., Wu, M.H. & Chang, T.S. (2009). Evaluation of depigmenting activity by 8-hydroxydaidzein in mouse B16 melanoma cells and human volunteers. *International Journal of Molecular Sciences*, Vol.10, No.10, (November 2009) pp. 4257-4266, ISSN 1422-0067

Takeuchi, S., Zhang, W., Wakamatsu, K., Ito, S., Hearing, V.J., Kraemer, K.H. & Brash, D.E. (2004). Melanin acts as a potent UVB photosensitizer to cause an atypical mode of cell death in murine skin. *Proceedings of the National Academy of Sciences of the United States of America*, Vol.101, No.42, (October 2004) pp. 15076-15081, ISSN 0027-8424

Thangasamy, T., Sittadjody, S., Lanza-Jacoby, S., Wachsberger, P.R., Limesand, K.H. & Burd, R. (2007). Quercetin selectively inhibits bioreduction and enhances apoptosis in melanoma cells that overexpress tyrosinase. *Nutrition and Cancer*, Vol.59, No.2, (2007) pp. 258-268, ISSN 1532-7914

Tran, T.T., Schulman, J & Fisher, D.E. (2008). UV and pigmentation: molecular mechanisms and social controversies. *Pigment Cell & Melanoma Research*, Vol.21, No.5, (October 2008) pp. 509-516, ISSN 1755-1471

Veierod, M.B., Weiderpass, E., Thorn, M., Hansson, J., Lund, E., Armstrong, B. & Adami, H.O. (2003). A prospective study of pigmentation, sun exposure, and risk of cutaneous malignant melanoma in women. *Journal of the National Cancer Instiute*, Vol.95, No.20, (October 2003) pp. 1530-1538, ISSN 0027-8874

Verschooten, L., Claerhout, S., Van Laethem, A., Agostinis, P. & Garmyn, M. (2006). New strategies of photoprotection. *Photochemistry and Photobiology*, Vol.82, No.4, (? 2006) pp. 1016-1023, ISSN 0031-8655

Villa, A., Viera, M.H., Amini, S., Huo, R., Perez, O., Ruiz, P., Amador, A., Elgart, G. & Berman, B. (2010). Decrease of ultraviolet A light-induced "common deletion" in healthy volunteers after oral Polypodium leucotomos extract supplement in a randomized clinical trial. *Journal of the American Academy of Dermatology*, Vol.62, No.3, (Mar 2010) pp. 511-513, ISSN 0190-9622

von Thaler, A.K., Kamenisch, Y. & Berneburg, M. (2010). The role of ultraviolet radiation in melanomagenesis. *Experimental Dermatology*, Vol.19, No.2, (February 2010) pp. 81-88, ISSN 0906-6705

Wang, H.T., Choi, B. & Tang, M.S. (2010). Melanocytes are deficient in repair of oxidative DNA damage and UV-induced photoproducts. *Proceedings of the National Academy of Sciences of the United States of America*, Vol.107, No.27, (July 2010) pp. 12180-12185, ISSN 0027-8424

Wang, K.H., Lin, R.D., Hsu, F.L., Huang, Y.H., Chang, H.C., Huang, C.Y. & Lee, M.H. (2006). Cosmetic applications of selected traditional Chinese herbal medicines. *Journal of Ethnopharmacology*, Vol.106, No.3, (July 2006) pp. 353-359, ISSN 0378-8741

Weller, R. (2003). Nitric oxide: a key mediator in cutaneous physiology. *Clinical Experimental Dermatology*, Vol.28, No.5, (September 2003) pp. 511-514, ISSN 0307-6938

Wenczl, E., Van der Schans, G.P., Roza, L., Kolb, R.M., Timmerman, A.J., Smit, N.P., Pavel, S. & Schothorst, A.A. (1998). (Pheo)melanin photosensitizes UVA-induced DNA damage in cultured human melanocytes. *Journal of Investigative Dermatology*, Vol.111, No.4, (October 1998) pp. 678-682, ISSN 0022-202X

Westerhof, W. (2006). The discovery of the human melanocyte. *Pigment Cell Research*, Vol.19, No.3, (June 2006) pp. 183-193, ISSN 0893-5785

Wittgen, H.G. & van Kempen, L.C. (2007). Reactive oxygen species in melanoma and its therapeutic implications. *Melanoma Research*, Vol.17, No.6, (December 2007) pp. 400-409, ISSN 0960-8931

Wood, J.M. & Schallreuter, K.U. (2008). A plaidoyer for cutaneous enzymology: our view of some important unanswered questions on the contributions of selected key enzymes to epidermal homeostasis. *Experimental Dermatology*, Vol.17, No.7, (July 2008) pp. 569-578, ISSN 0906-6705

Xiao, L., Matsubayashi, K. & Miwa, N. (2007). Inhibitory effect of the water-soluble polymer-wrapped derivative of fullerene on UVA-induced melanogenesis via downregulation of tyrosinase expression in human melanocytes and skin tissues. *Archives of Dermatological Research*, Vol.299, No.5-6, (August 2007) pp. 245-257, ISSN 0340-3696

Yamaguchi, Y., Takahashi, K., Zmudzka, B.Z., Kornhauser, A., Miller, S.A., Tadokoro, T., Berens, W., Beer, J.Z. & Hearing, V.J. (2006). Human skin responses to UV radiation: pigment in the upper epidermis protects against DNA damage in the lower epidermis and facilitates apoptosis. *The FASEB Journal*, Vol.20, No.9, (July 2006) pp. 1486-1488, ISSN 0892-6638

Yamakoshi, J., Otsuka, F., Sano, A., Tokutake, S., Saito, M., Kikuchi, M. & Kubota, Y. (2003). Lightening effect on ultraviolet-induced pigmentation of guinea pig skin by oral administration of a proanthocyanidin-rich extract from grape seeds. *Pigment Cell Research*, Vol.16, No.6, (December 2003) pp. 629-638, ISSN 0893-5785

Yamamura, T., Onishi, J. & Nishiyama, T. (2002). Antimelanogenic activity of hydrocoumarins in cultured normal human melanocytes by stimulating intracellular glutathione synthesis. *Archives of Dermatological Research*, Vol.294, No.8 (November 2002) pp. 349-354, ISSN 0340-3696

Yanase, H., Ando, H., Horikawa, M., Watanabe, M., Mori, T. & Matsuda, N. (2001). Possible involvement of ERK 1/2 in UVA-induced melanogenesis in cultured normal human epidermal melanocytes. *Pigment Cell Research*, Vol.14, No.2, (April 2001) pp. 103-109, ISSN 0893-5785

Yap, W.N., Zaiden, N., Xu, C.H., Chen, A., Ong, S., Teo, V. & Yap, Y.L. (2010). Gamma- and delta-tocotrienols inhibit skin melanin synthesis by suppressing constitutive and UV-induced tyrosinase activation. *Pigment Cell & Melanoma Research*, Vol.23, No.5, (October 2010) pp. 688-692, ISSN 1755-1471

Yoshimura, M., Watanabe, Y., Kasai, K., Yamakoshi, J. & Koga, T. (2005). Inhibitory effect of an ellagic acid-rich pomegranate extract on tyrosinase activity and ultraviolet-induced pigmentation. *Bioscience, Biotechnology, and Biochemistry*, Vol.69, No.12, (December 2005) pp. 2368-2373, ISSN 0916-8451

Panich, U., Kongtaphan, K., Onkoksoong, T., Jaemsak, K., Phadungrakwittaya, R., Thaworn, A., Akarasereenont, P. & Wongkajornsilp, A. (2010). Modulation of antioxidant defense by Alpinia galanga and Curcuma aromatica extracts correlates with their inhibition of UVA-induced melanogenesis. *Cell Biology and Toxicology*, Vol.26, No.2, (April 2010) pp. 103-116, ISSN 0742-2091

13

Adaptation to ER Stress as a Mechanism of Resistance of Melanoma to Treatment

Xu Dong Zhang, Peter Hersey, Kwang Hong Tay,
Hsin-Yi Tseng, Chen Chen Jiang and Li Dong
University of Newcastle
Australia

1. Introduction

A number of cellular stress conditions, such as nutrient deprivation, hypoxia, alterations in glycosylation status, and disturbances of calcium flux, lead to accumulation and aggregation of unfolded and/or misfolded proteins in the endoplasmic reticulum (ER) lumen and cause so-called ER stress. The ER responds to the stress conditions by activation of a range of stress-response signalling pathways to alter transcriptional and translational programs, which couples the ER protein folding load with the ER protein folding capacity and is termed the unfolded protein response (UPR).

The UPR of mammalian cells is initiated by three ER transmembrane proteins - activating transcription factor 6 (ATF6), inositol-requiring enzyme 1 (IRE1) and double-stranded RNA-activated protein kinase-like ER kinase (PERK) that act as proximal sensors of ER stress. Under unstressed conditions, the luminal domains of these sensors are occupied by the ER chaperone glucose-regulated protein 78 (GRP78). Upon ER stress, sequestration of GRP78 by unfolded proteins activates these sensors by inducing phosphorylation and homodimerization of IRE1 and PERK, and relocalization of ATF6 to the Golgi where it is cleaved by Site 1 and Site 2 proteases (S1P and S2P) leading to its activation as a transcriptional factor. The UPR is fundamentally a cyto-protective response, but excessive or prolonged UPR can result in cell death, predominantly by induction of apoptosis.

Nevertheless, most melanoma cell lines are insensitive, relative to cultured melanocytes and fibroblasts, to apoptosis induced by pharmacological ER stress inducers, suggesting that melanoma cells may have developed adaptive mechanisms to counteract the apoptosis-inducing outputs of the UPR, thus surviving ER stress conditions. This is supported by increased expression of GRP78, a commonly used indicator of activation of the UPR, in melanoma cells *in vivo*, which is associated with progression of the disease. It is conceivable that, like many other solid cancers, melanoma cells in a developing tumour without sufficient blood supply may undergo hypoxia, nutrient starvation and acidosis. In addition, accumulation of mutant proteins and increased glycolytic activity in cancer cells may also contribute to ER stress.

How the UPR switches between the pro-survival and pro-apoptotic signalling pathways remains a dilemma. It is conceivable that adaptive processes converge on mechanisms that inhibit apoptosis. In this chapter, we will discuss multiple mechanisms that are involved in resistance of melanoma cells to apoptosis induced by ER stress. These include persistent activation of the IRE1 branch of the UPR that is responsible for up-regulation of the anti-apoptotic Bcl-2 family protein Mcl-1, and dysregulation of CHOP, a transcription factor down-stream of the PERK branch of the UPR that otherwise triggers apoptosis by up-regulation of the BH3-only protein Bim. We will also present evidence showing important roles of activation of other survival pathways such as the MEK/ERK and PI3K/Akt pathways in adaptation of melanoma cells to ER stress.

Two fundamental questions that are directly relevant to clinical management of melanoma are how adaptation to ER stress impacts on responses of melanoma cells to treatment and whether induction of ER stress by therapeutic agents is beneficial or detrimental. Melanoma cells under pharmacological ER stress acquire resistance to apoptosis induced by microtubule-targeting drugs docetaxel and vincristine, suggesting that activation of the UPR protects melanoma cells against these agents. On the other hand, induction of apoptosis by a number of chemotherapeutic drugs, such as the DNA damaging drugs cisplatin and adriamycin, the proteasome inhibitor bortezomib, and the synthetic retinoid derivative fenretinide, is known to be associated with induction of ER stress. However, there is evidence showing that inhibition of the UPR effector GRP78 sensitizes melanoma cells to cisplatin and adriamycin. We will discuss possible explanations for these seemingly paradoxical observations in this chapter, and will propose that induction of ER stress by therapeutic agents is a double-edged sword. We will also present data demonstrating that targeting adaptive mechanisms to ER stress may be useful in the treatment of melanoma, especially in combination with agents that induce ER stress.

2. ER stress and the UPR

The ER is an organelle of a lacey network of cisternae that has essential roles in many cellular processes required for cell survival, growth and other functions. These include intracellular calcium homeostasis, protein folding and glycosylation, and lipid biosynthesis (Gaut & Hendershot, 1993). Moreover, because the ER releases calcium through ion channels in response to second messengers such as inositol triphosphate (IP3) and protein kinases, it is also regarded as a signalling organelle (Schröder & Kaufman, 2005).

ER stress is a condition under which intracellular or extracellular disturbances, such as nutrient deprivation, hypoxia, alterations in glycosylation status, disturbances of calcium flux, cause accumulation and aggregation of unfolded and/or misfolded proteins in the ER lumen (Ma & Hendershot, 2004; Ron & Walter, 2007; Schröder & Kaufman, 2005). Cells undergoing ER stress respond to protect themselves by activating the UPR, which alters transcriptional, translational, and post-translational programs, resulting in up-regulation of ER chaperones, general translational attenuation, and enhanced ER-associated degradation (ERAD) of misfolded and unfolded proteins. The signalling pathways of the UPR are initiated by three ER transmembrane proteins, ATF6, IRE1, and PERK (Ma & Hendershot, 2004; Ron & Walter, 2007; Schröder & Kaufman, 2005). Under unstressed conditions, the luminal domains of these sensors are occupied by ER chaperone proteins, in particular, GRP78. Upon ER stress, increased binding of GRP78 with misfolded and unfolded proteins causes removal of GRP78 from ATF6, IRE1, and PERK, thus resulting in release of these proximal ER stress sensors and activation the UPR (Fig. 1). GRP78 has therefore been termed the "master regulator" of the UPR (Hendershot, 2004; Lee, 2005).

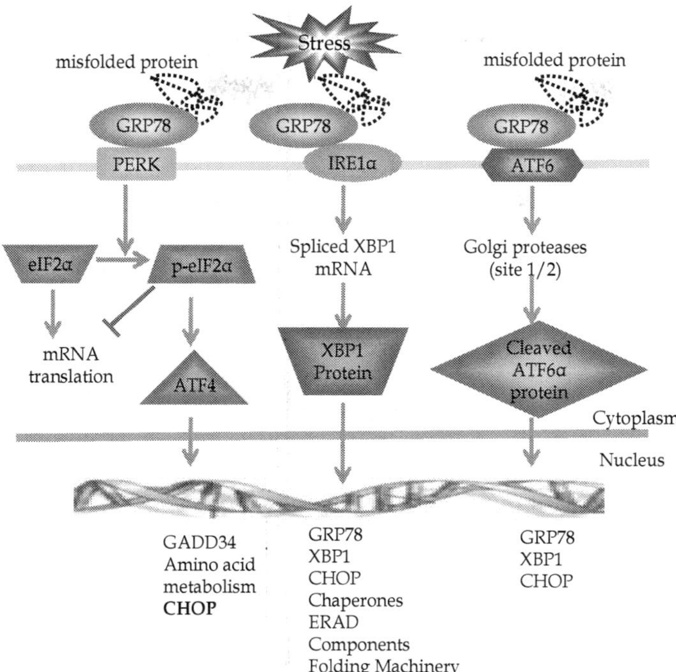

Fig. 1. A schematic illustration of signalling pathways of the UPR

2.1 IRE1α

IRE1α is an unusual protein in that it acts as both a serine/threonine protein kinase and an endoribonuclease (Ma & Hendershot, 2004; Ron & Walter, 2007; Schröder & Kaufman, 2005). The latter activity processes an intron leading to the catalytic removal of a 26-base intron from the mRNA of the gene, *X-box-binding protein 1* (*XBP1*). This splicing and re-ligation results in a translational frameshift to produce the active XBP1 protein, a basic leucine zipper (bZIP) family transcription factor that can bind to both the ER stress response element (ERSE) and the unfolded protein response promoter elements (UPRE), thus transcriptionally up-regulating a number of genes involved in the UPR (Lee, et al., 2003). In addition, IRE1α is also necessary for cleavage and post-transcriptional degradation of many other mRNAs encoding secreted proteins. This plays a part in reducing protein loading onto the ER (Hollien & Weissman, 2006).

As a protein kinase, IRE1α can form protein complexes with TNF receptor-associated factor 2 (TRAF2) and apoptosis signal-regulating kinase 1 (ASK1). This causes activation of ASK1 that in turn activates Jun N-terminal kinase (JNK) (Nishitoh, et al., 2002; Urano, et al., 2000). Moreover, binding of IRE1α to TRAF2 leads to activation of a number of other protein kinases implicated in immunity and inflammation (Urano, et al., 2000). IRE1α can also bind to the multi-domain pro-apoptotic Bcl-2 family proteins Bax and Bak (Hetz, et al., 2006). This association may cause activation of IRE1α, and thus modulating calcium flux and UPR signalling.

2.2 ATF6

ATF6 has two isoforms, α and β (Ma & Hendershot, 2004; Ron & Walter, 2007; Schröder & Kaufman, 2005). They are members of the bZIP transcription factor family and have conserved protein domain, but interestingly, divergent transcriptional activation domains. ATF6α is the better characterized of the two that shares many of the activities of IRE1α. Upon ER stress it is freed from the ER membrane and translocates to the Golgi compartment, where it is cleaved by the S1P/S2P serine protease to produce a transcription factor that binds to ERSE elements, thus activating genes encoding proteins involved in the UPR including XBP1, C/EBP homologous protein (CHOP), and ER chaperone proteins such as GRP78 and GRP94 (Okada, et al., 2002; Yoshida, et al., 2001).

2.3 PERK

PERK is a serine/threonine protein kinase. Oligomerization of PERK at the ER membrane leads to its autophosphorylation and activation (Ma & Hendershot, 2004; Ron & Walter, 2007; Schröder & Kaufman, 2005). Activated PERK phosphorylates the translation initiation factor, eukaryotic initiation factor 2 α (eIF2α), leading to its inactivation and attenuation of translation. However, selective mRNAs can be preferentially translated. The best characterized of these is the transcription factor ATF4 that activates the transcription of genes including CHOP, GRP78, and GRP94. PERK$^{-/-}$ cells and cells expressing eIF2α that cannot be phosphorylated are hypersensitive to ER stress-induced cell death, indicating the importance of signals initiated by PERK in protection of cells from ER stress (Harding, et al., 2000).

3. ER stress and cell death

Although ER stress activates the UPR that is essentially a cyto-protective response, prolonged or excessive activation of the UPR can result in cell death by inducing primarily apoptosis (Ma & Hendershot, 2004; Ron & Walter, 2007; Schröder & Kaufman, 2005). In some circumstances, ER stress can also trigger autophagy that contributes to degradation of excessive proteins and protects cells from apoptosis (Høyer-Hansen & Jäättelä, 2007), but similar to the UPR, excessive autophagy can lead to autophagic cell death (Codogno & Meijer, 2005). Moreover, ER stress has been shown to play a role in oncogene-induced senescence (Denoyelle, et al., 2006).

Induction of apoptosis by ER stress in most cell types involves many of the same molecules that have important roles in other apoptotic cascades including Bcl-2 family proteins and caspases (Boyce & Yuan, 2006; Ferri & Kroemer, 2001). However, how ER stress-induced apoptotic signalling is triggered may vary among different cell types and ER stress inducers in question.

3.1 The mitochondrial apoptotic pathway and ER stress-induced apoptosis

Involvement of the mitochondrial apoptotic pathway in ER stress-induced apoptosis has been well-documented (Boyce & Yuan, 2006; Ferri & Kroemer, 2001), although there have also been reports showing that, at least in some circumstances, ER stress can trigger apoptosis independently of mechanisms mediated by mitochondria (Rao, et al., 2002).

The mitochondrial apoptotic pathway is tightly regulated by interactions between pro- and anti-apoptotic Bcl-2 family proteins (Cory & Adams, 2002). Among them, anti-apoptotic proteins such as Bcl-2, Bcl-X$_L$, and Mcl-1 protect mitochondrial integrity, whereas pro-apoptotic members of the family promote the release of apoptogenic proteins such as cytochrome c, second mitochondria-derived activator of caspase (Smac)/direct inhibitor of apoptosis-binding protein with low pI (DIABLO) from mitochondria (Du, et al., 2000; Li, et al., 1997; Verhagen, et al., 2000). The pro-apoptotic proteins of the Bcl-2 family can be further divided into BH3-only proteins such as Bim, PUMA, and Noxa and their effectors, the multidomain proteins Bax and Bak. Activation of BH3-only proteins are essential in induction of apoptosis, as they act as "death ligands" to activate Bax and Bak by directly binding to them, or by indirectly displacing them from anti-apoptotic Bcl-2 family members. The interactions between BH3-only proteins and anti-apoptotic proteins are highly selective (Chen, et al., 2005). For example, while Bim and PUMA can tightly engage all the anti-apoptotic proteins, thus being particularly potent apoptosis initiator, Bad can only bind to Bcl-2 and Bcl-X$_L$, but not Mcl-1. In addition, Bid and Bim have been shown to be the only BH3-only proteins that can directly bind to and activate Bax (Kuwana, et al., 2005). Anti-apoptotic proteins of the family may also constitute more than one functional class. For instance, Mcl-1 was proposed to play a unique apical role, elimination of which is required at an early stage of induction of apoptosis (Nijhawan, et al., 2003).

The multidomain pro-apoptotic Bcl-2 family proteins Bax and Bak can localize to the ER membrane, where they bind to IRE1α, which has been shown to be required for activation of IRE1α and subsequent activation of XBP1 (Zong, et al., 2003). Loss of Bax/Bak leads to, at least in some cases, impairment of adaptation to ER stress (Hetz, et al., 2006). It appears therefore that Bax/Bak may have a pro-survival role in the ER stress response, presumably due to activation of the IRE1α/XBP-1 pathway. Indeed, ER localized Bax/Bak has been suggested to act as an adaptive mechanism under conditions of mild or transient ER stress, but as pro-apoptotic molecules under prolonged or strong ER stress conditions (Heath-Engel, et al., 2008; Hetz & Glimcher, 2008).

Involvement of Bax- and Bak-dependent mitochondrial apoptotic pathway strongly suggests that one or more BH3-only proteins play critical roles in ER stress-induced apoptosis. This is further supported by inhibition of ER stress-induced apoptosis with over-expression of Bcl-2 or one of its anti-apoptotic homologs (Boyce & Yuan, 2006; Ferri & Kroemer, 2001). Indeed, ER stress can up-regulate PUMA and Noxa in various types of cells (Armstrong, et al., 2007; Li, et al., 2006; Wang, et al., 2009). This has been shown to be p53-dependent or –independent presumably related to different types of cells used in varying studies and ER stress inducers in question. For example, p53-dependent up-regulation of PUMA and Noxa has been demonstrated in mouse embryo fibroblasts exposed to tunicamycin and thapsigargin (Li, et al., 2006), which are commonly used laboratory tools as ER stress inducers. Tunicamycin induces ER stress by inhibition of glycosylation, whereas thapsigargin, by inhibition of ER Ca^{2+} ATPases. In contrast, p53-independent activation of PUMA was observed in human osteosarcoma SAOS-2 cells, and colon cancer HCT116 cells subjected to ER stress (Reimertz, et al., 2003).

Another BH3-only protein that plays an important role in ER stress-induced apoptosis in certain circumstances is Bim. This was initially suggested by translocation of Bim to the ER upon induction of ER stress, and was further supported by the finding that ectopic expression of ER-targeted Bim induced apoptosis (Morishima, et al., 2004). More recently, Bim was found to be transcriptionally up-regulated in diverse types of cells under stress (Puthalakath, et al., 2007). This is mediated by binding of heterodimers of the transcription factors CHOP and C/EBPα to an unconventional promoter within the first intron of the Bim gene. In addition, ER stress triggers protein phosphatase 2A-mediated dephosphorylation of Bim, which prevents its ubiquitination and proteasomal degradation.

The BH3-only protein BIK is predominantly located to the ER, where it forms complex with GRP78. BIK has been shown to regulate Bax- and Bak-dependent release of calcium from the ER and mitochondrion-mediated apoptosis in cells under ER stress (Fu, et al., 2007; Mathai, et al., 2005). Another BH3-only protein that has been reported to be activated by ER stress is Bad, which is under physiological conditions phosphorylated and sequestered in the cytoplasm by the protein 14-3-3, but was dephosphorylated in response to several ER stress stimuli (Elyaman, et al., 2002; Szegezdi, et al., 2008).

Besides up-regulation/activation of pro-apoptotic Bcl-2 family proteins, down-regulation of anti-apoptotic Bcl-2 family members by ER stress also contribute to ER stress-induced apoptosis. Transcriptional repression of Bcl-2 by CHOP has long been reported (McCullough, et al., 2001), but this is not universally observed in all cell type (Puthalakath, et al., 2007). Induction of ER stress may also impinge on Bcl-2 phosphorylation and stability. This has been suggested to be mediated by protein phosphatase 2A (Lin, et al., 2006). Down-regulation of Mcl-1 has also been frequently observed. This is, at least in some cases, due to inhibition Mcl-1 mRNA translation (Fritsch, et al., 2007).

3.2 Caspases and ER stress-induced apoptosis

Activation of initiator caspases is a proximal event in induction of apoptosis by either the intrinsic (mitochondrial) or extrinsic (death receptor) apoptotic pathways. Although processing of caspase-8, -9, and -2 has been observed in cells under ER stress, which eventually leads to activation of effector caspases such as caspase-3 and -7, activation of caspase-12 in rodents and caspase-4 in human appears essential in ER stress-induced apoptosis (Ferri & Kroemer, 2001; Hitomi, et al., 2004).

Caspase-12 is located to the ER and is selectively activated by ER stress (Hitomi, et al., 2004). Caspase-12 deletion inhibits apoptosis induced by a variety ER stress inducers such as tunicamycin and thapsigargin. In contrast, over-expression of caspase-12 induces apoptosis. There is large body of evidence showing that caspase-12 is activated by ER stress up-stream of effector caspases, indicating it functions as an initiator caspase. However, caspase-12 is expressed only in rodents. Its human homologue is silenced by several mutations during evolution (Fischer, et al., 2002). Human caspase-4 is the closest homologue to murine caspase-12 and is at least partially located to the ER (Hitomi, et al., 2004). Caspase-4 has been shown to fulfil the function of caspase-12 in ER stress-induced apoptosis in some types of human cells (Hitomi, et al., 2004; Jiang, et al., 2007).

How caspase-12 and caspase-4 is activated in cells under ER stress remains to be determined. A number of biologic events have been shown to be associated with activation of caspase-12 in murine cells (Boyce & Yuan, 2006; Heath-Engel, et al., 2008; Nakagawa, et al., 2000; Urano, et al., 2000). First, caspase-12 activation has been linked to release of calcium from ER and consequent activation of calpain. Inhibition of calpain by chemical inhibitors and genetic approaches and chelation of intracellular calcium can block caspase-12 activation induced by various ER stress inducers; second, ER stress triggers recruitment of caspase-7 to the ER where it complexes with caspase-12 leading to its activation. GRP78 also exists at the complex and plays a role in inhibiting both caspase-7 and -12; and third, it has been suggested that caspase-12 is associated with TRAF2, but under ER stress, recruitment of the TRAF2/caspase-12 complex to IRE1α provides a scaffold for caspase-12 activation. However, if human caspase-4 is similarly activated as murine caspase-12 by ER stress remains to be clarified.

4. Adaptation of melanoma cells to ER stress

Although excessive or prolonged UPR can result in apoptosis, most melanoma cell lines are not sensitive to apoptosis induced by pharmacological ER stress inducers, tunicamycin and thapsigargin. This suggests that melanoma cells may have adapted to ER stress conditions by development of resistance mechanisms against ER stress-induced apoptosis.

There is ample evidence showing that the UPR is activated in various solid tumours due to both intrinsic and extrinsic factors (Lee, 2007; Ma & Hendershot, 2004). Increased expression of GRP78, a commonly used indicator of activation of the UPR, has been reported in a variety of cancers. In some cases, GRP78 expression is associated with tumour growth and resistance to chemotherapy (Lee, 2007; Ma & Hendershot, 2004). Consistently, GRP78 is also expressed at varying, but commonly higher levels in melanoma cells relative to melanocytes both *in vitro* and *in vivo* (Jiang, et al., 2009a; Zhuang, et al., 2009). In addition, the levels of GRP78 correlate with progression of the disease and other markers of prognosis such as tumour thickness and mitotic rate (Zhuang, et al., 2009). Similarly, the active form of XBP1 mRNA is expressed at higher levels in cultured melanoma cells (Jiang, et al., 2009a). Therefore, melanoma cells have adapted to ER stress, which appears to be imposed on melanoma cells at early stages of development, in that UPR has been shown to be activated at initiation stages of melanoma by the oncogenic form of HRAS (HRAS^{G12V}) (Denoyelle, et al., 2006).

It is conceivable that cells in a developing tumour without sufficient blood supply may undergo hypoxia, nutrient starvation and acidosis (Lee, 2007; Ma & Hendershot, 2004). In addition, mutated proteins in cancer cells may also contribute to ER stress. Another ER stress-inducing mechanism of cancer cells is increased glycolytic activity due to the Warburg effect. High levels of lactate dehydrogenase (LDH) are readily apparent in patients with melanoma, and the levels in sera are the single most powerful predictor of prognosis in metastatic disease (Balch, et al., 2009; Eton, et al., 1998). In support of the importance of increased glycolysis in induction of ER stress in melanoma, the levels of LDH5 are correlated with the levels of GRP78 in melanoma cells *in vivo* (Zhuang, et al., 2010).

5. Adaptive mechanisms of melanoma cells to ER stress

Adaptation to ER stress is believed to be an intrinsic consequence of low level activation of the UPR. However, it remains a paradox how the UPR switches between the pro-survival and pro-apoptotic signalling pathways. Nevertheless, adaptive processes converge on mechanisms that inhibit apoptosis. Because ER stress can induce apoptosis through multiple mechanisms, it is conceivable that adaptation of melanoma cells to ER stress is the consequence of activation of multiple anti-apoptotic mechanisms.

5.1 Up-regulation of Mcl-1 is critical for survival of melanoma cells upon ER stress

Mcl-1 is an anti-apoptotic Bcl-2 family protein that is of particular importance in melanoma, in that its expression increases with melanoma progression and is associated with poor prognosis (Zhuang, et al., 2007). Moreover, Mcl-1 is a major resistance mechanism of melanoma cells to apoptosis induced by a variety of apoptotic stimuli (Jiang, et al., 2008; Wang, et al., 2007). As a protein with a rapid turn-over rate, Mcl-1 expression is frequently regulated by post-translational mechanisms (Schwickart, et al., 2010; Warr & Shore, 2008; Zhong, et al., 2005). Nevertheless, an increase in the Mcl-1 protein levels often correlates with an increase in its mRNA levels, mostly due to enhanced transcription (Iglesias-Serret, et al., 2003; Warr & Shore, 2008). In addition, Mcl-1 can be regulated at the translational level. For example, the Mcl-1 protein levels have been shown to be markedly reduced by thapsigargin due to translational repression mediated by phosphorylation of eIF2α downstream of PERK (Fritsch, et al., 2007).

In contrast to down-regulation by ER stress in many other cell types, Mcl-1 along with Bcl-2 is up-regulated in melanoma cells by ER stress (Jiang, et al., 2008). Although up-regulated, Bcl-2 does not appear to be critical for protection of melanoma cells from ER stress-induced apoptosis, in that inhibition of Bcl-2 by siRNA has only a minimal effect on sensitivity of melanoma cells to ER stress-induced apoptosis, whereas over-expression of Bcl-2 can only delay the onset of apoptosis, but does not rescue melanoma cells from apoptosis induced by ER stress when Mcl-1 is deficient. On the other hand, siRNA inhibition of Mcl-1 readily enhances ER stress-induced apoptosis, and over-expression of Mcl-1 efficiently protects melanoma cells from apoptosis induced by tunicamycin or thapsigargin, even when Bcl-2 is inhibited. Therefore, Mcl-1, but not Bcl-2, plays a determining role in survival of melanoma cells under ER stress conditions. Indeed, while the Mcl-1 expression is associated with melanoma progression, the expression of Bcl-2 decreases during progression of melanoma (Zhuang, et al., 2007). Importantly, the levels of Mcl-1 in melanoma cells are correlated with the levels of GRP78, suggesting that the increase in Mcl-1 in melanoma may be a consequence of activation of the UPR and an adaptive mechanism of melanoma cells to ER stress (Zhuang, et al., 2009).

Up-regulation of the Mcl-1 protein in melanoma cells under ER stress is associated with an increase in the Mcl-1 mRNA, which is efficiently inhibited by actinomycin D, a general transcription inhibitor, indicating that a transcriptional increase is involved in ER stress-induced up-regulation of Mcl-1 (Jiang, et al., 2008). Analysis of the Mcl-1 promoter region identifies a binding site for the E26 transformation specific sequence (Ets)-1 that is activated by treatment with tunicamycin or thapsigargin (Dong, et al., 2011). Ets-1 is a member of the Ets family of transcription factors that play roles in many biologic processes such as cell growth and survival (Dittmer, 2003; Hahne, et al., 2008). Indeed, inhibition of Ets-1 by siRNA or mutations in the Ets-1 binding site blocks up-regulation of the Mcl-1 transcript by ER stress, and recapitulates the effect of inhibition of Mcl-1 on sensitization of melanoma cells to ER stress-induced apoptosis (Dong, et al., 2011). Therefore, Ets-1 is responsible for transcriptional up-regulation of Mcl-1 by ER stress in melanoma cells.

Ets-1 is expressed at high levels in many types of cancers and is involved in many biological processes in cancer cells such as cell growth and survival (Davidson, et al., 2001; Span, et al., 2002). In melanoma, the levels Ets-1 were similarly found to be higher than those in benign melanocytic lesions and melanocytes and to increase with progression of the disease (Rothhammer, et al., 2004; Torlakovic, et al., 2004). Although the role of Ets-1 in regulation of apoptosis may vary between different cell types, transcriptional up-regulation of Mcl-1 by Ets-1 in melanoma cells subjected to ER stress indicates that it is critical in protection of melanoma cells against ER stress-induced apoptosis (Dong, et al., 2011).

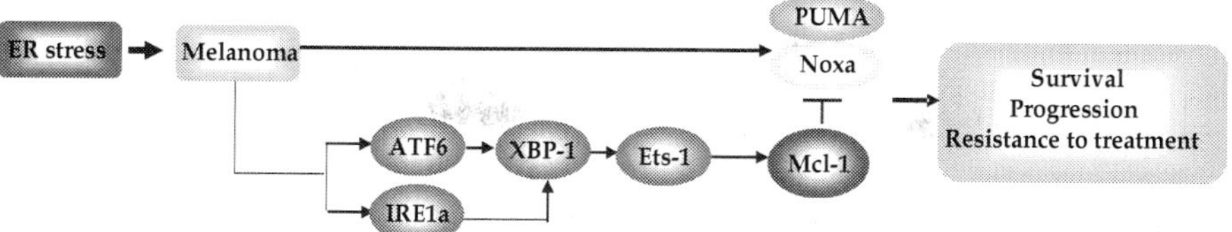

Fig. 2. A schematic illustration of Ets-1-mediated up-regulation of Mcl-1 downstream of XBP-1 in melanoma cells under ER stress

Importantly, Ets-1 is also transcriptionally up-regulated in melanoma cells upon induction of ER stress, which is partially inhibited in melanoma cells deficient in IRE1α or ATF6, indicating that these branches of the UPR are involved in the ER stress-triggered increase in Ets-1 in melanoma cells (Dong, et al., 2011). The convergence of the IRE1α and ATF6 pathways on XBP-1 suggest that XBP-1 may be involved in up-regulation of Ets-1 by the UPR. Indeed, inhibition of XBP-1 blocks ER stress-induced up-regulation of Ets-1 (Dong, et al., 2011). Thus, XBP-1 plays an important role in up-regulation of Ets-1, and subsequent up-regulation of Mcl-1 in melanoma cells subjected to ER stress.

Taken together, it appears that a signalling nodule of XBP1-Ets-1-Mcl-1 leading to transcriptional up-regulation of Mcl-1 is activated in melanoma cells upon activation of the UPR, which is important for protection of melanoma cells against ER stress-induced apoptosis by antagonizing pro-apoptotic Bcl-2 family proteins, such as PUMA and Noxa that are also increased by ER stress in melanoma cells (Fig. 2) (Jiang, et al., 2008).

5.2 Induction of GRP78 in adaptation of melanoma cells to ER stress

As the "master regulator" of the response of cells to ER stress, GRP78 plays an important role in survival of cells under ER stress (Lee, 2005, 2007). Multiple mechanisms have been reported to contribute to GRP78-mediated inhibition of apoptosis in cell under ER stress. These include its binding to unfolded/misfolded proteins to limit their aggregation, binding to calcium to maintain calcium homeostasis, and binding to caspase-12 and caspase-7 to inhibit their activity (Lee, 2005, 2007). In addition, GRP78 has been shown to promote cell proliferation and to be necessary for ER stress-induced autohpagy (Li, et al., 2008). Although the three branches of the UPR can all contribute to induction of GRP78, the ATF6 pathway plays a dominant role in regulation of GRP78 expression (Harding, et al., 2002; Zhang & Kaufman, 2004).

As a typical ER lumenal chaperone, GRP78 can also be expressed on the surface of various types of cancer cells including melanoma cells, in particular, when cells are under ER stress (Gonzalez-Gronow, et al., 2009; Lee, 2007). Relocation of GRP78 to the cell surface appears to be mediated its C-terminal ER retention motif, as deletion of the motif alters its cell surface presentation (Gonzalez-Gronow, et al., 2009). Cell surface GRP78 interacts with a number of cell surface proteins and soluble ligands such as activated α(2)-macroglobulin and acts as an initiator of intracellular signalling pathways, thus promoting cell survival and proliferation (Gonzalez-Gronow, et al., 2009; Zhang, et al., 2010).

Autoantibodies that react with GRP78 expressed on the cell surface can be detected in the sera of patients with prostate cancer, ovarian cancer and melanoma (Gonzalez-Gronow, et al., 2009). These autoantibodies are a negative prognostic factor in prostate cancer (Gonzalez-Gronow, et al., 2009). However, if they are of prognostic value in melanoma patients has not been established. Nevertheless, binding of autoantibodies to the cell surface GRP78 has been reported to promote tumour growth of a murine melanoma model (de Ridder, et al., 2010). Because its preferential expression on the cell surface of cancer cells, GRP78 has been suggested to be a tumour-associated antigen (Misra, et al., 2011).

5.3 Sustained IRE1α signalling may be essential for adaptation of melanoma cells to ER stress

No trigger for ER stress has been identified that selectively elicits only protective responses or apoptosis. However, the duration of activation of individual arms of the UPR plays an important role in determining cell fate in response to ER stress. The IRE1 pathway is rapidly attenuated after induction of ER stress even in the presence of ER stress inducers, whereas the ATF6 branch is also attenuated, albeit with slow kinetics. In contrast, the PERK pathway of the UPR persists for considerably longer periods, and is presumably responsible for induction of apoptosis in the absence of activation of IRE1 and ATF6 (Lin, et al., 2007; Rubio, et al., 2011). It appears that cyto-protective outputs of the initial combined activation of three arms of the UPR outweigh pro-apoptotic outputs. However, attenuation of IRE1 and ATF6 signalling create an imbalance that leads to apoptosis. Consistent with this, IRE1α - or ATF6-deficient cells demonstrate reduced survival rate in cells treated with ER stress inducers.

In agreement with this model, deficiency in IRE1α- or ATF6- renders melanoma cells sensitivity to apoptosis induced by ER stress. In contrast, melanoma cells deficient in PERK remain relatively resistant to ER stress-induced apoptosis (Hersey & Zhang, 2008). It has been found that elevated levels of GRP78 along with phosphorylated PERK and eIF2a, persisted for at least 36 hours in the presence tunicamycin and thapsigargin (Hersey & Zhang, 2008). This suggests that, in contrast to observations made in other cell types, IRE1 and ATF6 signalling in melanoma cells was not rapidly attenuated under prolonged ER stress. Therefore, a testable hypothesis is that perpetuation of IRE1 and/or ATF6 signalling with or without attenuation of the PERK pathway is an essential mechanism of adaptation of melanoma cells to ER stress.

How the duration of activation of the UPR pathways is regulated is not entirely clear; although it is known that negative feed-back mechanism exists to switch off UPR signalling once stress imposed on the ER is resolved (Zhang & Kaufman, 2004). Recently, it was found that rapid attenuation of the IRE1/XBP1 pathway is associated with binding of IRE1α with Bax inhibitor-1 (BI-1), an evolutionarily conserved ER-resident protein (Bailly-Maitre, et al., 2010; Lisbona, et al., 2009).

BI-1 was initially identified as an inhibitor of Bax-induced apoptosis that is a transmembrane protein functionally related to the BCL-2 family of proteins and is primarily located to the ER membrane (Xu & Reed, 1998). Although BI-1 has no obvious homology with Bcl-2-related proteins, it physically interacts with different members of this family such as BCL-2 and Bcl-X$_L$ (Xu & Reed, 1998). BI-1 has been known to protect cells from apoptosis induced by various stimuli, including ER stress (Robinson, et al., 2011). However, BI-1 deficient cells displays hyperactivation of IRE1α, leading to increased levels of activation of XBP-1 and upregulation of UPR target genes (Lisbona, et al., 2009). This is associated with the formation of a stable protein complex between BI-1 and IRE1α, decreasing its ribonuclease activity. If regulation of IRE1α by BI-1 is related to BAX and Bak that can also bind to IRE1α on the ER membrane is currently unclear, it is known however that the ER-associated RING-type E3 ligase bifunctional apoptosis regulator (BAR) interacts with BI-1 and promotes its proteasomal degradation (Rong, et al., 2011).

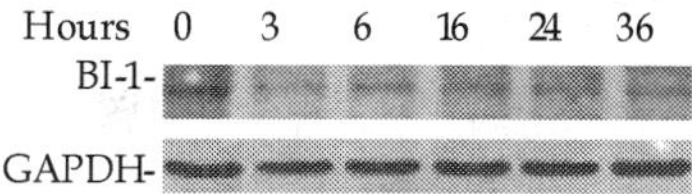

Fig. 3. ER stress down-regulates BI-1 in melanoma cells. Whole cell lysates from a melanoma cell line treated with TM (3µM) for indicated periods were subjected to Western blot analysis of BI-1 and GAPDH (as a loading control)

Interestingly, sustained activation of the IRE1/XBP1 pathway in melanoma cells upon induction of ER stress is associated with a decrease in the expression of BI-1 (Fig. 3), but whether there is a cause and effect relationship between two events remains to be studied. In addition, if down-regulation of BI-1 by ER stress is due to by enhancement in BAR-mediated proteasomal degradation is currently unknown.

5.4 Dysregulation of the CHOP/Bim axis in adaptation of melanoma cells to ER stress

CCAAT/enhancer binding protein homologous protein (CHOP), also known as growth arrest- and DNA damage-inducible gene 153 (GADD153) was first identified as a DNA-damage-inducible gene of the C/EBP family of transcription factors (Ron & Habener, 1992). CHOP is ubiquitously expressed at low levels, but its expression can be induced by various cellular stress conditions, such as DNA damage and nutrient depletion (Ron & Habener, 1992). Induction of CHOP has been shown to be essential for ER stress-induced apoptosis, in that CHOP-/- mice exhibit reduced apoptosis in response to ER stress (Oyadomari, et al., 2002; Oyadomari & Mori, 2004). Although the three pathways of the UPR can all mediate transcriptional up-regulation of CHOP, the PERK branch appears to play a dominant role in induction of CHOP in cells under ER stress (Oyadomari & Mori, 2004).

CHOP-induced apoptosis was initially shown to be associated with transcriptional repression of Bcl-2 expression (McCullough, et al., 2001). Up-regulation of the BH3-only proteins PUMA and Noxa in cells under ER stress has also been reported to be associated with CHOP (Li, et al., 2006). More recently, it was demonstrated that CHOP can transcriptionally up-regulate another BH3-only protein Bim in diverse types of cells (Puthalakath, et al., 2007). This requires formation of CHOP-C/EBPα heterodimers, which then bind to a non-conventional promoter within the first intron of the *Bim* gene. Inhibition of phosphorylation of Bim by protein phosphatase 2A (PP2A) also contributes the increased Bim expression in cells subjected to ER stress. Dephosphorylation of Bim by PP2A enhances the stability of the Bim protein. In addition, CHOP can up-regulate the death receptor, TNF-related apoptosis-inducing ligand (TRAIL) receptor 2 (TRAIL-R2), thus activating the death receptor pathway enhancing TRAIL-induced apoptosis in many cell types (Lin, et al., 2008; Yamaguchi & Wang, 2004).

Nevertheless, the CHOP/Bim axis-mediated apoptosis signalling does not appear to function effectively in melanoma cells, even though CHOP is strongly induced by ER stress along with activation of PERK and phosphorylation of eIF2α in the cells under ER stress (Fig. 4). Strikingly, while over-expression of CHOP does not confer sensitivity of melanoma cells to ER stress-induced apoptosis, inhibition of CHOP by siRNA resulted in low levels of apoptosis in the cells (Zhang, et al. unpublished data). These results suggest that, instead inducing apoptosis, CHOP may have a pro-survival role in melanoma cells, as it does in neurons (Halterman, et al., 2010). How the biological function of CHOP is switched from pro-apoptotic to pro-survival in melanoma cells remains, however, to be elucidated.

Induction of ER stress causes up-regulation of Bim mRNA in melanoma cells. However, the increase in Bim expression at the protein level appears to be transient, which is associated with an increase in phosphorylation of the protein (Fig. 4), in contrast to its dephosphorylation by ER stress in many other cell types. Increased phosphorylation of Bim is, at least in part, due to activation of the MEK/ERK pathway, in that inhibition of MEK by the small molecule inhibitor U0126 blocked Bim phosphorylation and increased the Bim expression at the protein level in melanoma cells subjected to tunicamycin (Zhang et al. unpublished data). The MEK/ERK pathway is known to be constitutively activated in melanoma cells (Jiang, et al., 2007). It is therefore conceivable that phosphorylation of Bim by ERK is dominant over its dephosphorylation by PP2A in melanoma cells when subjected to ER stress, thus leading to its rapid degradation by the proteasome system. Although the exact mechanism needs to be further clarified, dysregulation of the CHOP/Bim axis appears to play an important role in survival of melanoma cells under ER stress.

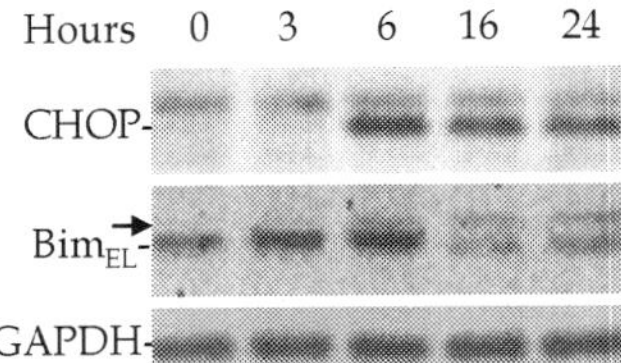

Fig. 4. ER stress induces changes in the expression CHOP and Bim in melanoma cells. Whole cell lysates from a melanoma cell line treated with TM (3μM) for indicated periods were subjected to Western blot analysis. The arrow heads points to bands of phosphorylated Bim_{EL}

Some other mechanisms that are involved in protection of melanoma cells from ER stress-induced apoptosis include activation of the PI3K/Akt signalling pathway and induction of the apoptosis repressor with caspase recruitment domain (ARC) protein (Chen, et al., 2008; Jiang, et al., 2009c). The list is expected to increase with better understanding of the mechanisms of induction of apoptosis by ER stress. Therefore, targeting multiple adaptive mechanisms may be needed to overcome resistance of melanoma cells to ER stress-induced apoptosis.

6. Adaptation to ER stress as a resistance mechanism of melanoma cells chemotherapeutic drugs

A growing body of evidence shows that induction of ER stress and subsequent activation of the UPR can alter chemosensitivity of cancer cells (Hersey & Zhang, 2008; Lee, 2007; Ma & Hendershot, 2004). On the other hand, induction of apoptosis is associated with induction of ER stress in many types of cancer cells by a number of different classes of chemotherapeutic drugs, such as the DNA-damaging agent cisplatin, the non-steroidal anti-inflammatory drug celecoxib, the proteasomal inhibitor bortezomib, and the general kinase inhibitor sorafenib, suggesting that induction of ER stress may be an important mechanism in killing of cancer cells by chemotherapeutic drugs (Hersey & Zhang, 2008; Hill, et al., 2009; Jiang, et al., 2009c; Lee, 2007; Ma & Hendershot, 2004; Martin, et al., 2010). On the other hand, melanoma cells have developed multiple adaptive mechanisms that render the cells largely resistant to ER stress-induced apoptosis, suggesting that adaptation to ER stress may contribute to resistance of melanoma cells to induction of apoptosis (Hersey & Zhang, 2008). Some adaptive mechanisms to ER stress, such as induction of GRP78 and Mcl-1, have been shown to play important roles in resistance of melanoma cells to various chemotherapeutic drugs (Hersey & Zhang, 2008; Jiang, et al., 2009a; Jiang, et al., 2009c).

6.1 GRP78 contributes to resistance of melanoma cells to cisplatin and adriamycin

Although cisplatin and adriamycin are conventionally regarded as DNA-damaging agents, they can induce ER stress in melanoma cells as shown by increased expression of GRP78 and activation of XBP-1 (Jiang, et al., 2009c). Whether induction of ER stress plays a part in induction of apoptosis by the drugs remains to be clarified, but GRP78 protects melanoma cells against cytotoxic effects of the drugs (Jiang, et al., 2009a). This is mediated, at least in part, by the inhibitory effect of GRP78 on activation of caspase-4. The latter is bound to and kept inactive by GRP78 in melanoma cells (Jiang, et al., 2007; Jiang, et al., 2009a). Inhibition of GRP78 by siRNA in melanoma cells subjected to ER stress frees caspase-4 and leads to its activation (Jiang, et al., 2007).

There was no correlation between the GRP78 expression levels and sensitivities of melanoma cell lines to cisplatin or adriamycin, suggesting that, besides GRP78, other mechanisms may also contribute to regulation of responses of melanoma cells to the drugs (Jiang, et al., 2009a). For example, expression of ATP-binding cassette (ABC) transporters and increased DNA repair are known to contribute to resistance of cancer cells against cisplatin and adriamycin (Frank, et al., 2005; Hall, et al., 2008). In addition, activation survival signalling pathways such as the PI3K/Akt and MEK/ERK pathways is a common cause for resistance of melanoma to apoptosis (Hersey, et al., 2006; Soengas & Lowe, 2003). Regardless, targeting GRP78 may be a useful strategy in sensitizing melanoma cells to these chemotherapeutic drugs.

6.2 Melanoma cells under ER stress are more resistance to microtubule-targeting durgs

Unlike cisplatin and adriamycin, the microtubule-targeting drugs docetaxel and vincristine do not trigger ER stress in melanoma cells as shown by their inability to induce GRP78 and the spliced XBP-1 mRNA. However, their cytotoxicity is attenuated in melanoma cells subjected to ER stress (Jiang, et al., 2009c). This was demonstrated by the observation that treatment with the ER stress inducer tunicamycin or thapsigargin before the addition of docetaxel or vincristine reduced the levels of apoptosis induced by the drugs. GRP78 does not appear to be involved in that sensitivity of melanoma cells to docetaxel- and vincristine-induced apoptosis cannot be enhanced by inhibition of GRP78. In contrast, activation of the PI3k/Akt pathway downstream of XBP-1-mediated signalling is critical in protection of melanoma cells against the drugs by preloaded ER stress (Jiang, et al., 2009c).

How Akt is activated by XBP-1 signalling in melanoma cells remains to be further studied, but it was recently shown that ER stress activated Akt in a zebrafish embryonic cell line through XBP-1-mediated up-regulation of insulin growth factor-1 (IGF-1) (Hu, et al., 2007). However, IGF-1/IGF-1 receptor signalling in melanoma cells originates mainly from exogenous IGF-1 because melanoma cells express no, or minimal, IGF-1 (Lee, et al., 2008; Rodeck, et al., 1991). Nevertheless, it is possible that XBP-1 may activate a factor or factors similar to IGF-1 that in turn causes activation of the PI3K/Akt pathway in melanoma cells under ER stress. In any case, it appears that activation of XBP-1 signalling as a consequence of adaptation to ER stress is an important resistance mechanism of melanoma cells to the microtubule-targeting drugs docetaxel and vincristine.

6.3 Melanoma cells under ER stress are more susceptible to apoptosis induced by the BH3 mimetic obatoclax

Small molecule mimics of BH3-only proteins are emerging as promising anti-cancer agents by inhibiting anti-apoptotic Bcl-2 family proteins. Obatoclax, also known as GX015-070, was identified by chemical library screening to bind the hydrophobic groove of anti-apoptotic Bcl-2 family proteins and antagonize their function (Nguyen, et al., 2007). Obatoclax can efficiently neutralize all anti-apoptotic Bcl-2 family proteins including Mcl-1, and has been reported to potently kill some types of cancer cells, such as myeloma cells, as a single agent, and to enhance apoptosis induced by various apoptotic stimuli such as TNF-related apoptosis inducing ligand (TRAIL) and the proteasome inhibitor bortezomib (Huang, et al., 2009; Konopleva, et al., 2008).

Because up-regulation of Mcl-1 is an important adaptive mechanism of melanoma cells to ER stress, it is conceivable that obatoclax may interrupt the adaptation by antagonizing Mcl-1. Indeed, obatoclax has been shown to potently overcome resistance of melanoma cells to apoptosis induced by the ER stress inducers tunicamycin and thapsigargin (Jiang, et al., 2009b). Besides its inhibitory effect on Mcl-1, obatoclax triggers further increases in the levels of the BH3-only protein Noxa in melanoma cells undergoing ER stress, which in turn cooperates with obatoclax in activating the mitochondrial apoptotic pathway (Jiang, et al., 2009b). Therefore, obatoclax is a potent agent that targets a major adaptive mechanism to ER stress in melanoma. Therefore, combinations of obatoclax and agents that induce ER stress may be a useful strategy in the treatment of melanoma.

6.4 Targeting GRP78 to sensitize melanoma cells to apoptosis induced by Fenretinide and Bortezomib

Fenretinide is a synthetic retinoid deriverative that has been shown to induce ER stress and apoptosis in melanoma cells (Hill, et al., 2009; Lovat, et al., 2008). Bortezomib is a peptide boronate inhibitor of the proteasome that is similarly known to induce apoptosis in melanoma cells that is associated with induction of ER stress (Hill, et al., 2009; Qin, et al., 2005). Activation of the UPR appears to protect melanoma cells from apoptosis induced by the drugs as inhibition of GRP78 by either siRNA knockdown or a GRP78-specific subtilise toxin produces synergistic induction of apoptosis (Martin, et al., 2010). In addition, inhibition of protein disulfide isomerase (PDI), an ER enzyme that catalyzes the formation and breakage of disulfide bonds within proteins as they fold and plays a role in protecting cells from ER stress, similarly enhanced induction of apoptosis in melanoma cells by fenretinide and bortezomib (Lovat, et al., 2008). It is conceivable that inhibition of other adaptive mechanisms such as up-regulation of Mcl-1 may also sensitize melanoma cells to apoptosis induced by the drugs.

7. Conclusion

Primary events in the development of melanoma are gradually being pieced together (Bennett, 2008; Hersey, et al., 2011), but a more complete picture of evolution of the disease and resistance of metastatic melanoma to treatment requires additional understanding of secondary events consequent on initiation of the malignancy. In this chapter, we have provided evidence showing that an important driver of secondary events is signals resulting from adaptation of melanoma cells to ER stress, which are not only important for resistance of melanoma cells to ER stress-induced apoptosis, but also render melanoma cells resistant to various chemotherapeutic drugs.

Although targeting adaptive mechanisms such as GRP78 and Mcl-1 have been shown to sensitize melanoma cells to apoptosis induced by a number of chemotherapeutic drugs, its effects on efficacy of other promising therapeutic agents such as inhibitors against the RAF/MEK/ERK and PI3K pathways need to be evaluated (Hersey, et al., 2011). Cross-talks between the UPR and the pathways are conceivable to play a role in regulation of sensitivity of melanoma cells to the inhibitors.

8. References

Armstrong, J.L., Veal, G.J., Redfern, C.P. & Lovat, P.E. (2007). Role of Noxa in p53-independent fenretinide-induced apoptosis of neuroectodermal tumours, *Apoptosis*, Vol. 12, No. 3, (Mar), pp. 613-622, ISSN 1360-8185

Bailly-Maitre, B., Belgardt, B.F., Jordan, S.D., Coornaert, B., von Freyend, M.J., Kleinridders, A., Mauer, J., Cuddy, M., Kress, C.L., Willmes, D., Essig, M., Hampel, B., Protzer, U., Reed, J.C. & Bruning, J.C. (2010). Hepatic Bax inhibitor-1 inhibits IRE1alpha and protects from obesity-associated insulin resistance and glucose intolerance, *J Biol Chem*, Vol. 285, No. 9, (Feb 26), pp. 6198-6207, ISSN 1083-351X

Balch, C.M., Gershenwald, J.E., Soong, S.J., Thompson, J.F., Atkins, M.B., Byrd, D.R., Buzaid, A.C., Cochran, A.J., Coit, D.G., Ding, S., Eggermont, A.M., Flaherty, K.T., Gimotty, P.A., Kirkwood, J.M., McMasters, K.M., Mihm, M.C., Jr., Morton, D.L., Ross, M.I., Sober, A.J. & Sondak, V.K. (2009). Final version of 2009 AJCC melanoma staging and classification, *J Clin Oncol*, Vol. 27, No. 36, (Dec 20), pp. 6199-6206, ISSN 1527-7755

Bennett, D.C. (2008). How to make a melanoma: what do we know of the primary clonal events?, *Pigment Cell Melanoma Res*, Vol. 21, No. 1, (Feb), pp. 27-38, ISSN 1755-1471

Boyce, M. & Yuan, J. (2006). Cellular response to endoplasmic reticulum stress: a matter of life or death, *Cell Death Differ*, Vol. 13, No. 3, (Mar), pp. 363-373, ISSN 1350-9047

Chen, L., Willis, S.N., Wei, A., Smith, B.J., Fletcher, J.I., Hinds, M.G., Colman, P.M., Day, C.L., Adams, J.M. & Huang, D.C. (2005). Differential targeting of prosurvival Bcl-2 proteins by their BH3-only ligands allows complementary apoptotic function, *Mol Cell*, Vol. 17, No. 3, (Feb 4), pp. 393-403, ISSN 1097-2765

Chen, L.H., Jiang, C.C., Watts, R., Thorne, R.F., Kiejda, K.A., Zhang, X.D. & Hersey, P. (2008). Inhibition of endoplasmic reticulum stress-induced apoptosis of melanoma cells by the ARC protein, *Cancer Res*, Vol. 68, No. 3, (Feb 1), pp. 834-842, ISSN 1538-7445

Codogno, P. & Meijer, A.J. (2005). Autophagy and signaling: their role in cell survival and cell death, *Cell Death Differ*, Vol. 12 Suppl 2, (Nov), pp. 1509-1518, ISSN 1350-9047

Cory, S. & Adams, J.M. (2002). The Bcl2 family: regulators of the cellular life-or-death switch, *Nat Rev Cancer*, Vol. 2, No. 9, (Sep), pp. 647-656, ISSN 1474-175X

Davidson, B., Risberg, B., Goldberg, I., Nesland, J.M., Berner, A., Trope, C.G., Kristensen, G.B., Bryne, M. & Reich, R. (2001). Ets-1 mRNA expression in effusions of serous ovarian carcinoma patients is a marker of poor outcome, *Am J Surg Pathol*, Vol. 25, No. 12, (Dec), pp. 1493-1500, ISSN 0147-5185

de Ridder, G.G., Gonzalez-Gronow, M., Ray, R. & Pizzo, S.V. (2010). Autoantibodies against cell surface GRP78 promote tumor growth in a murine model of melanoma, *Melanoma Res*, (Dec 15), ISSN 1473-5636

Denoyelle, C., Abou-Rjaily, G., Bezrookove, V., Verhaegen, M., Johnson, T.M., Fullen, D.R., Pointer, J.N., Gruber, S.B., Su, L.D., Nikiforov, M.A., Kaufman, R.J., Bastian, B.C. & Soengas, M.S. (2006). Anti-oncogenic role of the endoplasmic reticulum differentially activated by mutations in the MAPK pathway, *Nat Cell Biol*, Vol. 8, No. 10, (Oct), pp. 1053-1063, ISSN 1465-7392

Dittmer, J. (2003). The biology of the Ets1 proto-oncogene, *Mol Cancer*, Vol. 2, (Aug 20), p. 29, ISSN 1476-4598

Dong, L., Jiang, C.C., Thorne, R.F., Croft, A., Yang, F., Liu, H., de Bock, C.E., Hersey, P. & Zhang, X.D. (2011). Ets-1 mediates upregulation of Mcl-1 downstream of XBP-1 in human melanoma cells upon ER stress, *Oncogene*, (Mar 21), ISSN 1476-5594

Du, C., Fang, M., Li, Y., Li, L. & Wang, X. (2000). Smac, a mitochondrial protein that promotes cytochrome c-dependent caspase activation by eliminating IAP inhibition, *Cell*, Vol. 102, No. 1, (Jul 7), pp. 33-42, ISSN 0092-8674

Elyaman, W., Terro, F., Suen, K.C., Yardin, C., Chang, R.C. & Hugon, J. (2002). BAD and Bcl-2 regulation are early events linking neuronal endoplasmic reticulum stress to mitochondria-mediated apoptosis, *Brain Res Mol Brain Res*, Vol. 109, No. 1-2, (Dec 30), pp. 233-238, ISSN 0169-328X

Eton, O., Legha, S.S., Moon, T.E., Buzaid, A.C., Papadopoulos, N.E., Plager, C., Burgess, A.M., Bedikian, A.Y., Ring, S., Dong, Q., Glassman, A.B., Balch, C.M. & Benjamin, R.S. (1998). Prognostic factors for survival of patients treated systemically for disseminated melanoma, *J Clin Oncol*, Vol. 16, No. 3, (Mar), pp. 1103-1111, ISSN 0732-183X

Ferri, K.F. & Kroemer, G. (2001). Organelle-specific initiation of cell death pathways, *Nat Cell Biol*, Vol. 3, No. 11, (Nov), pp. E255-263, ISSN 1465-7392

Fischer, H., Koenig, U., Eckhart, L. & Tschachler, E. (2002). Human caspase 12 has acquired deleterious mutations, *Biochem Biophys Res Commun*, Vol. 293, No. 2, (May 3), pp. 722-726, ISSN 0006-291X

Frank, N.Y., Margaryan, A., Huang, Y., Schatton, T., Waaga-Gasser, A.M., Gasser, M., Sayegh, M.H., Sadee, W. & Frank, M.H. (2005). ABCB5-mediated doxorubicin transport and chemoresistance in human malignant melanoma, *Cancer Res*, Vol. 65, No. 10, (May 15), pp. 4320-4333, ISSN 0008-5472

Fritsch, R.M., Schneider, G., Saur, D., Scheibel, M. & Schmid, R.M. (2007). Translational repression of MCL-1 couples stress-induced eIF2 alpha phosphorylation to mitochondrial apoptosis initiation, *J Biol Chem*, Vol. 282, No. 31, (Aug 3), pp. 22551-22562, ISSN 0021-9258

Fu, Y., Li, J. & Lee, A.S. (2007). GRP78/BiP inhibits endoplasmic reticulum BIK and protects human breast cancer cells against estrogen starvation-induced apoptosis, *Cancer Res*, Vol. 67, No. 8, (Apr 15), pp. 3734-3740, ISSN 0008-5472

Gaut, J.R. & Hendershot, L.M. (1993). The modification and assembly of proteins in the endoplasmic reticulum, *Curr Opin Cell Biol*, Vol. 5, No. 4, (Aug), pp. 589-595, ISSN 0955-0674

Gonzalez-Gronow, M., Selim, M.A., Papalas, J. & Pizzo, S.V. (2009). GRP78: a multifunctional receptor on the cell surface, *Antioxid Redox Signal*, Vol. 11, No. 9, (Sep), pp. 2299-2306, ISSN 1557-7716

Hahne, J.C., Okuducu, A.F., Sahin, A., Fafeur, V., Kiriakidis, S. & Wernert, N. (2008). The transcription factor ETS-1: its role in tumour development and strategies for its inhibition, *Mini Rev Med Chem*, Vol. 8, No. 11, (Oct), pp. 1095-1105, ISSN 1389-5575

Hall, M.D., Okabe, M., Shen, D.W., Liang, X.J. & Gottesman, M.M. (2008). The role of cellular accumulation in determining sensitivity to platinum-based chemotherapy, *Annu Rev Pharmacol Toxicol*, Vol. 48, pp. 495-535, ISSN 0362-1642

Halterman, M.W., Gill, M., DeJesus, C., Ogihara, M., Schor, N.F. & Federoff, H.J. (2010). The endoplasmic reticulum stress response factor CHOP-10 protects against hypoxia-induced neuronal death, *J Biol Chem*, Vol. 285, No. 28, (Jul 9), pp. 21329-21340, ISSN 1083-351X

Harding, H.P., Calfon, M., Urano, F., Novoa, I. & Ron, D. (2002). Transcriptional and translational control in the Mammalian unfolded protein response, *Annu Rev Cell Dev Biol*, Vol. 18, pp. 575-599, ISSN 1081-0706

Harding, H.P., Zhang, Y., Bertolotti, A., Zeng, H. & Ron, D. (2000). Perk is essential for translational regulation and cell survival during the unfolded protein response, *Mol Cell*, Vol. 5, No. 5, (May), pp. 897-904, ISSN 1097-2765

Heath-Engel, H.M., Chang, N.C. & Shore, G.C. (2008). The endoplasmic reticulum in apoptosis and autophagy: role of the BCL-2 protein family, *Oncogene*, Vol. 27, No. 50, (Oct 27), pp. 6419-6433, ISSN 1476-5594

Hendershot, L.M. (2004). The ER function BiP is a master regulator of ER function, *Mt Sinai J Med*, Vol. 71, No. 5, (Oct), pp. 289-297, ISSN 0027-2507

Hersey, P., Smalley, K.S., Weeraratna, A., Bosenberg, M., Zhang, X.D., Haass, N.K., Paton, E., Mann, G. & Scolyer, R.A. (2011). Meeting report from the 7th International Melanoma Congress, Sydney, November, 2010, *Pigment Cell Melanoma Res*, Vol. 24, No. 1, (Feb), pp. e1-15, ISSN 1755-148X

Hersey, P. & Zhang, X.D. (2008). Adaptation to ER stress as a driver of malignancy and resistance to therapy in human melanoma, *Pigment Cell Melanoma Res*, Vol. 21, No. 3, (Jun), pp. 358-367, ISSN 1755-1471

Hersey, P., Zhuang, L. & Zhang, X.D. (2006). Current strategies in overcoming resistance of cancer cells to apoptosis melanoma as a model, *Int Rev Cytol*, Vol. 251, pp. 131-158, ISSN 0074-7696

Hetz, C., Bernasconi, P., Fisher, J., Lee, A.H., Bassik, M.C., Antonsson, B., Brandt, G.S., Iwakoshi, N.N., Schinzel, A., Glimcher, L.H. & Korsmeyer, S.J. (2006). Proapoptotic BAX and BAK modulate the unfolded protein response by a direct interaction with IRE1alpha, *Science*, Vol. 312, No. 5773,(Apr 28), pp. 572-576, ISSN 1095-9203

Hetz, C. & Glimcher, L. (2008). The daily job of night killers: alternative roles of the BCL-2 family in organelle physiology, *Trends Cell Biol*, Vol. 18, No. 1, (Jan), pp. 38-44, ISSN 1879-3088

Hill, D.S., Martin, S., Armstrong, J.L., Flockhart, R., Tonison, J.J., Simpson, D.G., Birch-Machin, M.A., Redfern, C.P. & Lovat, P.E. (2009). Combining the endoplasmic reticulum stress-inducing agents bortezomib and fenretinide as a novel therapeutic strategy for metastatic melanoma, *Clin Cancer Res*, Vol. 15, No. 4, (Feb 15), pp. 1192-1198, ISSN 1078-0432

Hitomi, J., Katayama, T., Eguchi, Y., Kudo, T., Taniguchi, M., Koyama, Y., Manabe, T., Yamagishi, S., Bando, Y., Imaizumi, K., Tsujimoto, Y. & Tohyama, M. (2004). Involvement of caspase-4 in endoplasmic reticulum stress-induced apoptosis and Abeta-induced cell death, *J Cell Biol*, Vol. 165, No. 3, (May 10), pp. 347-356, ISSN 0021-9525

Hollien, J. & Weissman, J.S. (2006). Decay of endoplasmic reticulum-localized mRNAs during the unfolded protein response, *Science*, Vol. 313, No. 5783, (Jul 7), pp. 104-107, ISSN 1095-9203

Høyer-Hansen, M. & Jäättelä, M. (2007). Connecting endoplasmic reticulum stress to autophagy by unfolded protein response and calcium, *Cell Death Differ*, Vol. 14, No. 9, (Sep), pp. 1576-1582, ISSN 1350-9047

Hu, M.C., Gong, H.Y., Lin, G.H., Hu, S.Y., Chen, M.H., Huang, S.J., Liao, C.F. & Wu, J.L. (2007). XBP-1, a key regulator of unfolded protein response, activates transcription of IGF1 and Akt phosphorylation in zebrafish embryonic cell line, *Biochem Biophys Res Commun*, Vol. 359, No. 3, (Aug 3), pp. 778-783, ISSN 0006-291X

Huang, S., Okumura, K. & Sinicrope, F.A. (2009). BH3 mimetic obatoclax enhances TRAIL-mediated apoptosis in human pancreatic cancer cells, *Clin Cancer Res*, Vol. 15, No. 1, (Jan 1), pp. 150-159, ISSN 1078-0432

Iglesias-Serret, D., Pique, M., Gil, J., Pons, G. & Lopez, J.M. (2003). Transcriptional and translational control of Mcl-1 during apoptosis, *Arch Biochem Biophys*, Vol. 417, No. 2, (Sep 15), pp. 141-152, ISSN 0003-9861

Jiang, C.C., Chen, L.H., Gillespie, S., Wang, Y.F., Kiejda, K.A., Zhang, X.D. & Hersey, P. (2007). Inhibition of MEK sensitizes human melanoma cells to endoplasmic reticulum stress-induced apoptosis, *Cancer Res*, Vol. 67, No. 20, (Oct 15), pp. 9750-9761, ISSN 0008-5472

Jiang, C.C., Lucas, K., Avery-Kiejda, K.A., Wade, M., deBock, C.E., Thorne, R.F., Allen, J., Hersey, P. & Zhang, X.D. (2008). Up-regulation of Mcl-1 is critical for survival of human melanoma cells upon endoplasmic reticulum stress, *Cancer Res*, Vol. 68, No. 16, (Aug 15), pp. 6708-6717, ISSN 1538-7445

Jiang, C.C., Mao, Z.G., Avery-Kiejda, K.A., Wade, M., Hersey, P. & Zhang, X.D. (2009a). Glucose-regulated protein 78 antagonizes cisplatin and adriamycin in human melanoma cells, *Carcinogenesis*, Vol. 30, No. 2, (Feb), pp. 197-204, ISSN 1460-2180

Jiang, C.C., Wroblewski, D., Yang, F., Hersey, P. & Zhang, X.D. (2009b). Human melanoma cells under endoplasmic reticulum stress are more susceptible to apoptosis induced by the BH3 mimetic obatoclax, *Neoplasia*, Vol. 11, No. 9, (Sep), pp. 945-955, ISSN 1476-5586

Jiang, C.C., Yang, F., Thorne, R.F., Zhu, B.K., Hersey, P. & Zhang, X.D. (2009c). Human melanoma cells under endoplasmic reticulum stress acquire resistance to microtubule-targeting drugs through XBP-1-mediated activation of Akt, *Neoplasia*, Vol. 11, No. 5, (May), pp. 436-447, ISSN 1476-5586

Konopleva, M., Watt, J., Contractor, R., Tsao, T., Harris, D., Estrov, Z., Bornmann, W., Kantarjian, H., Viallet, J., Samudio, I. & Andreeff, M. (2008). Mechanisms of antileukemic activity of the novel Bcl-2 homology domain-3 mimetic GX15-070 (obatoclax), *Cancer Res*, Vol. 68, No. 9, (May 1), pp. 3413-3420, ISSN 1538-7445

Kuwana, T., Bouchier-Hayes, L., Chipuk, J.E., Bonzon, C., Sullivan, B.A., Green, D.R. & Newmeyer, D.D. (2005). BH3 domains of BH3-only proteins differentially regulate Bax-mediated mitochondrial membrane permeabilization both directly and indirectly, *Mol Cell*, Vol. 17, No. 4, (Feb 18), pp. 525-535, ISSN 1097-2765

Lee, A.H., Iwakoshi, N.N. & Glimcher, L.H. (2003). XBP-1 regulates a subset of endoplasmic reticulum resident chaperone genes in the unfolded protein response, *Mol Cell Biol*, Vol. 23, No. 21, (Nov), pp. 7448-7459, ISSN 0270-7306

Lee, A.S. (2005). The ER chaperone and signaling regulator GRP78/BiP as a monitor of endoplasmic reticulum stress, *Methods*, Vol. 35, No. 4, (Apr), pp. 373-381, ISSN 1046-2023

Lee, A.S. (2007). GRP78 induction in cancer: therapeutic and prognostic implications, *Cancer Res*, Vol. 67, No. 8, (Apr 15), pp. 3496-3499, ISSN 0008-5472

Lee, J.T., Brafford, P. & Herlyn, M. (2008). Unraveling the mysteries of IGF-1 signaling in melanoma, *J Invest Dermatol*, Vol. 128, No. 6, (Jun), pp. 1358-1360, ISSN 1523-1747

Li, J., Lee, B. & Lee, A.S. (2006). Endoplasmic reticulum stress-induced apoptosis: multiple pathways and activation of p53-up-regulated modulator of apoptosis (PUMA) and NOXA by p53, *J Biol Chem*, Vol. 281, No. 11, (Mar 17), pp. 7260-7270, ISSN 0021-9258

Li, J., Ni, M., Lee, B., Barron, E., Hinton, D.R. & Lee, A.S. (2008). The unfolded protein response regulator GRP78/BiP is required for endoplasmic reticulum integrity and stress-induced autophagy in mammalian cells, *Cell Death Differ*, Vol. 15, No. 9, (Sep), pp. 1460-1471, ISSN 1350-9047

Li, P., Nijhawan, D., Budihardjo, I., Srinivasula, S.M., Ahmad, M., Alnemri, E.S. & Wang, X. (1997). Cytochrome c and dATP-dependent formation of Apaf-1/caspase-9 complex initiates an apoptotic protease cascade, *Cell*, Vol. 91, No. 4, (Nov 14), pp. 479-489, ISSN 0092-8674

Lin, J.H., Li, H., Yasumura, D., Cohen, H.R., Zhang, C., Panning, B., Shokat, K.M., Lavail, M.M. & Walter, P. (2007). IRE1 signaling affects cell fate during the unfolded protein response, *Science*, Vol. 318, No. 5852, (Nov 9), pp. 944-949, ISSN 1095-9203

Lin, S.S., Bassik, M.C., Suh, H., Nishino, M., Arroyo, J.D., Hahn, W.C., Korsmeyer, S.J. & Roberts, T.M. (2006). PP2A regulates BCL-2 phosphorylation and proteasome-mediated degradation at the endoplasmic reticulum, *J Biol Chem*, Vol. 281, No. 32, (Aug 11), pp. 23003-23012, ISSN 0021-9258

Lin, Y.D., Chen, S., Yue, P., Zou, W., Benbrook, D.M., Liu, S., Le, T.C., Berlin, K.D., Khuri, F.R. & Sun, S.Y. (2008). CAAT/enhancer binding protein homologous protein-dependent death receptor 5 induction is a major component of SHetA2-induced apoptosis in lung cancer cells, *Cancer Res*, Vol. 68, No. 13, (Jul 1), pp. 5335-5344, ISSN 1538-7445

Lisbona, F., Rojas-Rivera, D., Thielen, P., Zamorano, S., Todd, D., Martinon, F., Glavic, A., Kress, C., Lin, J.H., Walter, P., Reed, J.C., Glimcher, L.H. & Hetz, C. (2009). BAX inhibitor-1 is a negative regulator of the ER stress sensor IRE1alpha, *Mol Cell*, Vol. 33, No. 6, (Mar 27), pp. 679-691, ISSN 1097-4164

Lovat, P.E., Corazzari, M., Armstrong, J.L., Martin, S., Pagliarini, V., Hill, D., Brown, A.M., Piacentini, M., Birch-Machin, M.A. & Redfern, C.P. (2008). Increasing melanoma cell death using inhibitors of protein disulfide isomerases to abrogate survival responses to endoplasmic reticulum stress, *Cancer Res*, Vol. 68, No. 13, (Jul 1), pp. 5363-5369, ISSN 1538-7445

Ma, Y. & Hendershot, L.M. (2004). The role of the unfolded protein response in tumour development: friend or foe?, *Nat Rev Cancer*, Vol. 4, No. 12, (Dec), pp. 966-977, ISSN 1474-175X

Martin, S., Hill, D.S., Paton, J.C., Paton, A.W., Birch-Machin, M.A., Lovat, P.E. & Redfern, C.P. (2010). Targeting GRP78 to enhance melanoma cell death, *Pigment Cell Melanoma Res*, Vol. 23, No. 5, (Oct), pp. 675-682, ISSN 1755-148X

Mathai, J.P., Germain, M. & Shore, G.C. (2005). BH3-only BIK regulates BAX,BAK-dependent release of Ca2+ from endoplasmic reticulum stores and mitochondrial apoptosis during stress-induced cell death, *J Biol Chem*, Vol. 280, No. 25, (Jun 24), pp. 23829-23836, ISSN 0021-9258

McCullough, K.D., Martindale, J.L., Klotz, L.O., Aw, T.Y. & Holbrook, N.J. (2001). Gadd153 sensitizes cells to endoplasmic reticulum stress by down-regulating Bcl2 and perturbing the cellular redox state, *Mol Cell Biol*, Vol. 21, No. 4, (Feb), pp. 1249-1259, ISSN 0270-7306

Misra, U.K., Payne, S. & Pizzo, S.V. (2011). Ligation of prostate cancer cell surface GRP78 activates a proproliferative and antiapoptotic feedback loop: a role for secreted prostate-specific antigen, *J Biol Chem*, Vol. 286, No. 2, (Jan 14), pp. 1248-1259, ISSN 1083-351X

Morishima, N., Nakanishi, K., Tsuchiya, K., Shibata, T. & Seiwa, E. (2004). Translocation of Bim to the endoplasmic reticulum (ER) mediates ER stress signaling for activation of caspase-12 during ER stress-induced apoptosis, *J Biol Chem*, Vol. 279, No. 48, (Nov 26), pp. 50375-50381, ISSN 0021-9258

Nakagawa, T., Zhu, H., Morishima, N., Li, E., Xu, J., Yankner, B.A. & Yuan, J. (2000). Caspase-12 mediates endoplasmic-reticulum-specific apoptosis and cytotoxicity by amyloid-beta, *Nature*, Vol. 403, No. 6765, (Jan 6), pp. 98-103, ISSN 0028-0836

Nguyen, M., Marcellus, R.C., Roulston, A., Watson, M., Serfass, L., Murthy Madiraju, S.R., Goulet, D., Viallet, J., Belec, L., Billot, X., Acoca, S., Purisima, E., Wiegmans, A., Cluse, L., Johnstone, R.W., Beauparlant, P. & Shore, G.C. (2007). Small molecule obatoclax (GX15-070) antagonizes MCL-1 and overcomes MCL-1-mediated resistance to apoptosis, *Proc Natl Acad Sci U S A*, Vol. 104, No. 49, (Dec 4), pp. 19512-19517, ISSN 1091-6490

Nijhawan, D., Fang, M., Traer, E., Zhong, Q., Gao, W., Du, F. & Wang, X. (2003). Elimination of Mcl-1 is required for the initiation of apoptosis following ultraviolet irradiation, *Genes Dev*, Vol. 17, No. 12, (Jun 15), pp. 1475-1486, ISSN 0890-9369

Nishitoh, H., Matsuzawa, A., Tobiume, K., Saegusa, K., Takeda, K., Inoue, K., Hori, S., Kakizuka, A. & Ichijo, H. (2002). ASK1 is essential for endoplasmic reticulum stress-induced neuronal cell death triggered by expanded polyglutamine repeats, *Genes Dev*, Vol. 16, No. 11, (Jun 1), pp. 1345-1355, ISSN 0890-9369

Okada, T., Yoshida, H., Akazawa, R., Negishi, M. & Mori, K. (2002). Distinct roles of activating transcription factor 6 (ATF6) and double-stranded RNA-activated protein kinase-like endoplasmic reticulum kinase (PERK) in transcription during the mammalian unfolded protein response, *Biochem J*, Vol. 366, No. Pt 2, (Sep 1), pp. 585-594, ISSN 0264-6021

Oyadomari, S., Koizumi, A., Takeda, K., Gotoh, T., Akira, S., Araki, E. & Mori, M. (2002). Targeted disruption of the Chop gene delays endoplasmic reticulum stress-mediated diabetes, *J Clin Invest*, Vol. 109, No. 4, (Feb), pp. 525-532, ISSN 0021-9738

Oyadomari, S. & Mori, M. (2004). Roles of CHOP/GADD153 in endoplasmic reticulum stress, *Cell Death Differ*, Vol. 11, No. 4, (Apr), pp. 381-389, ISSN 1350-9047

Puthalakath, H., O'Reilly, L.A., Gunn, P., Lee, L., Kelly, P.N., Huntington, N.D., Hughes, P.D., Michalak, E.M., McKimm-Breschkin, J., Motoyama, N., Gotoh, T., Akira, S., Bouillet, P. & Strasser, A. (2007). ER stress triggers apoptosis by activating BH3-only protein Bim, *Cell*, Vol. 129, No. 7, (Jun 29), pp. 1337-1349, ISSN 0092-8674

Qin, J.Z., Ziffra, J., Stennett, L., Bodner, B., Bonish, B.K., Chaturvedi, V., Bennett, F., Pollock, P.M., Trent, J.M., Hendrix, M.J., Rizzo, P., Miele, L. & Nickoloff, B.J. (2005). Proteasome inhibitors trigger NOXA-mediated apoptosis in melanoma and myeloma cells, *Cancer Res*, Vol. 65, No. 14, (Jul 15), pp. 6282-6293, ISSN 0008-5472

Rao, R.V., Castro-Obregon, S., Frankowski, H., Schuler, M., Stoka, V., del Rio, G., Bredesen, D.E. & Ellerby, H.M. (2002). Coupling endoplasmic reticulum stress to the cell death program. An Apaf-1-independent intrinsic pathway, *J Biol Chem*, Vol. 277, No. 24, (Jun 14), pp. 21836-21842, ISSN 0021-9258

Reimertz, C., Kogel, D., Rami, A., Chittenden, T. & Prehn, J.H. (2003). Gene expression during ER stress-induced apoptosis in neurons: induction of the BH3-only protein Bbc3/PUMA and activation of the mitochondrial apoptosis pathway, *J Cell Biol*, Vol. 162, No. 4, (Aug 18), pp. 587-597, ISSN 0021-9525

Robinson, K.S., Clements, A., Williams, A.C., Berger, C.N. & Frankel, G. (2011). Bax Inhibitor 1 in apoptosis and disease, *Oncogene*, (Feb 7), ISSN 1476-5594

Rodeck, U., Melber, K., Kath, R., Menssen, H.D., Varello, M., Atkinson, B. & Herlyn, M. (1991). Constitutive expression of multiple growth factor genes by melanoma cells but not normal melanocytes, *J Invest Dermatol*, Vol. 97, No. 1, (Jul), pp. 20-26, ISSN 0022-202X

Ron, D. & Habener, J.F. (1992). CHOP, a novel developmentally regulated nuclear protein that dimerizes with transcription factors C/EBP and LAP and functions as a dominant-negative inhibitor of gene transcription, *Genes Dev*, Vol. 6, No. 3, (Mar), pp. 439-453, ISSN 0890-9369

Ron, D. & Walter, P. (2007). Signal integration in the endoplasmic reticulum unfolded protein response, *Nat Rev Mol Cell Biol*, Vol. 8, No. 7, (Jul), pp. 519-529, ISSN 1471-0072

Rong, J., Chen, L., Toth, J.I., Tcherpakov, M., Petroski, M.D. & Reed, J.C. (2011). Bifunctional apoptosis regulator (BAR), an endoplasmic reticulum (ER)-associated E3 ubiquitin ligase, modulates BI-1 protein stability and function in ER Stress, *J Biol Chem*, Vol. 286, No. 2, (Jan 14), pp. 1453-1463, ISSN 1083-351X

Rothhammer, T., Hahne, J.C., Florin, A., Poser, I., Soncin, F., Wernert, N. & Bosserhoff, A.K. (2004). The Ets-1 transcription factor is involved in the development and invasion of malignant melanoma, *Cell Mol Life Sci*, Vol. 61, No. 1, (Jan), pp. 118-128, ISSN 1420-682X

Rubio, C., Pincus, D., Korennykh, A., Schuck, S., El-Samad, H. & Walter, P. (2011). Homeostatic adaptation to endoplasmic reticulum stress depends on Ire1 kinase activity, *J Cell Biol*, Vol. 193, No. 1, (Apr 4), pp. 171-184, ISSN 1540-8140

Schröder, M. & Kaufman, R.J. (2005). ER stress and the unfolded protein response, *Mutat Res*, Vol. 569, No. 1-2, (Jan 6), pp. 29-63, ISSN 0027-5107

Schwickart, M., Huang, X., Lill, J.R., Liu, J., Ferrando, R., French, D.M., Maecker, H., O'Rourke, K., Bazan, F., Eastham-Anderson, J., Yue, P., Dornan, D., Huang, D.C. & Dixit, V.M. (2010). Deubiquitinase USP9X stabilizes MCL1 and promotes tumour cell survival, *Nature*, Vol. 463, No. 7277, (Jan 7), pp. 103-107, ISSN 1476-4687

Soengas, M.S. & Lowe, S.W. (2003). Apoptosis and melanoma chemoresistance, *Oncogene*, Vol. 22, No. 20, (May 19), pp. 3138-3151, ISSN 0950-9232

Span, P.N., Manders, P., Heuvel, J.J., Thomas, C.M., Bosch, R.R., Beex, L.V. & Sweep, C.G. (2002). Expression of the transcription factor Ets-1 is an independent prognostic marker for relapse-free survival in breast cancer, *Oncogene*, Vol. 21, No. 55, (Dec 5), pp. 8506-8509, ISSN 0950-9232

Szegezdi, E., Herbert, K.R., Kavanagh, E.T., Samali, A. & Gorman, A.M. (2008). Nerve growth factor blocks thapsigargin-induced apoptosis at the level of the mitochondrion via regulation of Bim, *J Cell Mol Med*, Vol. 12, No. 6A, (Dec), pp. 2482-2496, ISSN 1582-1838

Torlakovic, E.E., Bilalovic, N., Nesland, J.M., Torlakovic, G. & Florenes, V.A. (2004). Ets-1 transcription factor is widely expressed in benign and malignant melanocytes and its expression has no significant association with prognosis, *Mod Pathol*, Vol. 17, No. 11, (Nov), pp. 1400-1406, ISSN 0893-3952

Urano, F., Wang, X., Bertolotti, A., Zhang, Y., Chung, P., Harding, H.P. & Ron, D. (2000). Coupling of stress in the ER to activation of JNK protein kinases by transmembrane protein kinase IRE1, *Science*, Vol. 287, No. 5453, (Jan 28), pp. 664-666, ISSN 0036-8075

Verhagen, A.M., Ekert, P.G., Pakusch, M., Silke, J., Connolly, L.M., Reid, G.E., Moritz, R.L., Simpson, R.J. & Vaux, D.L. (2000). Identification of DIABLO, a mammalian protein that promotes apoptosis by binding to and antagonizing IAP proteins, *Cell*, Vol. 102, No. 1, (Jul 7), pp. 43-53, ISSN 0092-8674

Wang, Q., Mora-Jensen, H., Weniger, M.A., Perez-Galan, P., Wolford, C., Hai, T., Ron, D., Chen, W., Trenkle, W., Wiestner, A. & Ye, Y. (2009). ERAD inhibitors integrate ER stress with an epigenetic mechanism to activate BH3-only protein NOXA in cancer cells, *Proc Natl Acad Sci U S A*, Vol. 106, No. 7, (Feb 17), pp. 2200-2205, ISSN 1091-6490

Wang, Y.F., Jiang, C.C., Kiejda, K.A., Gillespie, S., Zhang, X.D. & Hersey, P. (2007). Apoptosis induction in human melanoma cells by inhibition of MEK is caspase-independent and mediated by the Bcl-2 family members PUMA, Bim, and Mcl-1, *Clin Cancer Res*, Vol. 13, No. 16, (Aug 15), pp. 4934-4942, ISSN 1078-0432

Warr, M.R. & Shore, G.C. (2008). Unique biology of Mcl-1: therapeutic opportunities in cancer, *Curr Mol Med*, Vol. 8, No. 2, (Mar), pp. 138-147, ISSN 1566-5240

Xu, Q. & Reed, J.C. (1998). Bax inhibitor-1, a mammalian apoptosis suppressor identified by functional screening in yeast, *Mol Cell*, Vol. 1, No. 3, (Feb), pp. 337-346, ISSN 1097-2765

Yamaguchi, H. & Wang, H.G. (2004). CHOP is involved in endoplasmic reticulum stress-induced apoptosis by enhancing DR5 expression in human carcinoma cells, *J Biol Chem*, Vol. 279, No. 44, (Oct 29), pp. 45495-45502, ISSN 0021-9258

Yoshida, H., Matsui, T., Yamamoto, A., Okada, T. & Mori, K. (2001). XBP1 mRNA is induced by ATF6 and spliced by IRE1 in response to ER stress to produce a highly active transcription factor, *Cell*, Vol. 107, No. 7, (Dec 28), pp. 881-891, ISSN 0092-8674

Zhang, K. & Kaufman, R.J. (2004). Signaling the unfolded protein response from the endoplasmic reticulum, *J Biol Chem*, Vol. 279, No. 25, (Jun 18), pp. 25935-25938, ISSN 0021-9258

Zhang, Y., Liu, R., Ni, M., Gill, P. & Lee, A.S. (2010). Cell surface relocalization of the endoplasmic reticulum chaperone and unfolded protein response regulator GRP78/BiP, *J Biol Chem*, Vol. 285, No. 20, (May 14), pp. 15065-15075, ISSN 1083-351X

Zhong, Q., Gao, W., Du, F. & Wang, X. (2005). Mule/ARF-BP1, a BH3-only E3 ubiquitin ligase, catalyzes the polyubiquitination of Mcl-1 and regulates apoptosis, *Cell*, Vol. 121, No. 7, (Jul 1), pp. 1085-1095, ISSN 0092-8674

Zhuang, L., Lee, C.S., Scolyer, R.A., McCarthy, S.W., Zhang, X.D., Thompson, J.F. & Hersey, P. (2007). Mcl-1, Bcl-XL and Stat3 expression are associated with progression of melanoma whereas Bcl-2, AP-2 and MITF levels decrease during progression of melanoma, *Mod Pathol*, Vol. 20, No. 4, (Apr), pp. 416-426, ISSN 0893-3952

Zhuang, L., Scolyer, R.A., Lee, C.S., McCarthy, S.W., Cooper, W.A., Zhang, X.D., Thompson, J.F. & Hersey, P. (2009). Expression of glucose-regulated stress protein GRP78 is related to progression of melanoma, *Histopathology*, Vol. 54, No. 4, (Mar), pp. 462-470, ISSN 1365-2559

Zhuang, L., Scolyer, R.A., Murali, R., McCarthy, S.W., Zhang, X.D., Thompson, J.F. & Hersey, P. (2010). Lactate dehydrogenase 5 expression in melanoma increases with disease progression and is associated with expression of Bcl-XL and Mcl-1, but not Bcl-2 proteins, *Mod Pathol*, Vol. 23, No. 1, (Jan), pp. 45-53, ISSN 1530-0285

Zong, W.X., Li, C., Hatzivassiliou, G., Lindsten, T., Yu, Q.C., Yuan, J. & Thompson, C.B. (2003). Bax and Bak can localize to the endoplasmic reticulum to initiate apoptosis, *J Cell Biol*, Vol. 162, No. 1, (Jul 7), pp. 59-69, ISSN 0021-9525